Making
Health, Illnes

The paper on which this book is printed meets the requirements of "ISO 9706:1994, Information and documentation – Paper of documents – Requirements for permanence".

ISBN: 90-420-1119-X

Printed in The Netherlands

Contents

Part 3 Healing Practices Today

Part 4 Making Sense of Living with Illness

Welcome to a *Probing the Boundaries* Project

Making Sense of: Health, Illness and Disease is an inter-disciplinary and multi-disciplinary research project which aims to explore the processes by which we attempt to create meaning in health, illness and disease. The project examines the models we use to understand our experiences of health and illness (looking particularly at perceptions of the body), and evaluates the diversity of ways in which we creatively struggle to make sense of such experiences and express ourselves across a range of media.

Among the themes explored by the project are:

- the 'significance' of health, illness and disease for individuals and communities
- the concept of the 'well' person; the preoccupation with health; the attitudes of the 'well' to the 'ill'; perceptions of 'impairment' and disability; the challenges posed when confronted by illness and disease; the notion of being 'cured'; chronic illness; terminal illness; attitudes to death
- how we perceive of and conduct ourselves through the experiences of health and illness
- 'models' of the body; the body in pain; biological and medical views of illness; the ambiguous relationship with 'alternative' medicine and therapies; the doctor-patient relationship; the 'clinical gaze'
- the impact of health, illness and disease on biology, economics, government, medicine, politics, social sciences; the potential influences of gender, ethnicity, and class; health care, service providers, and public policy
- the nature and role of 'metaphors' in expressing the experiences of health, illness and disease - for example, illness as 'another country'; the role of narrative and narrative interpretation in making sense of the 'journey' from health through illness, diagnosis, and treatment; the importance of story telling; dealing with chronic and terminal illness; the 'myths' surrounding health, illness and disease
- the relationship between creative work and illness and disease: the work of artists, musicians, poets, writers. Illness and the literary imagination - studies of writers and literature which take health, disability, illness and disease as a central theme

Dr Robert Fisher
Inter-Disciplinary.Net
http://www.inter-disciplinary.net

Introduction

Vera Kalitzkus and Peter L. Twohig

Health, illness and disease are topics well-suited to inter-, multi- and transdisciplinary inquiry. Increasingly, the study of health care demands some consideration of epidemiology, many different sciences, clinical practice, sociology, anthropology, literary criticism, history and philosophy, to name only a few. The result is that new conversations are initiated that situate health in broader social and cultural contexts. These new conversations draw connections between health, illness and disease and other issues, including those of politics, economics, culture, gender, race, identity and myriad others. One forum for these discussions are the yearly conferences on "Making Sense of: Health, Illness and Disease", organized by Rob Fisher (Learning Solutions), Oxford. The volume contains a selection of papers from the first conference in Oxford in June 2002, that – the steering committee believes – best present the inter-disciplinarity and the character of the inspiring event. It is our hope that these conversations will stimulate further inquiry.

The papers that follow utilize a variety of methodologies and approaches to pursue a wide range of topics in many different settings. The first part of the volume consists of papers with a broader overview and theoretical approaches. The second section explores in depth the cultural significance of narratives and metaphors of health, illness and disease. The third section critically examines healing practices at the point of care in contemporary society. The last section consists of papers focussing on patients' illness experiences.

This book acknowledges that there are many ways to 'make sense' of health, illness and disease, including the perspectives of people experiencing disease or illness, health care providers and cultural producers. All shape, in different and sometimes contradictory ways, the experience of health, illness and disease. Through expanding our inquiry beyond the traditional boundaries of biomedicine, we hope to draw attention to the many ways in which health is embedded in socio-cultural norms and the symbolic nature of health practices from multiple perspectives. Health, illness and disease are complex concepts forged not only in the hospital or in the clinic, nor solely through the health care professional and patient dyad but also through literature, the stories we tell, through media, public policy and contemporary clinical practice. This is to say that health cannot be viewed apart from other aspects of the social system. This interplay between health, illness and disease and other social institutions make these ideal topics for interdisciplinary inquiry.

What is the meaning of suffering or is there a meaning in suffering? *Harold Schweizer* reviews classical literature on suffering and concludes that "there is no other meaning to suffering than the acknowledgement of its meaninglessness." It is especially challenging to endure the meaninglessness of suffering. The task of literature therefore is to show us "how it is to suffer *without* meaning or justice." Literature can provide us with insights and enables empathy for suffering people, although this can never be more than an approximation to that life experience. Literature on suffering is therapeutic, Schweizer argues, in the sense that the sufferer recognises her own language of suffering and with that "the legitimacy of her own story of suffering."

Aspects of making sense of health, illness and disease on a different level are provided by *Gloria Onyeioziri* with her paper on "The Scholarship of Blindness." As a blind scholar she is concerned with the *perception* of the other as well as the *self-perception* as the other and analyzes the interpretation and understanding of "texts" by blind scholars. Onyeioziri discusses two theoretical models with specific reference on blindness and proposes a third model that – instead of focussing on the differences between the sighted and the blind, concentrates on the semiotic universe of blind scholarship. This model, she believes, comes closer to the lived experience of blind scholarship and could be used for a revised understanding and appreciation of blind scholarship by the sighted. With that she shows the intellectual, social and cultural factors involved in that context. Her insights are also applicable to other forms of otherness or disability.

Jayanta Bhattacharya examines the cultural construction of body concepts and practices in the light of the colonial history of India. As every society and historical setting produces their own specific construction of the body – and also a respective form of healing or medical system – he analysis the "construction of colonial medical hegemony at the level of the epistemological space of the body." His paper gives insights into the conflicting underlying cultural assumptions embedded in the biomedical perspective through a comparison with the body in Ayurveda, the traditional Indian medical system. Through this comparison, he reveals the lasting effect on the lived experience of people of colonial discourses.

Betty Bednarski examines the writings of Jacques Ferron, a family doctor of the 20th century from Quebec, Canada. She gives insights into the life of that doctor on three levels: exploring his biography, exploring his medical ideas and how he converged them through his literature and finally, she analysis the way Ferron incorporates his medical live into his fictional writings. Bednarski is explicitly concerned with the impact of Ferrons' oeuvre on medical professional readers. Throughout, Bednarski contrasts the clinical approach to "making sense" of health, illness and disease, with its immediacy, to that of the writer, who selects and shapes aspects of the experience to highlight particular elements. She notes that, paradoxically, the distance of the literary text can provide new insights into health care. Medical practitioners and students could learn from writings such as Ferron's to attend to the biographical, social, cultural as well as political context in which their profession is acting. They could become more sensitive to the human side, the context of illness instead of concentrating only on the biomedical defined disease they learn to identify. It could be a step on the way to merge the medical knowledge with the subjective side of illness – the lived experience.

Louise Penner's analysis of rhetorical strategies used in the writings of Florence Nightingale on contagion and contamination contextualises medical theories and shows how medical ideas and findings are never neutral, but rather linked to broader social and political questions in any historical period. Through her study, we are reminded to challenge the assumptions underlying contemporary health practices, to reveal their ideological underpinnings.

The *second part* of the volume extends the themes of the first part, through in-depth analyses of the meaning of narratives and metaphors for the experience of being ill and dealing with illness on a cultural level.

Catherine Garrett draws our attention to the spiritual realm in the experience of suffering and points out, how the divine evolves in narratives of chronic illness. But not only literature, also other forms of art works like sculptures or music can help us making sense of illness drawing our understanding to a deeper level. She describes illness narratives as healing discourses in contemporary society. It is a way of gaining back a sense of being part of a community and cared for as well as understood – an aspect also pointed out by Harold Schweizer. According to sociologist Clive Seale, narratives on grief and loss serve to reconstruct "the aging, dying and bereaved body and self through talk at the level of discursive consciousness" and achieve the "ritual inclusion as member of a moral community."[1] Garrett provides a roadmap to the vast literature on narratives through her typology. At the same time, she notes that for healing to be achieved, it must take place on various levels, including the individual, the social and the political.

Emma Govan analyses the depiction of sickness in theatre production and the affect of it on the audience using psychoanalytical theory. Her analysis is based on an examination of theatrical performances of severe illness, wherein sick actors acted sickness and the strong audience response highlights how "different dramas offer different lessons." Nevertheless, it became evident that in order to 'enjoy' suffering portrayed in the theatre, it has to be clear that the suffering is an illusion. Suffering in theatre plays can be cathartic for sufferers as well as their carers, as Schweizer argues in his paper in this volume. Such performances can disrupt the prevailing social and psychological repression of death and instead offer a tool for "learning" how to suffer through a public and shared event.

Sofie Vandamme ponders the use of metaphor in illness for dealing with it by exploring two examples: Susan Sontag and Jean-Luc Nancy. Sontag describes the non-metaphorical talk about illness as the only 'healthy' way to talk about it. On the contrary, Nancy makes clear that for him to live and cope with severe illness is only possible through the use of metaphor. For him there is no non-metaphorical understanding of illness, it cannot be separated from the contextual metaphorical understanding. Sontag seeks to liberate the sufferer from stigma and guilt. Yet, as Nancy convincingly shows in his writing about the experience of organ transplantation, in other cases the use of metaphor is helpful to make sense of the experience of illness, suffering and estrangement.

The *third section* of papers examine healing practises in contemporary society.

Peter Twohig et al. examine the ways in which cardiovascular evidence is incorporated into clinical practice. Working with family physicians in Nova Scotia, Canada, they analysed the ways in which family physicians attempt to apply cardiovascular recommendations in primary care. These findings are of importance for many debates within contemporary medicine, including the limits of evidence-based approaches, the confrontation between patient values and biomedical choices, the struggle to apply scientific evidence in real-world practice settings and the material condition of both individual patients and a health care system struggling under mounting costs.

Jamilla Mildorfs' paper continues the focus on general practice, through a sociolinguistic analysis of Scottish general practitioners' narratives on domestic violence. She shows the dilemma of GPs professional role as generalists who must deal with problems that transcend neatly defined biomedical conditions and solutions. Mildorfs' examination of the intersection between medical and psychosocial problems reveals how GPs attempt to restrict their task and sphere of responsibility to the biomedical model.

Two papers focus on the salutogenic resources of people in illness rather than on their suffering. *Bernie Warren* draws us into the world of clown doctors – specifically trained professional artists working in a clinical or health care setting – and shows us the value of laughter as medicine. The work of his own clown company "Fools for Health" in

Ontario, Canada, bears positive effects on the emotional state of patients, but also ameliorates the atmosphere and work of the therapy team as a whole. Clown doctors focus on the healthy aspects of patients while not denying their illness. In doing so, they can stimulate salutogenic resources in the patients with sometimes even improvements on the physical level. Another strength of clown doctors is their function as a trickster within the health care setting. Disturbing the clinical routine and sometimes braking up encrusted hierarchical positions and relationships, creates opportunities for new encounters between the doctors and patients, between patients and relatives as well as between the medical staff themselves.

Celia Bandman et al. describe their pilot program in a cancer centre setting that involves the work of her as a "medical humanist." Bandman, a writer, devotes herself to the task of mediating between the life worlds of the patients, nursing staff and doctors. Drawing on her expert use of language, using symbols and metaphors from literature and art, she is able to bridge the experience of patients and doctors thus creating 'new spaces' in between the two worlds. The medical humanist as well as the clown doctors find themselves in a marginal position within the health care system from where they are able to stimulate the inner resources of patients – old or young – as well as the medical stuff. Both papers show, how important it is for the health care system and the professionals to find some healing and relief also for themselves.

The final part of the book examines the direct experience of patients with illness. In order to make sense of health, illness and disease it is important to listen to the accounts of people actually living it.

The *fourth part* of this volume is concerned with the actual experience of living with illness, especially with chronic illness.

Susan Mills draws our attention to the fact that people live astonishingly well under conditions of chronic illness. While she acknowledges that many people with chronic illness endure hardship, she shifts our focus to the realm of coping with illness and toward a liberating analysis that experiencing chronic illness might also present an opportunity for personal growth and enhancement. In her review on literature and studies on that topic it becomes clear that living with chronic illness can make up a huge and dominating part of a persons self definition, but it does not have to be the only one and also not the dominating one. This serves as an important corrective to the prevailing view of chronic illness as a totalizing experience.

Jane Appletons' paper on research ethics is of central concern for all doing research in the field of suffering, illness and dying. Many of the contributions in this volume advocate for further explorations of the perspectives of those living with illness and disease. Appleton reminds us all that such research requires a sensitive approach and that exploring the voices of such people may be ethically contentious. Her paper asks for careful reflection on the part of the research about the ethical aspects and the possible effects of the research process on research participants.

In contrast to Mills' paper, that of *Emma Sayers and Miles Little* focuses on the difficulties arising after having survived a serious illness such as cancer. "The experience of cancer," they write, "brings uncomfortable insights into the fragility of life and the vulnerability of the body." Sayers and Little clearly articulate that this experience is one that changes the self and personality and quite often does not allow to return to the former self and former life. The existential upheaval has to be dealt with. Former patients suffer from lack of self-esteem, fatigue and guilt. They are expected to 'return to normal' and to be thankful for their survival. The existential angst among cancer survivors needs to be acknowledged in order to be overcome, the authors conclude.

The paper of *Vera Kalitzkus* is based on her research on organ transplantation from the viewpoint of donor families and transplant recipients in Germany. Organ transplantations transgress the boundaries between life and death as well as between individual persons. She explores how relatives of brain-dead organ donors and organ recipients live with these vague boundaries and make sense of their experience. As in the paper of Vandamme and Oderwald, Kalitzkus argues that organ transplantations awaken a great number of cultural assumptions and metaphors that people either have to deal with or can use as a means to making sense of their experience. Still, the positive picture of transplantation medicine painted in the public discourse needs revision in order to acknowledge the conflicts and psychological burdens attached to the transplantation experience. The problems of survivors as shown in the last paper is also applicable for patients living with organ transplants – even more so as they know that their time will be a limited one. For both sides of organ transplantation the need to deal with death and bereavement becomes evident.

Notes

[1] Clive Seale, *Constructing Death. The Sociology of Dying and Bereavement* (Cambridge: Cambridge University Press, 1998), 33.

Bibliography

Seale, Clive. *Constructing Death. The Sociology of Dying and Bereavement*. Cambridge: Cambridge University Press, 1998.

Part 1

Theoretical and Historical Approaches

The Question of Meaning in Suffering

Harold Schweizer

When philosophers and writers claim that there is no source of knowledge and meaning other than through suffering – "Until we are sick we understand not," writes Aeschylus; "Suffering is the sole origin of consciousness," writes Dostoevsky – they imply that suffering results in an ethical, perhaps even a spiritual, understanding.[1] Thus they attribute an exemplary authority to suffering. All other stories pale in comparison. The narrative of suffering is therefore the most authoritative, the archetypal narrative: the story of Job, of Oedipus, of Hamlet, of Faust. An understanding of these stories, such is the implication, should lead to ethical or spiritual insights, hence the pedagogic value attributed to them. And yet, what is baffling about the authority of such archetypal stories is that the consciousness and understanding resulting from suffering remains tormenting and deeply uncertain. Perhaps precisely because of that uncertainty the story of suffering is always retold or imitated by other narratives, read and re-read by readers across generations.

This essay is an inquiry into the literary dimensions of suffering. Rather than a conception of meaning as transcendental signified, I propose that the meaning of suffering consists in its narrative temporality, or the processes of its articulation over time and between subjects. Often curtailed by economic and scientific imperatives, such an understanding of suffering aims to legitimize suffering in its complex or indeterminable signification. A literary narrative, I argue, creates a social space within which suffering can be articulated in all its irreducible complexities. Or to say this differently, the task of literature is not to produce meaning but to represent the process and difficulty of the quest for meaning. But precisely in this sense literature is therapeutic. In its pages the sufferer finds her language, and in this language the legitimacy of her endurance of, and protest against, suffering – a legitimacy which is frequently denied in the name of diagnosis or meaning.

In order to identify some aesthetic and ethical dimensions in the emergence of meaning out of suffering, I examine two exemplary narratives of suffering: Albert Camus' *The Plague* and Kafka's story "In the Penal Colony." While traditional narratives, such as Camus' *The Plague* demonstrate that we can bear the question of suffering to remain unanswered, Kafka's story implies that we cannot bear to have it unasked.

1. Suffering and Literature

What is the particular relevance of literary discourse to an inquiry into the question of how we experience illness and disease? It may appear from the outset that a literary contribution to such an inquiry might somehow miss the point. First and foremost, surely, we must ask how we can alleviate suffering. Perhaps, if there is time at the end of the day, one may turn to a novel or poem to read about suffering. But that seems perhaps a questionable luxury. There is no time at the end of the day. What then can a literary perspective on these fundamental aspects of human experience contribute?

Our concept of suffering is narrative or literary, that is to say, we make sense of suffering in terms of generic literary distinctions. Briefly summarized: one can conceive of pain as lyrical or monologic and of illness and suffering as temporal and thus as narrative and dialogic. To that effect Charles Darwin writes in his *Genesis of Species*:

> Only during consciousness does [suffering] exist, and only in the most highly organized men does it reach its acme. The author has been assured that the lower races of men appear less keenly sensitive to physical suffering than do more cultivated and refined human beings. Thus only in man can there really be any intense degree of suffering, because only in him is there that intellectual recollection of past moments and that anticipation of future ones, which constitute in great part the bitterness of suffering. The momentary pang, the present pain which beasts endure though real enough, is yet, doubtless, not to be compared as to its intensity with the suffering which is produced in man through his high prerogative of self-consciousness.[2]

While Darwin's additional remarks that "lower races of men appear less keenly sensitive to physical suffering than do more cultivated and refined human beings" may strike us as potentially legitimizing the torture and suppression of the "lower races," a temporal consciousness and its attendant narrative articulation do appear as markers of refined reflection, producing no less than such works as Greek tragedy, the Book of Job, or Shakespeare's *King Lear*. But the distinction between pain and suffering need not lead to a privileging of suffering over pain, or of sustained narrative reflection over the a-temporal experience of pain which Darwin associates with beasts. The experience of pain may have produced the lyric's solipsistic hermeticism, the literature of fragmentation, the theater of cruelty: Paul Celan, T.S. Eliot, Antonin Artaud. The primitive and the avant-garde, in other words, may share deeper implications of the a-temporality of pain: the infinite, the universal. Perhaps these are realms prior or past to the more sociable narratives of suffering.

But it is difficult to separate pain from suffering, just as disease and illness blend into each other. The traditions referred to above are not easily distinguishable. There is fragmentation and aporia in Greek tragedy just as there is narrative coherence in Beckett's *Waiting for Godot*. There are inexplicable complications and repetitions in prolonged experiences of suffering just as there are narrative developments in the otherwise unpredictable, repetitive occurrences of pain. What is to be gained, however, from such literary classifications of the expressions of suffering is perhaps a deeper, more complex understanding of the particular difficulties in experiencing what we call suffering. For it is not easy to suffer. When we say that it is not easy to suffer, we are referring to more than the presence of pain, the etiology of a disease, or the evolution of an illness. The problem with suffering is that it has to be endured, and endurance is not just time passing. For the sufferer, endurance is "the bitterness of suffering," it is reflection and anticipation which are accompanied by a sense of injustice and protest.

2. The Injustice of Suffering

In Kafka's story "The Penal Colony" a soldier has been strapped onto a meticulously constructed torture machine which writes with a set of mechanized needles the sentence of the condemned man into his flesh. As in Kafka's story, something is being inscribed on my body when I suffer, and even if I eventually understand my sentence – cancer, muscular dystrophy, rheumatoid arthritis, lupus, Alzheimer's – I do not know why I am condemned. In Kafka's story, the full and final understanding of the sentence occurs only at the point of death as if to suggest that such understanding can only be physical, not mental, as if such understanding of the sentence that condemns me to death was to bear out the German phrase "*Etwas am eigenen Leibe erfahren*" (to experience something on one's own body). Kafka's German uses precisely this phrase – "Er erfährt es ja auf seinem Leib"[3] – when the explorer asks the officer who operates the machine:

> Does he know his sentence?" "No," said the officer, eager to go on with his exposition, but the explorer interrupted him: "He doesn't know the sentence that has been passed on him?" "No," said the officer again …, "There would be no point in telling him. He'll learn it on his body."[4]

Although the knowledge gained from suffering is indubitable, the law by which suffering is imposed is "very ingenious," as the explorer exclaims – but it is utterly illegible. When the officer shows the explorer "the guiding plans" for the prisoner's torture, the explorer cannot decipher them – "... all he could see was a labyrinth of lines crossing and re-crossing each other .... 'Read it,' said the officer. 'I can't,' said the explorer."[5] When the officer eventually spells out the sentence – "'BE JUST!'"[6] – it is likely meant as a caustic allegory of the injustice of suffering. The script for the prisoner's torture, as the officer explains, "'can't be a simple one, it's not supposed to kill a man straight off....'"[7]

Even if Kafka's allegorical story dramatizes the grotesque randomness and indecipherable logic of suffering, in our own quotidian or clinical circumstances the etiology of suffering is no less ironic and incomprehensible. For a diagnosis, too, is a sentence. Although the patient understands the sentence that condemns her, although she understands her diagnosis or her disease, she does not understand why she is condemned. When the oncologist pronounces the dreaded verdict, the patient does not therefore suffer from cancer. She suffers the injustice of her sentence. And similarly, when the teacher tells her students that Hamlet suffers from doubt or Oedipus from hubris, he does not tell them why they suffer. Doubt is not the meaning of *Hamlet*. Nor is sin the meaning of Job's suffering, even if his four eager counselors agree unanimously that Job suffers because of sin. But they suffer from impatience. They don't want to hear about the suffering of Job and thus they prolong it. Such a story as Job's, or Hamlet's, is not about the attainment of a particular, determinable meaning contained in one diagnostic pronouncement. The story of suffering is the struggle for meaning. It is the struggle with the question, "Why am I condemned?"

The question, "Why am I condemned?" implies protest and moral complaint. This protest echoes in such common expressions as, "How could this have happened to me?", "How will I bear this pain?", "When will I be better?" Proceeding from past to future, the sequence or temporality implied in such questions outlines a narrative that I have not authorized and whose meaning I cannot decipher. Something is being inscribed on me. I am a condemned man. Why am I condemned? We begin to understand that the question about the meaning of suffering is an ethical question. It is about justice. It is prompted by the protest and moral outrage in suffering. It is this question of justice that underwrites the ethos of tragic literature. Here suffering is rarely proportionate to its cause, often claims its victims indiscriminately, and always implies the protest that somehow it "should not" have happened. In spite of eminently human or natural causes, any sufferer who is prompted to such protest declares allegiance, ultimately, to a metaphysics wherein the protest against suffering seeks its legitimacy with a God who could have averted it.

So fundamental, indeed primitive, seems to be the association of suffering with protest that its universal representative in Camus' *The Plague* is a small child whose innocence underscores this fundamental, moral dimension of suffering:

> For the first time he opened his eyes and gazed at Rieux, who was standing immediately in front of him. In the small face, rigid as a mask of grayish clay, slowly the lips parted and from them rose a long, incessant scream, hardly varying with his respiration, and filling the ward with a fierce indignant protest, so little childish that it seemed like a collective voice issuing from all sufferers there.[8]

"Hardly varying with his respiration," the scream is imbedded in the rhythm of breathing and writing alike: it engenders a spectrum of narratives of suffering ranging from Father Paneloux's theodicy to Dr. Rieux's existential pragmatism. Indeed, that in the child's scream all childishness seems to be lost and its protest given over to represent a "collective voice" suggests that such narratives of suffering, redemptive or pragmatic, originate in a scream, and that in all such narratives all childishness is lost.[9]

If to articulate the child's "indignant protest" is the cause and purpose of the narrative, how then can such intention not abrogate the injustice of the child's suffering? How can it do justice to the injustice of suffering? These questions address the perhaps insurmountable difficulties, both aesthetic and ethical, of a narrative of suffering. If it must articulate the sufferer's reflection and anticipation, her bitterness, her hope, or her resignation, how would such articulation, such verbal extension of her cry, constitute justice?

In a tentative answer to these questions, I suggest that a narrative can offer nothing but its own aesthetic as a forum for the articulation of the protest against suffering. The possibility and the performance of narrative as such, its legitimization and dissemination in culture, are first answers to the question of how suffering acquires meaning. Indeed, there is no other meaning to suffering than the acknowledgment of its meaninglessness.[10] The possibility of a literature that performs this acknowledgment is thus already a partial answer to the question of the meaning of suffering. The making of meaning, as the child's scream implies, must be transferred to and continued in another's voice – Dr. Rieux's, for example, or the reader's.

3. Suffering and Ethics

The possibility of a response to suffering is fundamentally humanizing. In the narrative of suffering, the empty, inhuman immanence of suffering receives a name, a plot, and a destination. But frequently, prolonged, chronic, or unremitting suffering empties time of its content, reduces the sufferer's experience to sheer repetition, and the sufferer simply endures the vast, formless expanses of time. Within this immeasurable dimension, she becomes a stranger to herself, a spectacle to others, a statistic for the records. She is dehumanized. She disappears in the mute materiality of her body. "They had already seen children die…" we read in *The Plague*, "the pain inflicted on these innocent victims had always seemed to them what in fact it was: an abominable thing. But hitherto they had felt its abomination in, so to speak, an abstract way…."[11] To condemn the sufferer to her body, to deny her the narrative of suffering, is to reduce the human to mere fact.

Such reduction of the human is refused in Camus' *The Plague* whose representative protagonist, Dr. Rieux, stands "immediately in front" of the child as if to stand for the human in the midst of the inhumanity of suffering, as if to exemplify the protest against the reduction of the human to the inhuman. In Dr. Rieux's frontal facing of the child's suffering seems embodied what Emmanuel Levinas identifies as the only meaning of suffering, which is

> the suffering for the useless suffering of the other, the just suffering in me for the unjustifiable suffering of the other, [and which] opens suffering to the ethical perspective of the inter-human. In this perspective there is a radical difference between *the suffering in the other*, where it is unforgivable to *me*, solicits me and calls me, and suffering *in me*, my own experience of suffering, whose constitutional or congenital uselessness can take on a meaning, the only one of which suffering is capable, in becoming a suffering (inexorable though it may be) of someone else.[12]

While suffering per se is meaningless, the only meaning, according to Levinas, is to choose it on behalf of another, thus to confront the gratuitousness of suffering with a purpose, its blind accident with an intention, its fact with a value. This scenario underscores the fundamental importance of a dialogic setting for the engendering of the meaning of suffering. Such meaning comes about, as Levinas suggests, only in the most intimate encounter: "It cannot give itself out as an example, or be narrated in edifying discourse. It cannot, without becoming perverted, be made into a preachment."[13] Experiences of suffering are always incomparable. No one's pain can serve as an example for another's. While

The Plague's main protagonist, Dr. Rieux, enacts the making of meaning by unflinchingly "standing immediately in front of" the suffering child, the same obligation is also that of the writer or reader who places him or herself "immediately in front" of the text that extends the child's cry. Even if this bodily or verbal facing of the sufferer does not result in his cure, Dr. Rieux's position exemplifies a helplessness that is ethical in that it acknowledges suffering itself. "Otherwise," as Stanley Cavell writes, "I am not emptied of help, but withholding it."[14]

> Now and then Rieux took his pulse – less because this served any purpose than as an escape from his utter helplessness .... And then, at one with the tortured child, he struggled to sustain him with all the remaining strength of his own body. But, linked for a few moments, the rhythms of their heartbeats soon fell apart, the child escaped him, and again he knew his impotence.[15]

When Rieux sums up the book as

> the record of what had to be done, and what assuredly would have to be done again in the never ending fight against terror and its relentless onslaught, despite their personal afflictions, by all who, while unable to be saints but refusing to bow down to pestilences, strive their utmost to be healers[16]

– *The Plague,* as any other narrative, will thus not be a record with curative properties. Rather it is the record of its own recurring necessity, a circular, interminable protest, however ineffectual, which is the narrative of suffering. To be a healer or a writer – and Camus' analogies between the two is explicit in the role of Rieux as both doctor and narrator – means to address tirelessly the same onslaught of suffering without hope for a final cure. Indeed, a cure is only as temporary as one's respite in the closure of a book such as *The Plague*. Beyond its closures, the question of the meaning of suffering will have to be taken up again as the responsibility for the making of meaning. It is a question that outlives its temporary aesthetic closure, just as "the plague bacillus never dies or disappears for good ... it can lie dormant for years and years ...."[17]

The necessity of story telling thus arises anew with each outbreak of suffering, each demanding that reader or writer place themselves "immediately in front," as it were, to hear and witness suffering so that in that very hearing and witnessing meaning – since it does not reside in suffering itself – can be affirmed. Hence Levinas's claim that the perspective of true empathy as an "inescapable obligation brings us close to God in a more difficult, but also more spiritual, way than does confidence in any kind of theodicy."[18] When thus Father Paneloux at the dying child's bedside "sank on his knees" and cried, "'My God, spare this child!'" – "...all present found it natural..."[19] for here all theodicy seems left behind in favor of a more natural spirituality. Even if closeness to God seems for Dr. Rieux not at issue, his angry complaint, "'That child, anyhow, was innocent, and you know it as well as I do,'" accuses the same God whom Paneloux had vainly implored. Neither Paneloux's nor Rieux's knowledge, despite their differences, amounts to a theodicy but rather to that "more difficult, but also more spiritual," empathy enjoined by Levinas.

4. Meaningless Suffering

The task of literature is not to yield meaning like a diagnosis (though we often request just this in our impatience) but to articulate how it is to suffer *without* meaning or justice. Such a story is Kafka's "In the Penal Colony." While in traditional narratives, such as Greek tragedy or the Book of Job, the question of meaning leaves open the possibility of an answer – even if such an answer may have to be given as another question – in Kafka the absence of that question at the moment of suffering is the most fundamental negation of hope. But it is a negation, as Walter Benjamin writes, that may yield to a deeper, spiritual insight: "Thus as Kafka puts it, there is an infinite amount of hope, but not for us. This statement really contains Kafka's hope; it is the source of his radiant serenity."[20]

The explorer, whose visit to the penal colony occasions the officer's elaborate demonstrations of the prisoner's torture machine, and who seems thus to be put in the position of reader or addressee of the story, remains throughout little more than indifferent to the suffering of the prisoner. Having "accepted merely out of politeness the Commandant's invitation to witness the execution of a soldier...,"[21] he is diametrically opposed to Dr. Rieux's ethical confrontation with suffering. Although periodically roused to indignation, the explorer retains his indifference to the prisoner's suffering whose physiognomy is described as resembling that of an animal, a "stupid-looking wide mouthed creature with bewildered hair and face,"[22] and who undergoes his punishment with the muteness of a beast. The prisoner is, in Levinas's terms, exemplary of "the 'pain-illnesses' of beings who are psychologically deprived, retarded, impoverished in their social life and impaired in their relation to the other person" and thus subject to "pure pain."[23]

The apparatus itself appears to function as an allegory – one among many – of the sublimely gratuitous logic of suffering, the "immanent structure of suffering" as Levinas would call it.[24] The apparatus is "effective in itself even though it stands alone in this valley."[25] Those to whom it is administered experience the pain of man as beast – a pain that does not enter into the social space implied in the narrative temporality of suffering. Much of the ghostly irony of the story derives from the Commandant's aesthetic admiration of the functioning of the machine at the expense of any concern for the suffering of the prisoner. The lack of such concern emphasizes the autonomous, immanent nature of pain. Kafka's meticulous efficiency of style, moreover, bears resemblance to the apparatus. Like the explorer who only *intends* his protest, Kafka's style only *intends* to provide that narrative space in which pain could be coaxed outside of its immanence into the more extensive dimensions of suffering. But the all too efficacious descriptions of the prisoner's pain, the Commandant's excessive aesthetic interest, and the explorer's good intentions, all keep this immanent realm of pain sealed off from human intervention.

Rather than with fear and pity, we thus read Kafka's story with fascination. All, including the reader, attend the scene of suffering as a spectacle. If "we must learn to reveal ourselves, to allow ourselves to be seen," as Stanley Cavell points out, then here all refuse. "When we do not, when we keep ourselves in the dark," Cavell continues, "the consequence is that we convert the other into a character and make the world a stage for him."[26] This then, is the diametrical opposite of the scene with the dying child in Camus' *The Plague* where, in Levinas's phrase, "...my orientation toward the other can lose the avidity proper to the gaze only by turning into generosity, incapable of approaching the other with empty hands."[27] In Kafka's story, all hands seem empty of such generosity. Our gaze remains avid, perhaps all the more so because what is fascinating in the suffering of another is not only the gratuitousness of the sufferer's fate, but also the accident of our own fortuitous exemption. To ask about the meaning of another's suffering would thus also mean to ask about our own fate. Fascination keeps our own fate in the dark.

The absence of human intervention in Kafka's story, as Camus writes in his essay "Hope and the Absurd in the Work of Franz Kafka," informs Kafka's Kierkegaardian paradox: "'Earthly hope must be killed; only then can one be saved by true hope....'"[28] Kafka's refusal to allow for the complaint or protest possible in the *social* dimensions of suffering may thus imply the insufficiency of those human dimensions to convey meaning and that, if there is meaning in suffering, it cannot be provided in "earthly" terms.

5. Suffering and Reading

In so called traditional literary works, the suspension of an answer about the meaning of suffering leads to the acknowledgment that we live with questions more than with answers. But beyond this cozy hermeneutical commonplace, even traditional narratives of suffering demonstrate how terrible it is to live with questions. "If I had called and he had answered me," Job cries, "yet I would not believe that he had harkened unto my voice. For he breaketh me with a tempest, and multiplieth my wounds without cause."[29] Our benevolent proclivity for questions rather than for answers disregards the severity of what it means to live with *real* questions, that is, with the possibility of real hope and of real despair. To convey such questions and such hope or despair is the mark of a literature of suffering. Good literature is hence an education in gravity, in learning how to behave in the presence of real questions.

How then does one behave in the presence of the question: Why am I condemned? Why do I suffer? Why do I have this illness? While these questions can be addressed to no one but to God, the question of how one behaves is addressed to the reader, as it is to the medical practitioner. One behaves with patience. It is perhaps no coincidence that this word intimates a solidarity with the patient, on whom patience has been imposed. Our ethics, following Levinas or Camus, is to choose what the sufferer cannot choose. One could understand this patience as the outsider's conscious and articulate participation in the patient's time of waiting. "All were waiting,"[30] we read in *The Plague*:

> They had already seen children die – for many months now death had shown no favoritism – but they had never yet watched a child's agony minute by minute, as they had now been doing since daybreak. Needless to say, the pain inflicted on these innocent victims had always seemed to them to be what in fact it was: an abominable thing. But hitherto they had felt its abomination in, so to speak, an abstract way; they had never had to witness over so long a period the death-throes of an innocent child.[31]

Something remarkable happens in this time. The hope of receiving an answer is embodied by the presence of the reader, the visitor, the physician. In them the question is deposited like a secret. The secret is shared but not revealed. By articulating this waiting for an answer, by not avoiding the question about the meaning of suffering, the solitary, unsharable experience of the sufferer has been filled with language and has thus been made accessible for empathy. The language of literature, like the theater in Cavell's discussion of *King Lear*, becomes "a place within which our hiddenness and silence and separation are accounted for, it gives us a chance to stop."[32]

The Kafkaesque sufferer, who does not ask the question of meaning, who does not ask, "Why do I suffer?" and for whom the visitor seems hardly present, relegates the reader to go on in his hiddenness and silence and separation. Such a reader is the explorer, whose German designation, "Reisender," seems to render more accurately the casualness of his involvement. He is a bystander not a witness. Mildly interested in the apparatus itself, "leaning back in his chair and crossing his legs,"[33] the explorer is Baudelaire's (or Eliot's) "hypocrite lecteur! mon semblable, – mon frère!" "...for he traveled only as an observer, with no intention at all of altering other people's methods of administering justice." The explorer's protest is faint and speculative at best. Although "[t]he injustice of the procedure and the inhumanity of the execution were undeniable,"[34] he eventually responds to the Commandant's request for moral support: "I can neither help nor hinder you."[35] If a reader of Kafka were, unlike the explorer, to *suffer* anonymity and distance, then such impotence would reveal – in Cavell's words – "my separateness from what is happening to them; that I am I, and here. It is only in this perception of them as separate from me that I make them present. That I make them other, and face them."[36] Empathy, in other words, is possible in the space *between* distance and identification, or *between* helplessness and sacrifice. For empathy is not synonymous with any of these terms: it is neither distance nor identification, neither helplessness nor sacrifice. It is in that space in-between, rather, where we may imagine the possibility of the meaning of suffering.

Notes

[1] See Arthur Schopenhauer, *The World as Will and Representation*, trans. E.F.J. Payne, 2 vols. (New York: Dover Publications, 1966): "If our life were without end and free from pain, it would possibly not occur to anyone to ask why the world exists, and why it does so in precisely this way, but everything would be purely as a matter of course" (vol. 2: 161). Richard Sewall makes a similar point quoting Aeschylus: "'Wisdom comes alone through suffering'" and Dostoevsky: "'Suffering is the sole origin of consciousness.'" See *The Vision of Tragedy* (New Haven: Yale University Press, 1980), 180. David Bakan assigns pain a central significance in respect to culture, social institutions, and religion: "In the thought of a number of classical social theorists – Bentham, Adam Smith, and others – pain is a given and constitutes the basis for explaining the complex interactions of men and their arrangements." See *Disease, Pain, and Sacrifice* (Chicago: The University of Chicago Press, 1968), 58. Keats interprets Aeschylus's proverbial phrase (above) into, "'Sorrow is wisdom," and "'Until we are sick, we understand not'", quoted in

Hermione de Almeida, *Romantic Medicine and John Keats* (Oxford: Oxford University Press, 1991), 307. Theodor Adorno claims that all forms of social action are fundamentally against suffering. See *Negative Dialectics*, trans. E.B. Ashton (New York: Seabury Press, 1973), 203. Elaine Scarry points out that "pain and the imagination are each other's missing intentional counterpart, and ... they together provide a framing identity of man-as-creator...." See *The Body in Pain: The Making and Unmaking of the World* (New York: Oxford University Press, 1985), 169.

[2] Charles Darwin, *Genesis of Species* (1871), quoted by Stephen Jay Gould, "Nonmoral Nature," <http://www.stephenjaygould.org/librarygould_nonmoral.html> (26 December, 2002).

[3] Franz Kafka, *Das Urteil und andere Erzählungen* (Frankfurt: Fischer Taschenbuch Verlag, 1971), 103.

[4] Franz Kafka, *The Metamorphosis, In the Penal Colony, and Other Stories*, trans. Willa and Edwin Muir (New York: Schocken Books, 1975), 197.

[5] Ibid., 202.

[6] Ibid., 219.

[7] Ibid., 202.

[8] Albert Camus, *The Plague*, trans. Stuart Gilbert (New York: Random House, 1948), 194.

[9] See Harold Schweizer, "Against Suffering: A Meditation on Literature," *Literature and Medicine* 19, no. 2 (Fall 2000), 229-240.

[10] Harold Schweizer, "Job or the Meaninglessness of Suffering," in *Suffering and the Remedy of Art* (Albany: State University of New York Press, 1997), 59-76.

[11] Camus, 192-193.

[12] Emmanuel Levinas, *Entre Nous: On Thinking of the Other*, trans. Michael B. Smith and Barbara Harshav (New York: Columbia University Press, 1998), 94.

[13] Ibid., 99.

[14] Stanley Cavell, *Disowning Knowledge: In Six Plays of Shakespeare* (New York: Cambridge University Press, 1991), 109.

[15] Camus, 194.

[16] Ibid., 278.

[17] Ibid.

[18] Levinas, 94.

[19] Camus, 195.

[20] Walter Benjamin, "Some Reflections on Kafka," in *Illuminations*, trans. Harry Zohn (New York: Schocken Books, 1968), 144.

[21] Kafka, 191.

[22] Ibid.

[23] Levinas, 93.
[24] Ibid., 240.
[25] Kafka, 210.
[26] Cavell, 104.
[27] Levinas, *Totality and Infinity*, trans. Alphonso Lingis (Pittsburgh: Duquesne University Press, 1969), 50.
[28] Camus, "Hope and the Absurd in the Work of Franz Kafka," in *The Myth of Sisyphus*, trans. Justin O'Brien (Harmondsworth: Penguin Books, 1977), 120.
[29] The Book of Job, KJV (9:16-17).
[30] Camus, *The Plague*, 194.
[31] Ibid., 192-193.
[32] Cavell, 104.
[33] Kafka, 195.
[34] Ibid., 206.
[35] Ibid., 213.
[36] Cavell, 109.

Bibliography

Adorno, T.W. *Negative Dialectics*. Trans. E.B. Ashton. New York: Seabury Press, 1973.

Almeida, Hermione de. *Romatic Medicine and John Keats*. Oxford: Oxford University Press, 1991.

Bakan, David. *Disease, Pain and Sacrifice*. Chicago: The University of Chicago Press, 1968.

Benjamin, Walter. "Some Reflections on Kafka." In *Illuminations*. Trans. Harry Zohn. New York: Schocken Books, 1968.

Camus, Albert. *The Plague*. Trans. Stuart Gilbert. New York: Random House, 1948.

Camus, Albert. "Hope and the Absurd in the Work of Franz Kafka." In *The Myth of Sisyphus*. Trans. Justin O'Brien. Harmondsworth: Penguin Books, 1977.

Cavell, Stanley. *Disowning Knowledge: In Six Plays of Shakespeare*. New York: Cambridge University Press, 1991.

Darwin, Charles. *Genesis of Species* (1871). Quoted by Stephen Jay Gould. "Nonmoral Nature." <http://www.stephenjaygould.org/librarygould.nonmoral.html> (26 December, 2002).

Kafka, Franz. *Das Urteil und andere Erzählungen*. Frankfurt: Fischer Taschenbuch Verlag, 1971.

Kafka, Franz. *The Metamorphosis, In the Penal Colony, and Other Stories*. Trans. Willa and Edwin Muir. New York: Schocken Books, 1975.

Levinas, Emmanuel. *Entre Nous: On Thinking of the Other*. Trans. Michael B. Smith and Barbara Harshav. New York: Columbia University Press, 1998.

Levinas, Emmanuel. *Totality and Infinity*. Trans. Alphonso Lingis. Pittsburgh: Duquesne University Press, 1969.

Scarry, Elaine. *The Body in Pain. The Making and Unmaking of the World.* New York: Oxford University Press, 1985.

Schopenhauer, Arthur. *The World as Will and Representation*. Trans. by E.F.J. Payne, 2 vols. New York: Dover Publications, 1966.

Schweizer, Harold. "Against Suffering: A Meditation on Literature." *Literature and Medicine* 19, no. 2 (Fall 2000): 229-240.

----------. "Job or the Meaninglessness of Suffering." In: *Suffering and the Remedy of Art*. Albany: State University of New York Press (1997): 59-76.

Sewall, Richard. *The Vision of Tragedy*. New Haven: Yale University Press, 1980.

Note on Contributor

Harold Schweizer is Professor of English and Chair of the Department of English at Bucknell University, USA.

The Scholarship of Blindness and the Blindness of Scholarship

Gloria Nne Onyeoziri

What happens when a blind person decides to be a scholar? This question presupposes several parentheses. I am placing in parentheses the difference between *being* a scholar as an existential choice by a free agent (or least an agent) and being perceived as a scholar by others. The other parenthesis involves adding the words black, African and woman to blind scholar. These are differences that I would ignore at the peril of my own identity and of claiming a shared experience that may not exist or resemble what I imagine it to be. Nevertheless, I do want to focus tentatively on the notion of the blind scholar and share my reflections on that notion.

The relationship between blindness and scholarship may be approached as a largely practical issue but also leads to a critical rethinking of the way blindness itself is conceived as a form of mediation between the perceiver and the perceived, the senses and sense, the visible and visionary. William Paulson demonstrates that the cognitive difference between the sighted and the unsighted has long been a matter of "psychological speculation." He also shows that the discussion of blindness did not lead to a coherent body of thought since blindness was a convenient notion serving various philosophical and epistemological purposes.[1] Yet the common assumption was that the primary conceptual difference between the sighted and the unsighted follows the perceptual divide between the "referential and non-referential functions of language,"[2] as if the blind existed in a world of purely ordered signifying chains unconnected with the perceptual world. This assumption leaves a number of questions unanswered. First of all it does not account for the role of non-visual perception in building the bridge between the concept and its referent. In particular, the voice as a link between language and the sensual world (especially the voice of the Other as speaker) is not explained. Whereas Enlightenment and post-Enlightenment speculation emphasized the restoration of sight as a return to the normal, little is said here and elsewhere of the loss of sight as a semiotic transformation leading to new ways of encoding and decoding signs, while not necessarily excluding continued reference to visual forms through the functioning of memory. Finally, the blindness/seeing divide as a dichotomy between the referential and non-referential ignores the possibility of translating from the visual to the verbal. In order to explore these problems, I would like to suggest two models that have been used to explain the possibility of blind agency and a third model that comes a little closer to my own experience.

What I will refer to as the overcoming model seems at first glance quite practical and even a little heroic. The overcoming model poses two fundamental problems. Firstly, the blind scholar can *only* function in a pseudo-heroic mode, because her success will always be seen as exceptional, extraordinary and therefore unconnected not only with the experience of people with similar disabilities but also in relation to all people having had different experiences of the success/failure dichotomy that dominates most contemporary societies. Secondly, the scholarship itself is necessarily defined as a partial vacuum, a lack that is being compensated for little by little but which stands guard at the outset of any intellectual endeavour as the defining authority. Perhaps even more fundamental is the fact that if one's work begins as a response to a lack which distinguishes whatever is obtained as attained to, it will always be marked out as a substitution or alternative to the original, always ideal, function which is always present as the desired though impossible goal – the thing lacked which has been accommodated but never truly replaced.

Applying this model to blindness poses its own particular conditions. To consider the concrete example of non-verbal communication, the overcoming model would have to presuppose a sort of lopsided pragmatics. Although Jacob Mey, for example, in his general introduction to pragmatics, often uses telephone conversations in order to simplify his illustrations, he also recognizes that the pragmatic deprived of the visual is in fact a special case requiring greater study.[3] In a face-to-face conversation, the sighted speaker (S) sends message A, B, C to his/her unsighted receiver (UR), but only A reaches its target while B and C are lost somewhere in the canal of communication (Jakobson's terminology). S is not considered responsible for this loss since the overcoming model functions only through the effort of UR who is cast in the pseudo-heroic role of overcomer. UR works with A and something like B he/she has guessed from contextual clues and then sends back a message which responds to a modified version of A, B, C while adding non-verbal elements which S is likely to be more cognizant of than he/she is. Since S's ABC coincide with what is understood to be the normal communication quotient, S is not expected to anticipate UR's reinterpretation of B and C. This model, like any model based on what the French historian Henri-Jacques Stiker presents as the historically determined notion of rehabilitation, "implies returning to a prior situation, a situation that existed for the able, but one only postulated for the others."[4] In the case of blindness this is particularly problematic in that the chimeric return to the "prior situation" involves not only UR's own ability but also his or her access to S's dis-abling and dis-qualifying gaze.

The second model, which has a long cultural and philosophical history, is a rhetorical word-game in which the figurative sense of vision or seeing as an ability to understand the Other is exploited. In a catachresis, which can be found in ancient literature and the Bible, the unwise person is called blind, whereas the physically blind person acquires the reputation of being able to see what the sighted cannot. This can be witnessed in the Oedipus story where the blind Tiresias saw prophetically what the sighted king could not see. Oedipus's loss of sight may be understood as a return to a balanced order in which physical blindness and conscious insight coincide.

A more recent example of the inversion model is Paul de Man's essay "The Rhetoric of Blindness: Jacques Derrida's Reading of Rousseau." In this context, blindness is the impossibility of coming to the insight the critic's own discourse has created: "their language could grope towards a certain degree of insight only because their method remained oblivious to the perception of this insight."[5] We could dissociate this figure from physical blindness except that the reading de Man offers of blindness and insight returns to visual privation in the form of Derrida's critique of Rousseau's privileging of music (as "a pure system of relations") over painting as a sensory and referential presence. De Man feels that Rousseau only used traditional Eighteenth Century vocabulary of representation as a rhetorical device to exhibit its own openness to ambivalence: "The rhetorical character of literary language opens up the possibility of the archetypal error: the recurrent confusion of sign and substance."[6] What de Man considers Derrida's blindness with regard to Rousseau maintains the metaphor of the blind interpreter, while allowing us to forget that the privileging of substance over sign also guarantees the interpretative superiority of the sighted who alone can confuse a sign's presence for its meaning.

The rhetorical model of blind scholarship may be criticized as a romanticized and impractical ideology, offering few practical solutions of real problems and attributing an at best fleeting role to the "vision" of the blind. But its greatest weakness lies precisely in the ease with which the metaphor (as a challenge to the conventional wisdom of speech) slips back into catachresis – at once holding up the possibility of a universal blindness and quietly hinting at the persistence of a renewed secondary claim to the substance of sight simply because there is no other means of accounting for the ambiguity of language. Naomi Schor remarks, "The catachresis of blindness cannot be dissolved by ideological fiat."[7] This trap of the figurative is, I believe, a continuation, through accidental omission, of the traditional sacralisation of the blind person as described by Paulson: "Far from remedying the exclusion of the blind, compensatory faculties such as prophecy or poetic inspiration confirm their separation – their links to the gods rather than to the profane doings of men."[8]

As a third model, I would like to suggest that although scholarship by the blind cannot exist in a cultural, social or intellectual vacuum and cannot ignore the existence of forms of communication to which it does not have access, it can accord primacy to the semiotic universe it inhabits and assume the functionality of those systems among which it navigates. This is not to claim "visionary" superiority, nor to "wish away the complications of an embodied life,"[9] but to consider the "advantages" of the sighted as a secondary issue irrelevant to the description of the blind scholar's perceptual, communicative and cognitive life.

If we start by assuming the blind researcher's semiotic field of inquiry to be a set of texts, we can establish an initial hypothesis that the blind scholar does not actually differentiate between an object of research and the place in which research occurs. This holds true whether one adopts a structuralist view of the text as immanence or a post-structuralist view according to which the text is a construction of some pre-textual reality (the meaning of which will always remain inaccessible except through the structure of the text). In the former case, where the only object of study is the text itself, no external trappings are added to the coded message coming to the blind researcher as a stark serialized code. In the second case, in the necessary absence of common ancillary codes contributing to the text's constructive function (visualizations, illustrations, diagrams, non-verbal elements of performance), the direct navigation of the text as a linear code imposes itself as the only representation of reality and the only form the object may assume.

However, even when the text is reduced to its "bare bones" as a form of communication, it remains a complex problem in itself, involving intertwined and interactive relationships between the implied author, the narrative voice, the reader and the referential Other (consciences and beings to which the text attributes actions, qualities and perspectives). The blind reader (whether through a Braille text or a recording) becomes a peculiar actant amid these complex relationships in the sense that she will not generally peruse the pages of a book but has to sit down to listen to the text in its linear totality and becomes a sort of captive listener-audience (pleonasm for emphasis); this resembles more a radio play than the private and self-centred act of reading, or the public effect of theatre which surrounds the spectator with multiple series of coordinated signals. But a radio play is designed to be exclusively auditory for all participants whereas the blind person's "radio play" was not designed for the unsighted and usually contains visual encoding. By visual encoding I am referring to a verbal message that, without necessarily designating a visual image as a part of its signifying chain, presupposes practical familiarity with a known visual form, icon or cliché. Whereas an example of visual signification would be a television commercial that reads: "If you don't like *this*, and you prefer *this*, you will want to buy *this*."

The blind reader must in turn reverbalize this visual encoding through interpretation, thus creating a further level of hermeneutic processing. The blind scholar as actant "witnesses" the text as a verbal act (both in the sense of an action and of the act of a play), rewrites a sort of "procès-verbal," but reporting on representational details and turning visualization back into words that describe images by attempting to ascribe verbal meaning to them. The radicalness of this actantial role will depend to some extent on the degree to which residual memory of vision may provide image-models to support interpretative hypotheses. Those models become more abstract and less currant over time. This would explain why temporary blindness and regained sight have taken precedence in both literary and theoretical discourse over a more radically code-transforming permanence of blindness.[10]

The blind reader who listens to her text can never forget, while listening to the text, the voice and interpretation of the oral narrator who thus becomes a new actant. Vastly increasing the level of indeterminacy of the message's reception and processing, this fact introduces another level of interaction. Not only is an oral reproduction of the text an interpretation in itself, but the blind reader can also take up a position critical of the interpretation, imagining her own voice as an alternative version of the author's imagined voice as what is being betrayed, occulted or supported by the oral narrator. The oral narrator may also coincide with or implicitly clash with the "written" narrator who was already inscribed into the text as a construction anticipating an oral narrator but not with the purpose in mind of communicating the text to a blind reader.

The primacy model does not only imply a particular set of relationships at the level of the performance involved in the process of communication, but also particular re-formulations of the experience of time and space. I have already insisted on the fact that visual encoding must be re-verbalized. This constitutes a space-to-discourse translation that does not necessarily eliminate the element of the spatial in discourse but reasserts the primacy of the verbal. Further, in all forms of research in the humanities, visual presentation is rarely if ever separated from the verbal act of representation. Print-type and page formatting carry connotations (for example as modern or old-fashioned). Many novels weave paintings, maps, family trees and photos into the text's fabric. Usually the blind scholar does not even feel the book in its materiality since her book is on cassettes. Many works add graphs, tables and illustrations assumed to be necessary for the understanding of the work and even of the conceptualisation of the object of discussion.

One could see the visual elements of communication as a source of a weakness or lack on the blind scholar's part, which can be only partially compensated for through a limiting selection of texts and the assistance of oral narrators who describe the visual elements. An explanation closer to the rhetorical model would say that the visual material acts as a supplement to a verbal code thereby revealed in its inadequacy and incompleteness: the blind reader once again becomes the archetypal seer who reveals to the sighted world the lacunae and "blind spots" of its own language. In day-to-day practice these explanations influence the thinking of both blind and sighted. One could suggest however that either reading "around" the visual or reading a translated version of the visually encoded text is just another form of decoding. Is a text in translation a degraded or imperfect rendering of the *original* or simply another version of what was already an incomplete act of communication? George Steiner, for example, devotes the first chapter of his work on translation (*After Babel*) to problems of understanding texts written in one's own language.[11] The assumption that the blind reader needs to have recourse to a picture's "translation" to understand the text further presupposes that "complete reading" accessible to an imaginary group of "complete" readers for whom either subjective interpretation is rendered unnecessary by the innate clarity of the communication process or whose subjective interpretative choices correspond exactly to all possible contexts of meaning surrounding the text. It is difficult to imagine how such a perfect correspondence could be demonstrated any more easily than it could be demonstrated that a blind reader has understood a text "completely" through auditory signs combined with the translation of visual signs into a second auditory signifying chain.

Interaction with the text is more a spatio-temporal than purely spatial experience. Much scholarship begins in the margins of other texts. Writing in the margins of texts is a practice that implies an ability to rewrite the text, to extend its dimensions both semantically and spatially without seriously interfering with the linear progression of reading. Other more rigorous and demanding forms of intertextual production, such as index cards or computer-based notes reflect a firmer retention of moments of interaction with the text and would appear, in their verbal nature, to be more accessible to the blind scholar. But the notes strengthen verbal memory not essentially because they store information in an encapsulated form (though they may succeed in doing that) but because they make information available to the accelerated gaze of the scanning eye.

The blind scholar as note-taker conceives of the textual margin in a unique way. To read, analyse and comment on a novel from a critical perspective for example, she maintains a global mental margin, a mental space of commentary that allows her to maintain a sense of the whole story (so that new marginal notes can be placed not at random but in a memorable location) while expanding the stock of pertinent details. The Braille or recorded notes that help to fix ideas in space and time are simply another version of the same process. By a long series of reading, remembering and rewriting, the number of specific references is reduced to the new story commonly referred to as a critical work. Aside from the labour-intensive nature of this work (which is yet to be recognized in economic terms), I believe that blind scholarship is in itself a particular mode of conceptualization. Whereas Proust's involuntary memory cannot be intentionally solicited but produces a vision of totality when called forth by contingent sensations, the blind scholar's marginal return tests the limits of intentional memory while slowly and painfully repeating its necessarily obsessive linear path through the text.

The practical realities of institutionalised scholarship and institutionalised disability dictate that the overcoming and rhetorical models will continue to influence the way in which blind scholarship is perceived and perceives itself. It would also be unrealistic to discount the role that changes in technology may play in future years in the resolution of many practical difficulties (or in adding new difficulties). Because the primacy model is so little understood and seems to have informed very little serious investigation, the Other tends to break in on us at points in a process that is different from its own, and thus to find us incomplete in a way that reflects more on the social isolation of our existence than on any insightful or meaningful communication. Perhaps when more work can be done in the direction I have suggested, I will not have to feel that if I do not practice reading my Braille text 20 or 30 times, I will not be seen as a scholar in the same right as my sighted colleagues. That would indeed be a light at the end of a tunnel we seem to share.

Notes

[1] William Paulson, *Enlightenment, Romanticism and the Blind in France* (Princeton University Press, 1987).

[2] Paulson, 19.

[3] Jacob Mey, *Pragmatics: An Introduction* (Oxford, Blackwell Press, 1993), 198.

[4] Henri-Jacques Stiker, *A History of Disability* (Ann Arbor: University of Michigan Press, 1999), 122.

[5] Paul de Man, *Blindness and Insight: Essays in the Rhetoric of Contemporary Criticism* (New York: Oxford University Press, 1971), 103.

[6] De Man, 135.

[7] Naomi Schor, "Blindness as Metaphor," *differences: A Journal of Feminist Cultural Studies* 11.2 (1999): 83.

[8] Paulson, 9.

[9] David Mitchell, Preface to H.-J. Stiker's *A History of Disability*, ix.

[10] See Schor's account of her temporary experience of blindness, 82-83.

[11] George Steiner, *After Babel: Aspects of Language and Translation* (London: Oxford University Press, 1975).

Bibliography

De Man, Paul. *Blindness and Insight: Essays in the Rhetoric of Contemporary Criticism.* New York: Oxford University Press, 1971, 102-141.

Holub, Robert. "Indeterminacy." in *Encyclopedia of Contemporary Literary Theory: Approaches, Scholars, Terms,* edited by Irena Makaryk, 562-532. Toronto: University of Toronto Press, 1993.

May, Jacob. *Pragmatics: An Introduction*. Oxford: Blackwell Press, 1993.

Mitchell, David. Preface to *A History of Disability* by Henri-Jacques Stiker. William Sayers, trans. Ann Arbor: University of Michigan Press, 1999, i-xxi.

Paulson, William. *Enlightenment, Romanticism and the Blind in France.* Princeton: Princeton University Press, 1987.

Schor, Naomi. "Blindness as Metaphor." *differences: A Journal of Feminist Cultural Studies* 11, 2 (1999): 76-105.

Steiner, George. *After Babel: Aspects of Language and Translation.* London: Oxford University Press, 1975.

Stiker, Henri-Jacques. *A History of Disability*. William Sayers, trans. Ann Arbor: University of Michigan Press, 1999.

Note on Contributor

Gloria Onyeoziri is an associate professor of French at the University of British Columbia. She is a specialist in African and Caribbean literatures and has published on Aime Cesaire, Aminata Sow Fall, Chinua Achebe, Ousmane Sembene, Henri Lopes, and Ahmadou Kourouma as well as such topics as literary semantics, irony and African women's writing. She recently co-authored an interdisciplinary study of Jean-Dominique Bauby's The Diving Bell and the Butterfly which appeared in the journal Literature and Medicine.

The Body: Epistemological Encounters in Colonial India

Jayanta Bhattacharya

In a revealing paragraph Elizabeth Grosz comments, "Every body is marked by the history and specificity of its existence. It is possible to construct a biography, a history of the body, for each individual and social body." In doing so, she notes, "The history would include not only all the contingencies that befall a body, impinging on it from the outside," but any such history "would also have to include the 'raw ingredients' out of which the body is produced."[1] My effort would be to delve into some of the unfamiliar nuances of the context-specific 'Indian body' at the epistemological level encountering dislocating colonial epistemological incursions moored in particular socio-economic roots.

A recent article in an authoritative medical journal has problematized – as well as de-essentialized, too, to a great extent – the prevailing universalization of medications and treatments. The author, who herself is a physician, comments, "Uncertainty influences all medical decision making." She continues, "Thus developing firm recommendations about specific providers for particular diagnoses or procedures is difficult." And, the most worrisome problem of "generalizability occurs when receptor polymorphisms and other inherent racial differences cause different responses to the same drugs."[2] This is a rather sad story. Roselyne Rey focuses on this problem in a more involved way. "Rather than incriminating a medical corps … subject to the same political, religious, and ideological currents as the rest of society," she urges, one "must question the conditions under which medicine is actually practised."[3] Beyond these castigations we would talk about happier days when everything on this green earth was becoming *universal* and/or *universalizable*. We would talk about an incomplete narrative of the 'colonial' body and the construction of colonial medical hegemony at the level of the epistemological space of the body. Colonial enterprise in medicine needed a colonized body for its own *medical* body's *becoming* to be more complete, comprehensive and authoritative.[4] It is through engaged encounters with the Other, with the otherness of the Other, that one comes to a more informed, textured understanding of the traditions to which 'We' ourselves belong. It is in our genuine encounters with what is other and alien (even in ourselves) that we can further our own self-understanding.[5]

As a cautionary note, epistemological inquiry employed in this essay should not be intended to replace the ontological essence of that structure. The body has come to be recognized as a terrain on which struggles over control and resistance are fought out in contemporary societies.[6] The assumption of classical positivist sociology, that the body belongs primarily to biology, has collapsed and the meaning of the body has become a problem for linguistic, cultural and social analysis. The contemporary discourse on the body has emerged as one of the major manifestations of a crisis in the intellectual politics and epistemology of Western social thought based on the rejection of subjectivity and any epistemological claim of access, however mediated, to objective social or historical reality.[7] The history of biomedicine proper is a record of the progress of medicine in time over certain favoured cultural areas in space. During this journey biomedicine got rid of all extra-scientific connotations to reach its acme. The material of a geo-cultural area when it involves human processes is better illuminated against the background of the cognitive categories produced internally. Indigenous subjectivity (focused through Ayurveda in India) opted for *wellness* with its own speculative logic metaphors ethical matrix, 'un-scientific' pathology/therapeutics/ expertise, *intersubjective* network of physician-patient-community. Gradually it metamorphosed into the search for biomedical *cure* endowed with its amazing therapeutic results, ingrained philosophical vision, almost accurate localization of disease through anatomical pathology, and transformation of patient's language into medical history taking, new techniques of therapeutics and overall *clinicalization*.[8]

All disease is semantic, is a symbol or a sign, which reveals a particular meaning. In a society of the seventeenth century Macbeth's body (for healing of scrofula by 'royal touch') was a metaphor. It was also a political reality that needed a 'social body' to operate on. With transition to the nineteenth century, new remedies, therapeutic devices and anatomo-patho-physiological knowledge of the body replaced the rituals that served to restore the corporeal integrity of the monarch. Foucault notices the opening up of the 'concrete individual' and the 'silent body' to the 'clinical gaze' and the 'language of rationality' for the first time in Western history.[9] The new scientific healing emphasized objectivity in the collection of data, largely dispensing with the patient's narrative in favour of specific measurements of biological activity.[10] There appeared a fast receding horizon of the *enigma* of the body – through which we could focus on "extra-theoretical spheres of validity" in scientific discourses.[11] The different corporeal ambiguities – as perceived in pre-colonial India as well as in different cultures – began to be sublated by the mimetic force of scientific rhetoric.

At this juncture let me cite two contrasting Indian (Bengali) examples which, *spatially* separated but *temporally* related, reveal an interesting perception of the body, health and disease in colonial India. A peasant of Birbhum region of Bengal writes to a person (to whom he owed some amount of money), "I went to town wreaking evils against you, so I am contacted with an alien disease. You should know it … and on getting cured I must repay the whole of debt whatever I owe to you."[12] This is an account of the 'social body' articulating its own logic, metaphor and ethical demands. A differing contemporary 'elite' account is provided by Dwijendranath, the eldest brother of Rabindranath Tagore. "Treatment by any means is a wild goose chase! So better not to say anything about *kaviraji chikitsa* (Ayurvedic treatment) – even the shimmering rays of nineteenth century knowledge has failed to penetrate its windows." Dwijendranath continues, "Modern medicine starts with dissecting a corpse, Ayurveda starts with elaborating on relationship between the body and mind." But inspired by 'modernity' he uses innovatively the categories of Ayurveda like *vayu, pitta*, *shlesma* (wind, bile, and phlegm) to interpret the superiority of Western intellect. Finally he concludes, "By the raging light and scorching heat of English education orthodoxies began increasingly to be banished from metropolis to the fringe of villages."[13] We can see the emergence of the 'medical body' as distinct from the 'social body'. But here is a subtle difference in conceptualisation between the body *as diseased* in biomedicine, and the body *in disease* in Ayurvedic perception that transforms finally into the 'diseased body' (a hybrid) in metropolitan Bengali perception. In the former it is the disengaged circumscribed biological body, while in the later one it is *embedded* in its environs. In *Caraka Samhita* we find, "Environment is important: it is vital to be in tune with the special qualities pertaining to each of the seasons."[14] To the colonizer, therefore, India came to be internally and inherently fissured in a time-scale. Space and time assumed morphological differentials leading to the production of ontologically different types of knowledge about the body. This trajectory took epistemologically different paths, too.[15] The colonial metropolitan account of the body/health/disease was accorded the privilege of 'authentic' knowledge and for the construction of colonial modernity *time* was privileged over *space*. The dominant representation of the body in modernity has been provided by the biomedical discourses, which became, in the nineteenth century, a science of universal bodily processes.[16] To emphasize, "The community also colonizes the life world of an individual in the same way as the state colonizes the life-world of a community."[17]

The emergence, codification and legitimisation of this phenomenon was to become perhaps the founding moment for the study of indigenous medicine and the construction of colonial medical hegemony in India. Interestingly, the concept of the biological body supposed to be uniform across spaces was seen to be dislocated/displaced when Western medical practice encountered a colonial space. Asymmetries and inequalities were retained in the hybrid interaction of the conceptions of the body produced within modern Western medicine and Ayurveda. In particular, while the context-responsive patterns of certain Indian ways of knowledge (particularly Ayurveda) were assimilated into the overall structure of the knowledge of the body in Western medicine – through the formation of "germ theory" and the "tropical medicine" sub-discipline – without threatening the subjectivity that was constructed and displayed within Western medicine, the constitutive principles of the knowledge of the body in Ayurveda were translated into and, in the end, displaced by those of Western medicine.[18]

In tropical medicine, an emergent new branch of Western medical discourses, "[t]he body was firmly located in India, and yet it was scientifically observable only through the knowledges and practices of colonial medicine."[19] The British attitudes towards the Indian environment and the process of imperial expansion were mutually constitutive: the one shaped and was in turn shaped by the other.[20] These ran from individual protective measures (for the White body) through to total ecological *management* schemes that required complete reshaping of the environment. Farley comments, "Tropical medicine was an important part of empire building and empire maintenance … the basic goal of tropical medicine was to render the tropical world fit for white habitation and white investment."[21] It was also a space for opening up of the vexed question of identity formation and the foregrounding of terrains of resistance.

This paper has three movements with significant amounts of overlap. The first examines the formation of colonial modernity and its interaction with the heterogeneous 'Indian body'. The second movement focuses on the conception of the body in Ayurveda. The final movement provides an account of the construction of hegemony and the splitting up of a hybrid space as a site of resistance.

1. Colonial Modernity

While talking about colonial medicine in India we are to ask: what was colonial about the colonization of the body? For the purposes of this essay, I would like to use "entrenched modernity or modern to suggest that all that is imaginable under the term 'modern' is not exhausted by what we have as the embodied form."[22] So there was in the knowledge emerging in the modern era a surplus left untapped after what got embodied. "Psychically, modernity is about identity … unfulfilled identity looks uncannily like recoiling from the flawed, illegitimate reality of the present."[23] But what became essential and strategic of colonialism is not entailed in the logic of Enlightenment. The mode of the colonial construction of modernity is, therefore, detachable from modernity though it came in the baggage of colonialism.[24] Colonial modernity instituted a science-civilization-progress framework and a *secular social hierarchy*.[25] But unlike European modernity, this colonial modernity was categorically shorn of *self-critique*. Eventually, colonial science was not a copy of the original in Europe, rather an uncanny double.[26] Within colonial discourse, colonial subjectivity is fixed in relation to an overriding subject, the ideal rational *subject*, being presented as the agent of history, the colonizer.[27] An illuminating example can be cited here. William H. Welch, an

American physician, asks in 1921: "Why is kala-azar almost confined to the natives and sprue to the foreign population? … There is still a mystery concerning some of the cases of splenomegaly, which do not seek to fall within any of the recognized categories."[28] In another observation, "The body rendered knowable by physiology, pathology, and visible in diseases … was required to also materialize itself as the body located in the knowledge of Indian conditions and disposition."[29] Europeans came to regard themselves as exotica on foreign soil: feelings of superiority and vulnerability were two sides of the same imperial coin.[30] Such an ambivalent position led to the production of knowledge where *similarity* was always superseded by *difference* and science became the measure for gauging progress toward modernity. The idea of modernity and modernization has always been value-laden and seen to be inextricably linked with the idea of *progress* and *improvement* recasting subjectivity with unique connotations.[31] The taxonomies of natural history, by constructing secularised notions of the 'modern' and the inferiority of non-Western societies produced a conception of civilization whose differing levels secured a place for the English as its apex.[32] But unlike other agencies of the colonial state, medicine operated through *uncoercive* management of desire, rather than a coercive one at other moments. It was "by teaching us to employ the methods of reason, universal modernity enables us to identify the forms of our own particular modernity."[33] Earlier colonial discourses, marked by difference, focused on a semiotic of grotesque and infectious bodies of the colonized.[34] It gradually transcended into the concept of the 'normalized body'.[35] In this dynamic there was a violent "functional change in a sign system … The change in signification-function supplements the previous one."[36] That historical change took place in both material and abstract spaces, indissolubly tied together in social space and the praxis that gave its form.

We can try "to learn something about the violence of our hermeneutic."[37] We languaged humans are rarely out of the community of words; the community of words is *never* out of us. Community is also the semiotic setting of life among humans, our inescapable sociality. It is *sign*-use that initiates an open-ended process of semiosis. It is interesting to note that the *indexical* parts of these semiotic symbolic assertions, expressed *metonymically* through actions in the life-world, can be appropriated to reconstitute/make/break the existing ones explained mytho-historically. Thus, without changing the prevailing icons of an indigenous society cultural hegemony can be constructed insidiously.[38]

I would modestly distinguish between the use we make of our bodies and the way our bodies function and would emphasize the way elements of physiology and anatomy can be taken up into the symbolic domain. The British came to India with this new concept-in-evolution of the body typically assumed to be a material entity subject to empirical rules of biological science, existing prior to the mutability and flux of cultural changes and diversity and characterized by unchangeable inner necessities. “It was the universality of the body and of physical pain, first mapped in surgical theaters and … in physiology laboratories, that provided science and medicine its authority” beyond the domain of the body “to talk about traumatic suffering of mind.”[39] Utility came to be an important yardstick in this notion of authority and progress and consequently banished India to the near-bottom rung of civilization, and then sentenced India to tutelage.[40] The concept of the body was made to evolve around this pivotal theme of utility (with science as the organizing metaphor) in sharp contrast to the Indian body image with its *embeddedness*.[41] This investigation enables us to rediscover one of the conditions of the emergence of the human sciences: the great 19th century effort in discipline and normalization.[42] Moreover, medicine itself acted in different contexts as a metonymy of power – colonial power in India.[43]

Precolonial understandings and interpretations of “health” and “illness” underwent metamorphosis to be concordant with the symptomatic approach taken by modern medicine. “Now the phenomenon of the social body is the effect not of a consensus but of the materiality of power operating on the very bodies of individuals.”[44] Quite clearly, we need to distinguish between normative rules of ‘medicalization’ and those practices and beliefs that are contingent. “Norms are relative to each other in a system, at least potentially. Their co-relativity within a social system tends to make this system an organization, that is, a unity in itself, if not by itself and for itself.”[45] The focus on the colonial era reveals a fact that illustrates quite nicely the localization of a Western movement in an altogether *different* context within the colonial sphere. I would try to posit it within the framework of heteronormativity and domesticity, the social body and subject-positions. “Miles away from the master-slave dialectics, the post-colonial debates discuss the subsumed contradictions, disjunctions and ambivalences.”[46] What is required in this context is to *foreground* the specificity of *locales* – the accretions of culture and history – that may invite unique readings on “common” themes. I am speaking then of complicating analysis, rather than positioning it within the fiction of autochthonous development.

Against this backdrop, it would be ingenuous to simply imagine away the West as a site of validation and performance. Needless to say, it is no longer even possible to conceive of a pristine theoretical and cultural world of non-Westerness, unmarked by a history of asymmetric interactions. It is difficult to move away from or criticize the discourse of the West by using a Western-led theory. My effort is not really a strategy for ‘improving’ the West, but primarily one of re-centering the non-West – the ‘marginal’. Again, this marginal is also internally differentiated, its fault lines and fissures variously articulated with the discourses of dominance.

2. The Body and Ayurveda

Ayurveda, besides being a medical treatise in itself, is part of a greater Indian logical tradition.[47] As shown by Bimal K. Matilal, the logical pattern and framework intensively used by *Caraka* was not "refutative enthymemes." It only established a proposition which happened to be 'logically contradictory' to the thesis of the 'demonstration'.[48] It is uniquely opposed to the 'exclusionary' and 'unitary' mode of 'positivist' reason practiced particularly during the 19th century. In Ayurveda, a discourse on the *world* (natural history) is contained within a discourse on *man* (medicine). *Biogeography* is absorbed into *therapeutics*. The objective or spatial reference, the environment, is incorporated within the subjective or practical reference.[49] Such a conception of illness is very different from a 'germ' conception where health is the absolute absence of the disease-causing agent and therefore health and illness are absolute opposites and could not possibly be metaphorized by one and the same image of natural or supernatural power. Here the religious and uncircumscribed language concerning disease and the technique of therapeutics were thought of and experienced as a unified field – a different form of cognition with its own logic and inferences. In this discourse, nature and man are two ontologically conjoined categories to explore into epistemology of the body/disease/nature. Nature in Ayurveda (as an *ontological given*) is the macrocosm wherein man resides as microcosm. Nature is, however, a topos, a place. We turn to this topic to order discourse, to compose our memory. It is figure, construction, artefact, movement, displacement.

In this discourse, the body becomes the tenuous drawbridge in the intersubjective network of physician-patient-community-nature.[50] Without the benefit of knowledge of physiology and anatomy, also of pathology, the physician (or doctor) had no other means of studying the affected parts of the body or the organic operation of the vital functions. Alternatively, "he could make no local diagnosis of the disease."[51] It should be mentioned that an "empirical approach to learning human anatomy by dissection, involving direct, firsthand observation of the body was fundamental to the Ayurvedic medical knowledge."[52] But over time "direct observation of a decaying corpse, considered polluting by Brahmins and the upper classes" was abandoned.[53] Specific Indian societal textures and stratifications, quite evidently, had its lasting impact on the epistemology of medicine and the body. So at the therapeutic level, the physician had to make out a doubly appropriate relationship: to render the environment appropriate to the needs of the patient and, conversely, to render the regimen of the patient appropriate to the ecological condition. He had to depend more on speculative logical diagnosis and *prognosis* of a disease rather than on clinical and curative ones. It is important to note Ayurveda defines health as *swasthya* to be established in one's self. In such low-technology systems there is a *shared distribution* of knowledge, which is based partially on the rich store of *prior experience* that participants bring to a contingent moment. The very fact of living as an *embodied subject* gives a particular character to the ontology of experience which emphasizes the degree to which social interactions are embodied, taking place in *concrete* space and time. In this situation bodies are marked by the *social* and this becomes an integral part of identities. Experience thus becomes intersubjective and embodied – not individual and fixed. But with the transformation from low to high technology, a change occurs as to who controls the information relevant to the management of the body *as* diseased (not the body *in* disease). In contrast to precolonial intersubjectivity the new mode of prescribing "provides a language of intersubjectivity among the community of physicians."[54] Coming to Ayurveda, "The masters in this science say that the place is of two kinds: the land and the body." The human body and the earth are both irrigated by fluids. The drainage of the human body and the cultivation of drained land are a *single* theme in Ayurveda.[55]

In this tradition a microcosmic man is conceived of as the localized part of macrocosmic nature. Medicine was the most important of all the physical sciences which were cultivated in ancient India, was directly and intimately connected with the *Samkhya* and *Vaisesika* physics and was probably the origin of the logical speculations subsequently codified in *Nyayasutras*.[56] It is explicitly taught in Ayurveda that its validity can be attributed to the fact that it was composed by trustworthy persons and that it can only be learned by trusting in their authority. Curiously enough, along with the rigorously logical speculative framework grounded in Ayurveda, the place of authority with regard to learning was equally ensconced in the same treatise.

Unlike Western logic, Indian logic is insistent on excluding terms that have no referential content from logical discourse. Also, (a) the role of *affect* as opposed to sanitized *cognition*, (b) *epistemological* issues grounded on grammar rather than on mathematics (as in the Western tradition), and (c) truth-validity unit in logical discourse (opposed to validity only) were the areas where new 'positivist' logic insinuated to reconstruct the logical frame and *sign*-system.[57] It is epitomized in Claude Bernard's remark on experimental physiology, "Philosophy … would be harmful to the scientist proper."[58] But to read this text hermeneutically we should "avoid reading back into the ancient medieval Sanskrit texts ideas and terms from the post-scientific revolution period."[59] Confronted with the difficulty of translation Dasgupta noted the problem. He could only give one sense of a word, which in the original Sanskrit has been used in a variety of senses, which the word has.[60] In Indian pre-colonial perception knowledge of the meaning of words is not only a tool to remove ignorance, but also a way to identify with *Sabda Brahman*.[61] Ayurveda is steadfast in insisting that medicine should always be centred on the person rather than on the disease. The philosophical emphasis on the wholeness of the person is reflected in the comprehensiveness of the diagnostic examination. The person in Ayurveda is conceived of as simultaneously living in and partaking of different orders of being – physical, psychological, social and, to add, metaphysical. The boundaries between these orders are fluid; the dividing line between psyche and soma or between soma and nature is much weaker than is the case with Western concepts of the person. [62] A fundamental postulate in Ayurveda is that the body, the physical part of the person, is in perpetual flux with nature, the physical part of the cosmos, for ceaseless transformations of matter through a dense circulation of symbols with a *polysemy* of meaning. The *floating signifiers* become an explanatory principle for this indigenous thought.[63] As a result the body and embodiment often intertwined to unfold a semiotic function where the body and person were perceptive of and expressive of one another. The body (*sharira*) consists of gross (*sthula*), subtle (*linga*) and causal (*karma*) bodies. In the discourses of health and illness the gross body is singled out and reverted to the state of harmony/equilibrium with other bodies. So with respect to the biomedical concept it was not the body per se, rather the bodily *being-in-the-world.* Situated in this transcendental nature of thinking and awe about authority of texts/person, Indian knowledge systems encountered colonial ones set in time-clock life style getting legitimised in the dominating social ethos.[64]

3. Construction of Hegemony

The Western image of the body is sharply differentiated from the rest of the objects in the universe. In an acute observation, "from at least the time of Descartes, the living body" is understood in medicine to be a kind of "animated corps," since "dissection was the primary means of aggregating facts about human biology."[65] Reading the other's body becomes a way, too, to be in contact with the whole cultural universe in which that body is immersed and by which it is moulded. To the colonizer, therefore, the study of India was made part of a larger scholarly enterprise in which this creation and dissemination of knowledge and at the same time the unequal asymmetric power relationships of imperialism helped shape the categories within which that knowledge was produced.[66] Faced with the impossible task of figuring the colonized Other and entrenched in alterity's unrepresentability, colonial medical discourses of that period dwell, with symptomatic insistence, on a semiotic of grotesque and infectious bodies as discussed above.[67] The question came up: how could the colonizing subject imagine the radical alterity of the native without introjecting its forms, that is, without being seduced or infected by the traits of its difference? "British people's conceptions of their own biomedical identities were formulated within a global context, as part of their own response to the experience of colonial disease."[68] It occurred in an *asymmetrically overdetermined* space where a continual exchange of metonymic (>) and metaphoric (<) signifiers/surpluses was taking place.

Metonymic knowledge of this bio-medical model at the root of medical epistemology necessarily regards the body as an object. Some important additions to the 'art of diagnosis' began to entail asymmetric change in the entire premise of: (a) doctor-patient relationship, and (b) medicine-society interactive zones. Listening with *stethoscope* revolved round a technique of *making-present* the spatial assignation of the invisible/inaudible advancing the ease, accuracy and acuteness of diagnosis.[69] The 'inside' of the body was involuted by the new emergent physician's glance and spread thin across the graphs and tables of anatomical knowledge. In an insightful remark, "Philosophical enquiry and applied science appeared to have raised Western thought to a commanding height from which the thought system of others could be confidentially measured."[70] As Luciene Febvre shows – even the words like 'system', 'deduction' etc. are absent from 16th century vocabularies.[71]

The narrow physical emphasis of Western medicine, it is claimed, has a powerful effect on individual subjectivity. By locating pathology in the individual and treatment in private settings divorced from everyday life, biomedicine weakens alternative accounts of the social sources of suffering and health.[72] Biomedicine de-socializes disease, and thereby authorizes the particular 'truth' that diseases are biological events, arising through impersonal, natural laws, rather than social ties and interests.[73] As it banishes experiential knowledge as an epistemological category to be replaced by abstraction, so experience is restricted to zero.[74] Long conceived in Western medicine as if they were machines, human bodies have actually become 'technological artefacts'. It was in sharp contrast to Ayurvedic examination solely based on feeling one's pulse and a careful particular mode of history taking only. Along with auscultation (with stethoscope) and percussion, use of dyes like Leishman's stain to locate the incriminating 'germ' or bacteria under microscope, insidiously led to *objectification* of a patient's body – *epistemologically* in the form of knowledge of the link between the social person and his or her illness.[75] New marks of authority and identification – distinctly different, yet insidiously masquerading, from pre-colonial marks – began circulating in the terrain on which opposed terms met, sometimes understood to remain in tension, at other moments collapsing upon one another. But beyond this, the repeatability of the marks, harnessed by various social agencies, seem to generate tirelessly new contexts of legitimacy. Biomedicine thus helped construct the individual as an autochthonous subject who exists against a background of facts and material objects. "This form of subjectivity … advances colonial rule. It subverts pre-colonial forms of consciousness, instils habits of … efficiency and work discipline," and finally, "paves the way for wage labour and other forms of colonial capitalism."[76]

In this changing paradigm of subject-positions, rather than asking how metaphors instantiate image schemas it is more apt to begin with the lived experience from which we derive schemas as abstract products of analytic abstraction. Here we need to talk about connections and affinities to avoid the production of one's own and another's experience as a resource for another closed narrative.[77]

Coming to the domain of practical therapeutics, particularly aided by the use of microscope and stethoscope, it proffered excellent results generating an eerie feeling about its healing potential. Imbued in *extra*-corporeal source of disease and divine healing power, the Indian population was perplexed by its consequences conveyed through its new scientific idioms and modes of communications.[78] During this sea change *symptoms* ceased to be *signs*, they became the *disease itself*.

This sort of biomedical model contains an implicit prerogative of authority based on professional knowledge in which the practitioner is in control of the body of the patient. Biomedicine and its practitioners deal with malfunctioning organs or other systems of the body and with symptoms thereof, not with "the body" as such. So the medical body is passive, and disciplined and *normalized* as well; any active capacities it may display are regarded as internal to its physiology, and these can be revealed to external observers as objective knowledge. All these epiphenomenona acted together whereby the hitherto existing patient as *embodied subject* became the *object* of colonial biomedicine. Consequent of this reconstituted perception, a permanent rupture began to insinuate in the man-nature perception. There were frequent epidemics of malaria and cholera as a result of new constructions of railways and high road. So in popular Indian perception *nature* metamorphosed into an incriminating *object*, which was quite in tune with the aspiring imperialist project.[79]

Interestingly enough, colonial medicine made a *heterologic* move to usurp the surplus meaning of the "spirituality of health" wherein a space for science-as-magic was opened. The *trope* of romantic aesthetics was conjoined with the *wonder* of curiosity to insinuate into this perception of local knowledge world. Floating signifiers being substituted by circumscribed scientific metonymies led to where "[c]ontingent figures of chances masqueraded deceptively as figures of necessity" and "metonymies are assimilated with metaphors with which they are contiguously associated."[80] The body became the *written* surface and the *writing* instrument for the emergent medical hegemony. It also became the absolute limit of the space where colonial medical hegemony was narrativized into a logic of care/cure.

One simple example: Gananath Sen, one of the most eminent Ayurvedic practitioners of that period, writes,

> I am here to appeal to your justice to give Ayurveda its share of consideration in the great work of Renaissance set upon you by a kind Providence and benign Government … We mean to employ the lever of our Western education to turn over these ruins.[81]

He turns quickly to discover examples of "germ theory of disease" even in ancient Ayurvedic texts. Self-evidently metaphoric Ayurvedic knowledge failed to sustain without being legitimised/reconstructed by metonymic biomedical knowledge – both operating at the level of epistemological space of the body. Here "germ theory" acted as a *metonymy* of power. In tandem, practical therapeutics and biomedical discourses acted in the same way achieving ontological consistency. Another example in this regard would be lamentation of Kanailal Dey, a distinguished physician of the late nineteenth century, for excluding indigenous herbal drugs in the latest list of drugs by the Government of India, "The Govt. of India have no doubt that other indigenous drugs would be employed in the Medical Depots if they could be obtained pure … price not exceeding that at which they can be imported."[82] One must note (a) the contentment in getting recognition from the colonial state, and (b) to come to terms with dominant market forces. Still another example: while getting some financial assistance from government, one of the Bengali magazines, dealing with health in an indigenous way, comments:

> Possibly it is known to many that we have received some amount of money from Bengal and Bombay governments etc. for propagating *Caraka* and *Susruta*. And the news of that aid has been loudly publicized too in all the newspapers. So, in this case, 'aided by government' becomes coterminous with sycophantic *kavirajas* (Ayurvedic physicians) around government in popular perception.[83]

It is to be noted that the epistemological root of Ayurveda was constituted in precolonial social milieu. But it was getting dislocated and displaced in the new socio-economic context when the emergence of market was a formidable phenomenon to cope with. The question arises: how does one adhere to one's local identity while living in a dislocating cultural milieu? Identity is not composed of a fixed set of memories but lies in the dialectical ceaseless activity of remembering and forgetting, assimilating and discarding. "…we find ourselves in the moment of transit where space and time cross to produce complex figures of difference and identity, past and present, inside and outside, inclusion and exclusion."[84] Here we can see the figures of doubling, the part objects of a metonymy of colonial desire which alienates the modality and normality of those dominant discourses in which they emerge as "inappropriate" colonial subjects. There is a resultant split of the colonial discourse. As it split open it "lost its autonomy and originality in the indigenisation of its authority" leading to a "space opened for the renegotiation of science's status as truth."[85] The metropolitan and the subaltern acted in differing ways for renegotiation of the body and subject-positions in this split-open *hybrid space*.

4. Conclusion

Such was a feature of the "Indianity" of the body, and also of health and illness. It existed, often liminally, with its subversive strategies and insinuating spaces of manoeuvring in an unequal struggle against hegemonizing the 'social body'. Uprooted in indigenous knowledge systems, healing practices were left with no source of cognitive and epistemological encounters with the West. The severance of the body's social roots, its dematerialization as a figment of discourse started to build up an entirely different story-in-the-making. It was the 'social body' where colonization operated resulting in the production of (a) a truncated cosmography and (b) logocentric social scripts. It yielded a hyphenated relation between norm and its transgression, inclusive of microsocial processes within which the self is created and maintained. Again, this same space was a competing area for the homogenizing 'unitary' nationalist discourse, too. In any specific colonial discourse the *metaphoric*/narcissistic and the *metonymic*/aggressive positions will function simultaneously, strategically poised in relation to each other.[86] It is the appearances of power within which the subjects of the discourses are constructed. This body, then, becomes a represented body. But it also reflects the representation of the community, reified 'social body', which thus acquires another type of cohesion and ontological consistency.[87] To come back from the erased margin of dissolution, this body insinuates within the interstices of the hybrid of *practical* therapeutics and *ontology* of health connoting subjectivity in popular conceptualisation. "It is from within the hegemonic space of this technological reason, then, a sign of unreason irrupts."[88] A new narrative of a "Third Worldly" health concept *signified* through social assistance-neighbourliness-community-physician paradigm does wait to be explored. It is distinct from the "First Worldly" concept of service-doctor-commodity-state-individual paradigm.

Health and the body, in today's world, have become increasingly the objects of seduction/interpellation by semiotically loaded hyperreal and metonymic signifiers. The body becomes plastic: a lifestyle accessory, a thing to be sculpted, shaped and stylised. Transnational capitalism demands flexible bodies for flexible accumulation and the organization of the body on an unprecedented scale.[89] Despite this fact we find before us a corporeity, which is marginalized as a consequence of the affirmation of new technologies. Still there exist dramatically a corporeity and a generativity on the forefront in cultures where the experience of maternity is central to women's life, a person in disease is still a concern for the community to which he belongs. But that is a separate account to be narrated at length elsewhere

A few points are for quick considerations. In an authoritative textbook of internal medicine traditional therapeutics is recognized for subsumption within modern pharmacopoeia. It remarks intriguingly, "Although many unconventional therapies are not supported by rigorous clinical trials, 'alternative' is not synonymous with unproven."[90] It is the mainstream attempt to represent the alterity's unrepresentability through the grand narrative of the Same, the trajectory of which we have explored in this inadequate treatise. There is a cautious note, too, "many alternative therapeutics complement rather than supplant conventional medicine."[91]

We are assured! But still we try to find out areas of contestations living inside this discourse – the text. We can try to replace the stifling monologues of Self and Other with a genuinely dialogic and dialectical history that can account for the formation of different selves and the construction of different epistemologies.[92] Subversive resistance through hybrid space (and hybrid vocabulary not discussed here) not only implies (a) a changing native culture but it also indicates (b) the impossibility of generating a sovereign hegemonic existence untouched by native culture. A clear distinction between authentic and contaminated was necessary to reject the similarities between the East and the contemporary colonial West in colonial India. We find in 'Public Works Code' (Ch. V, section 1, paragraph 3), "The health and comfort of troops (European) are to be held as paramount considerations to which all others must give way."[93] That very narrative is being rewritten assimilating these distinctions through performative and constative manoeuvres of invisible hegemonic paradigms and discourses.

To de-essentialize this universalised epistemological/ontological preoccupations we have to search for different epistemologies, corporeities and selves. One has to emphasize that power-knowledge never succeeds in completely overcoming the body. The body always exceeds the power frame that attempts to control it. This exceeding is possible partly because of the internal conflicts and contradictions among the various discourses that attempt to control the body.

Notes

[1] Elizabeth Grosz, *Volatile Bodies* (Indianapolis: Indiana University Press, 1994), 142.
[2] Barbara J. McNeil, "Hidden Barriers to Improvement in the Quality of Care," *New England Journal of Medicine*, Vol. 345, 22 (2001), 1612-1620. Also numerous debates and articles around similar themes can be

found in various issues of *British Medical Journal* and *Annals of Internal Medicine*, besides *NEJM.*

[3] Roselyne Rey, *The History of Pain,* transl. L. E. Wallace et al. (Cambridge Massachusetts: Harvard University Press, 1995), 328-29.

[4] Michael Worboys, "Manson, Ross, and Colonial Medical Policy," in *Disease, Medicine, and Empire: Perspectives on Western Medicine and the Experience of European Expansion*, ed. Roy MacLeod and Milton Lewis (London: Routledge, 1988), 21-37.

[5] Richard J. Bernstein, *The New Constellation: The Ethical-Political Horizon of Modernity/Postmodernity* (Massachusetts: MIT Press, 1995), 66-67.

[6] Philip Hancock et al., Introduction, *The Body, Culture and Society* (Buckingham: Open University Press, 2000), 1.

[7] Terence Turner, "Bodies and Anti-Bodies: Flesh and Fetish in Contemporary Social Theory," in *Experience and Embodiment: The Existential Ground of Culture and Self*, ed. Thomas J. Csordas (London: Cambridge University Press, 1994), 29.

[8] Robert A. Arnowitz, *Making Sense of Illness: Science, Society, and Disease* (New York: Cambridge University Press, 1998), 130-136, 143-144.

[9] Michel Foucault, *The Birth of the Clinic* (New York: Vintage Books, 1973), xiv.

[10] Guenter B. Risse, "Medical Care," in *Companion Encyclopedia of History of Medicine, Vol. 1*, ed. W. F. Bynum and Roy Porter (New York: Routledge, 1993), 45-77.

[11] Hans-Georg Gadamer, *The Enigma of Health* (Cambridge: Polity Press, 1996), 2. Though he has used this theorization with respect to 'normal sciences' per se, it is quite relevant here for its insight.

[12] Panchanan Mandal, *Chithipatre Samajchitra (Social Picture through Letters)* (Visva Bharati archives).

[13] Dwijendranath read this essay at the 8th session of Kambulitola Education Society, Calcutta on 24th August 1891.

[14] Dominik Wujastyk, *The Roots of Ayurveda* (India: Penguin, 1998), 7.

[15] T. J. S. Patterson, "The relationship of Indian and European Practitioners of Medicine from the Sixteenth Century," in *Studies on Indian Medical History,* ed. G. J. Muelenbeld and Dominik Wujastyk (Delhi: Motilal Banarasidas, 2001), 111-120.

[16] Hancock, 6.

[17] Veena Das, *Critical Events* (Delhi: Oxford University Press, 1999), 16.

[18] Richard Wolff, Editor's Comments, *Rethinking Marxism*, Vol. 13, 2 (2001).

[19] Gyan Prkash, *Another Reason* (Delhi: Oxford University Press, 1999), 136.

[20] Mark Harrison, *Climates and Constitutions* (Delhi: Oxford University Press, 1999), 2.

[21] John Farley, *Bilharzia: A History of Imperial Tropical Medicine* (New York: Cambridge University Press, 1991), 14-71.
[22] Javeed Alam, "Modernity and its Philosophic Vision," in *The Making of History*, ed. Panikkar et al., (Delhi: Tulika, 2000), 497. For a somewhat corroborative view, see Charles Taylor, *Sources of the Self: The Making of Modern Identity* (Cambridge: Cambridge University Press, 1992).
[23] Zygmunt Baumann, "Parvenu and Pariah: Heroes and Victims of Modernity," in *The Politics of Postmodernity,* ed. Lames Good and Irving Velody (London: Cambridge University Press, 1998), 23.
[24] Alam, 407.
[25] Ashis Nandy, "The Intimate Enemy," in *Exiled at Home* (Delhi: Oxford University Press, 1998). In his observation through institution of secular social hierarchy *cognition* was insulated from *affect.*
[26] Gyan Prakash, 5.
[27] Homi K. Bhabha, *The Location of Culture* (New York: Routledge, 1994), 171-197.
[28] This was a paper presented at the 1st Chinese Medical Conference, September 15-22, 1921 and included in *Pathological Problems in the Orient, Dedication Ceremonies and Medical Conference*, (Peking: Peking Union Medical College, 1922), 377-381 (Visva Bharati archives).
[29] Prakash, 127. In a different setting Warwick P. Anderson notes, "In magnifying microbes as social actors, American physicians made Philipino bodies … the objects of ceaseless medical inspection and regulation. It was the beginning of modern tropical medicine." "Immunities of Empire: Race, Disease, and the New Tropical Medicine, 1900-1920," *Bulletin of the History of Medicine,* 70, 1 (1996), 94-111.
[30] Mark Harrison, "'The Tender Frame of Man': Disease, Climate, and Racial Difference in India and the West Indies, 1760-1860," *Bulletin of the History of Medicine*, 70, 1 (1996), 68-93.
[31] Alain Renaut, *The Era of the Individual: A Contribution to a History of Subjectivity*, trans. M. B. DeBevoise and F. Philip (Delhi: MLBD, 2000), 3-57.
[32] Thomas R. Metcalf, *Ideologies of the Raj* (Delhi: Cambridge University Press, 1998), 3.
[33] Partha Chatterjee, "Talking about our Modernity in Two Languages" in *The Partha Chatterjee Omnibus* (Delhi: Oxford University Press, 1999).
[34] For example see a poem of 1890 on grotesque aboriginal woman by J. Burton Stephens cited in Ross Woodrow's "Race and Image" website <http://www.newcastle.edu.au/department/fad/fi/woodrow/race.htm>
[35] Mark Harrison, *Climates and Constitutions*, 111-152, 215-224.
[36] Gayatri C. Spivak, "Deconstructing Historiography," in *Subaltern Studies iv*, ed. Ranajit Guha (Delhi: Oxford University Press, 1999), 331-333.
[37] Harold Schweizer, "To Give Suffering a Language," in *Literature and Medicine*, 14, 2 (1995), 210-221.

[38] Diane P. Mines, *From Homo Hierarchicus to Homo Faber: Breaking Convention Through Semiosis*, paper presented at the 1996 American Anthropological Association meeting in San Francisco, USA.
[39] Allan Young, "Sufferings and the Origins of Traumatic Memory," in *Social Suffering,* ed. Arthur Kleinman et al. (Delhi: Oxford University Press, 2000), 245-260.
[40] James Mill, *The History of British India* (first published in 1817, reprinted, Associated Press: New Delhi, 1972). Also, Eric Stokes, *The English Utilitarians and India* (Oxford: Clarendon Press, 1959).
[41] Sudhir Kakar, *Shamans, Mystics and Doctors* (Delhi: Oxford University Press, 1982).
[42] Georges Canguilhem, *On the Normal and the Pathological* (Dordrecht: Reidel Publishing Company, 1978), 178.
[43] A huge cache of *Tattvabodhini Patrika (Journal for Awakening of Knowledge)*, published during early and mid-19th century, reveals Bengali metropolitan attitudes toward biomedicine (Visva Bharati archives).
[44] Michel Foucault, *Power/Knowledge* (New York: Pantheon Books, 1977), 55-62.
[45] Canguilhem, 153.
[46] Deepak Kumar, *Science and the Raj* (Delhi:, 1997), 17.
[47] Surendranath Dasgupta, *A History of Indian Philosophy*, Vol. 2 (Delhi: MLBD), 273-436.
[48] Bimal Krishna Matilal, *Logic, Language and Reality* (Delhi: MLBD, 1977), 3.
[49] Francis Zimmermann, *The Jungle and the Aroma of Meat* (Delhi: MLBD, 1999), 20-21.
[50] Kakar (1998).
[51] Zimmermann, 20.
[52] Kenneth G. Zysk, *Ascetism and Healing in Ancient India* (Delhi: MLBD, 2000), 37.
[53] Ibid, 35.
[54] For a better understanding see, Gananath Obeyesekere, "Science, Experimentation, and Clinical Practice in Ayurveda," in *Paths to Asian Medical Knowledge*, eds. Charles Leslie and Allan Young (Delhi: Munshiram Manoharlal, 1993), 160-176.
[55] Zimmermann, 22-23.
[56] Dasgupta, 273.
[57] Geraldine H. Forbes, *Positivism in Bengal: A Case Study in the Transmission and Assimilation of an Ideology* (Kolkata: Papyrus, 1999), 111-136.
[58] Claude Bernard. *The Introduction to the Study of Experimental Medicine*. Tr. A. S. Weber, (Paris: J. B. Bailliere et Fils, 1865). 87-88.
[59] Wujastyk, 35.
[60] Dasgupta, 337.

[61] H. G. Coward and K. K. Raja (eds.), *Encyclopedia of Indian Philosophies,* Vol. 5 (Delhi: MLBD, 2001), 54.
[62] Kakar, 219-251.
[63] Jose Gil, *Metamorphose of the Body*, trans. Stephen Muecke, (Minneapolis: University of Minnesota Press, 1995), 93-104.
[64] Sumit Sarkar, *Writing Social History* (Delhi: Oxford University Press, 1986), 182-357. For the epistemological root of Ayurveda see T. J. S. Patterson, ibid, 111-120.
[65] Margaret Lock, "Displacing Suffering: The Reconstruction of Death in North America and Japan," in *Social Suffering*, ed. Arthur Kleinman et al. (Delhi: Oxford University Press, 2000), 207-244.
[66] Metcalf, 1-2.
[67] Gyan Prakash, 128. He argues: "The emergent regime of knowledge conjured up of the image of a spectral body composed of unhygienic habits and superstitious beliefs."
[68] Alan Bewell, *Romanticism and Colonial Disease* (Baltimore: John Hopkins University Press, 1999), 19.
[69] C. Peter W. Warren, "The History of Diagnostic Technology for Diseases of the Lungs," *Canadian Medical Association Journal*, Nov. 2, 9 (1999), 161.
[70] Stanley J. Tambiah, *Magic, Science, Religion and the Scope of Rationality* (New York: Cambridge University Press, 1990), 86.
[71] Ibid, 86 (quoted).
[72] For important studies see Arthur Kleinman, *Patients and Healers in the Context of Culture* (Berkley: University of California Press, 1980), and *The Illness Narrative* (New York: Basic Books, 1988).
[73] Bjoren Hofmann, "The Technological Invention of Diseases," *Journal of Medical Ethics: Medical Humanities* 27 (2001), 10-19.
[74] Claude Alvares, *Homo Faber: Technology and Culture in India, China and the West 1500-1972* (Bombay: Allied Publishers, 1979).
[75] Otto Lene, "Medicine, Disease, and Culture," *Ethnologia Scandinavica*, 23 (1993), 25-35.
[76] Paul Brodwin, *Medicine and Mortality in Haiti* (New York: Cambridge University Press, 1996), 54.
[77] Donna Haraway, "Situated Knowledges: The Science Question in Feminism and the Privilege of Partial Perspective," *Feminist Studies* 14 (1998), 577-590.
[78] For some illuminating studies on various aspects of encounters between indigenous healing practices in India and 'cosmopolitan' medicine, see Brahmananda Gupta, "Indigenous Medicine in Nineteenth- and Twentieth-century Bengal" in ed. Charles Leslie *Asian Medical Systems: A Comparative Study* (Delhi: MLBD, 1998), 368-378.
[79] Satpal Sangwan, "From Gentlemen Amateurs to Professionals: Reassessing the Natural Science Tradition In Colonial India 1780-1840,"

in Richard Grove et al. (eds.), *Nature and the Orient* (Delhi: Oxford University Press, 1992), 210-236.
[80] Jonathan Culler, *The Pursuit of Signs* (London: Routledge, 1981), 220-222.
[81] Gananath Sen, *Hindu Medicine* (an address delivered at the Hindu University Foundation Ceremony, Benaras), Calcutta, 1916 (Visva Bharati archives).
[82] Kanailal Dey, *Indigenous Drugs of India* (Calcutta, 1896) (Visva Bharati archives).
[83] Editorial of *Chikitsa Smmilani* (Union of Medical Treatments), 1892. Compiled by Pradip Basu, *Samayiki* (Calcutta: Ananda Publishers, 1998), 124.
[84] Homi K. Bhabha in his Interview in *Artforum*, 33, 7 (1995).
[85] Gyan Prakash, 72.
[86] Bhabha, *The Location of Culture* (New York: Routledge, 1998), 171-197.
[87] Gil, 290.
[88] Sundar Kali, "Mythicising the White Man," in *History and the Present*, eds. Partha Chatterjee and Anjan Ghosh (Delhi: Permanent Black, 2002).
[89] Hancock, 3.
[90] Harrison's *Principles of Internal Medicine* (New York: McGraw Hill, 2001), 49.
[91] Ibid, 49.
[92] Kumkum Sangari, "The Politics of the Possible," in *Interrogating Modernity* (Calcutta: Seagull Books, 1993), 247.
[93] W. J. Moore, *Health in the Tropics* (London: John Churchill, 1862), 65 (Visva Bharati archives).

Bibliography

Alam, Javeed, "Modernity and its Philosophic Vision." In *The Making of History*, ed. by K.N Panikkar, Terence J. Byres and Utsa Patnaik, 405-439. New Delhi: Tulika, 2000.

Alvares, Claude. *Homo Faber: Technology and Culture in India, China and the West 1500-1972.* Bombay: Allied Publishers, 1979.

Anderson, Warwick P. "Immunities of Empire: Race, Disease, and the New Tropical Medicine, 1900-1920." *Bulletin of the History of Medicine,* 70, 1 (1996): 94-111.

Basu, Pradip. *Samayiki.* Calcutta: Ananda Publishers, 1998.

Baumann, Zygmunt. "Parvenu and Pariah: Heroes and Victims of Modernity." In *The Politics of Postmodernity,* ed. by Good Lames and Velody Irving, 23-35. London: Cambridge University Press, 1998.

Bernard, Claude. *The Introduction to the Study of Experimental Medicine.* Translated by A. S. Weber. Paris: J. B. Bailliere et Fils, 1865.

Bernstein, Richard J. *The New Constellation: The Ethical-Plitical Horizon of Modernity/Postmodernity.* Massachusstes: MIT Press, 1995.

Bewell, Alan. *Romanticism and Colonial Disease.* Baltimore: John Hopkins University Press, 1999.

Bhabha, Homi K. *The Location of Culture.* New York: Routledge, 1998.

Brodwin, Paul. *Medicine and Mortality in Haiti.* New York: Cambridge University Press, 1996.

Canguilhem, Georges. *On the Normal and the Pathological.* Dordrecht: Reidel Publishing Company, 1978.

Chatterjee, Partha. "Talking about our Modernity in Two Languages." In *The Partha Chatterjee Omnibus*, 262-285. New Delhi: Oxford University Press, 1999.

Coward, Harold. G. and Raja, K. Kunjunni. (eds.). *Encyclopedia of Indian Philosophies*, Vol. 5, 51-82. Delhi: MLBD, 2001.

Culler, Jonathan. *The Pursuit of Signs.* London: Routledge, 1981.

Das, Veena. *Critical Events.* Delhi: Oxford University Press.

Dasgupta, Surendranath, *A History of Indian Philosophy*, Volume 2, 273-436. Delhi: MLBD.

Dey, Kanailal. *Indigenous Drugs of India.* Calcutta, 1896 (Visva Bharati archives).

Farley, John. *Bilharzia: A History of Imperial Tropical Medicine.* Cambridge: Cambridge University Press, 1991.

Febvre, Luciene. *The Problem of Unbelief in the Sixteenth Century: The Religion of Rabelais.* Quoted in Stanley J. Tambiah (1990).

Forbes, Geraldine H. *Positivism in Bengal: A Case Study in the Transmission and Assimilation of an Ideology*. Kolkata: Papyrus, 1999.

Foucault, Michel. *The Birth of the Clinic: An Archeology of Medical Perception.* New York: Vintage Books, 1994.

Foucault, Michel. *Power/Knowledge.* New York: Pantheon Books, 1980.

Gadamer, Hans-Georg. *The Enigma of Health.* Cambridge: Polity Press, 1996.

Gil, Jose. *Metamorphoses of the Body.* Translated by Stephen Muecke. Minneapolis: University of Minnesota Press, 1995.

Grosz Elizabeth. *Volatile Bodies.* Indianapolis: Indiana University Press, 1994.

Gupta, Brahmananda, "Indigenous Medicine in Nineteenth- and Twenteenth-Century Bengal." In *Asian Medical Systems: A Comparative Stusdy*, ed. by Charles Leslie, 368-378. Delhi: MLBD, 1993.

Hancock, Philip, Bill Hughes, Elizabeth Jagger et al. *The Body, Culture and Society.* Buckingham: Open University Press, 2000.

Haraway, Donna. "Situated Knowledges: The Science Question in Feminism and the Privilege of Partial Perspective." *Feminist Studies* 14 (1998): 577-590.

Harrison, Mark. *Principles of Internal Medicine.* New York: McGraw Hill, 2001.

Harrison, Mark. *Climates and Constitutions.* Delhi: Oxford University Press, 1999.

Harrison, Mark. "'The Tender Frame of Man': Disease, Climate, and Racial Difference in India and the West Indies, 1760-1860." *Bulletin of the History of Medicine*, 70, 1 (1996): 68-93.

Hofmann, Bjoren. "The Technological Invention of Diseases." *Journal of Medical Ethics: Medical Humanities* 27 (2001): 10-19.

Kakar, Sudhir. *Shamans, Mystics and Doctors.* Delhi: Oxford University Press, 1998.

Kali, Sundar. "Mythicising the White Man." In *History and the Present*, ed. by Partha Chatterjee and Anjan Ghosh, 44-70. New Delhi: Permanent Black, 2002.

Kleinman, Arthur. *Patients and Healers in the Context of Culture.* Berkley: University of California Press, 1980.

Kleinman, Arthur. *The Illness Narrative.* New York: Basic Books, 1988.

Kumar, Deepak. *Science and the Raj.* Delhi: Oxford University Press, 1997.

Lock, Margaret, "Displacing Suffering: The Reconstruction of Death in North America and Japan." In *Social Suffering*, ed. by Arthur Kleinman, Veena Das and Margaret Lock, 207-240. New Delhi: Oxford University Press, 2000.

Mandal, Panchanan. *Chithipatre Samajchitra (Social Picture through Letters).* (Visva Bharati archives).

Matilal, Bimal Krishna. *Logic, Language and Reality.* New Delhi: Motilal Banarasidas, 1977.

McNeil, Barbara J. "Hidden Barriers to Improvement in the Quality of Care." *New England Journal of Medicine*, 345, 22 (2001): 1612-1620.

Metcalf, Thomas R. *Ideologies of the Raj.* New Delhi: Cambridge University Press, 1998.

Mill, James. *The History of British India.* First published in 1817, reprinted. New Delhi: Associated Press, 1972.

Mines, Diane P. *From Homo Hierarchicus to Homo Faber: Breaking Convention Through Semiosis.* Paper presented at the 1996 American Anthropological Association meeting in San Francisco, USA.

Moore, W. J. *Health in the Tropics*. London: John Churchill, 1862 (Visva Bharati archives).

Nandy, Ashis. *Exiled at Home.* New Delhi: Oxford University Press, 1998.

Obeyesekere, Gananath. "Science, Experimentation, and Clinical Practice in Ayurveda." In *Paths to Asian Medical Knowledge*, ed. by Charles Leslie and Allan Young, 160-176. Delhi: Munshiram Manoharlal, 1993.

Otto, Lene. "Medicine, Disease, and Culture." *Ethnologia Scandinavica*, Vol. 23, 1993. 25-35.

Patterson, T. J. S. "The relationship of Indian and European Practitioners of Medicine from the Sixteenth Century." In *Studies on Indian Medical History*, ed. by Gerrit Jan Muelenbeld and Dominik Wujastyk, 111-120. Delhi: MLBD, 2001.
Prkash, Gyan. *AnotherReason*. New Delhi: Oxford University Press, 1999.

Rey, Roselyn. *The History of Pain*. Translated by L. E. Wallace, J. A. Cadden and S.W. Cadden. Cambridge: Harvard University Press, 1995.

Risse, Guenter B. "Medical Care." In *Companion Encyclopedia of History of Medicine*, Volume 1, ed. by W. F. Bynum and Roy Porter, 45-77. New York: Routledge, 1993.

Sangari, Kumkum. "The Politics of the Possible." In *Interrogating Modernity*, ed. by Tejaswini Niranjana, P. Sudhir and Vivek Dhareswar, 242-272. Calcutta: Seagull Books, 1993.

Sangwan, Satpal. "From Gentlemen Ameteurs to Professionals: Reassessing the Natural Science Tradition In Colonial India 1780-1840." In *Nature and the Orient*, ed. by Grove, Richard, Vinita Damodaran and Satpal Sangwan, 210-236. Delhi: Oxford University Press, 1992.

Sarkar, Sumit. *Writing Social History*. Delhi: Oxford University Press, 1986.

Schweizer, Harold. "To Give Suffering a Language." *Literature and Medicine*, 14, 2 (1995): 210-221.

Sen, Gananath. *Hindu Medicine* (an address delivered at the Hindu University Foundation Ceremony, Benaras), Calcutta, 1916 (Visva Bharati archives).

Spivak, Gayatri C. "Deconstructing Historiography." In *Subaltern Studies iv*, ed. by Ranajit Guha, 330-363. New Delhi: Oxford University Press, 1999.

Tambiah, Stanley J. *Magic, Science, Religion and the Scope of Rationality*. New York: Cambridge University Press, 1990.

Warren, C. Peter W. "The History of Diagnostic Technology for Diseases of the Lungs." *Canadian Medical Association Journal*, Nov. 2, 9 (1999), 161.

Worboys Michael. “Manson, Ross, and Colonial Medical Policy.” In *Disease, Medicine, and Empire: Perspectives on Western Medicine and the Experience of European Expansion*, ed. by Roy MacLeod and Milton Lewis, 21-37. London: Routledge, 1988.

Wujastyk, Dominik. *The Roots of Ayurveda*. India: Penguin, 1998.

Young, Allan. “Sufferings and the Origins of Traumatic Memory.” In *Social Suffering*, 245-260.

Zimmermann, Francis. *The Jungle and the Aroma of Meat.* Delhi: MLBD, 1999.

Zysk, Kenneth G. *Ascetism and Healing in Ancient India.* Delhi: MLBD, 2000.

Note on Contributor

By profession a medical practitioner, the author is an independent scholar. He is recently enrolled as a doctoral fellow of medical anthropology in North Bengal University, West Bengal, India.

Acknowledgement

For some initial thoughts I am indebted to (1) a draft of Anirban Das – later published in *Rethinking Marxism*, volume 13, no. 2 (Summer 2001), and to (2) an essay by Ajit Chaudhury on “Synthetic Hegemony” published in *margins*, 3rd issue, Calcutta.

Putting Medicine in its Place: The Case of Physician-Writer Jacques Ferron

Betty Bednarski

1. Introduction

Any consideration of the ways in which medical professionals "make sense" of their experience of health, illness and disease must necessarily take into account the phenomenon of the physician-writer. The purpose of this paper is to shed light on that phenomenon by examining the case of Quebec's Jacques Ferron (1921–1985), a much-celebrated literary figure who was also a family doctor. Ferron is the author of a prodigious body of work, which contains powerful fictions of illness and much outspoken commentary on medicine. His writing has been the object of intense scrutiny by literary scholars, both in Canada and internationally, but few have written about the incorporation of medical narratives into that work.[1] Nor have medical scholars seen the significance of Ferron's literary treatment of medical themes. There has been as yet little serious analysis of his discourse on medicine, and nothing to indicate that he has found an audience among the broad community of physician-readers who would seem to be his natural interlocutors.[2] This study grows out of a desire to bring Ferron the writer to the attention of a medical readership, as well as to the attention of scholars in the history of medicine and those exploring the relationship between medicine and literature.[3] It should be read as an introduction. I see it myself as a kind of summary. It will point to some – just some – of the ways in which this particular medical professional has "made sense" of medicine through writing, and at the same time give an indication of where more ambitious explorations might lead.

I approach Ferron's "making sense" in three distinct but interconnected ways. The first approach is essentially biographical. I will concentrate to begin with on the man himself, on his life, and on the coexistence in this life of two activities – the literary and the medical – , on what I call the "uneasy partnership" between the physician and the literary man. Ferron was one of Quebec's most prolific writers. He is the author of over thirty books – novels, essays, short-stories, plays – and, if one counts the vast personal correspondence and the letters and opinion pieces published in newspapers and magazines, of literally hundreds of other, smaller texts. But this writer had studied medicine at Laval University in the early 1940s. He had done a stint as a doctor in the Canadian Army, then worked as a country doctor in a remote fishing village in the Gaspé. For thirty-five years he kept up a busy family practice in Longueuil, on the south shore of the St. Lawrence River, opposite Montreal, even finding time to work for several long stretches alongside psychiatrists in Montreal mental hospitals. I will be attempting to understand the relationship between these activities as Ferron himself saw it, as he himself interpreted it, asking: How did Ferron reconcile literature and medicine? Did he reconcile them, in fact? How did they fit together? How did he cope? I will refer mainly to autobiographical comment (often made in the course of interviews) and to the autobiographical fictions that constitute the greater part of Ferron's literary output in the last ten years or so of his life.[4]

My second approach will be to focus on Ferron's ideas on medicine itself. Here, we will see Ferron "interpreting" medicine in the most direct and straightforward way. Like any doctor, he had attitudes of his own, formed judgments, held views. And being a writer, he was able to articulate them clearly, often eloquently. What exactly did he think about medicine? About its effectiveness, its claims? About doctors themselves? About patients? Or about particular illnesses and their treatment? What were some of the debates he engaged in? What, explicitly, did he say? I say "explicitly" because, while these questions may seem at first to be very straightforward, I am conscious of a risk we run. It is dangerous to ask outright of a literary text, and in particular of a work of fiction, "What does this writer think?" It is possible to find an answer to the question (though it's preferable not to ask it in those terms), but it is not to be found where the "naïve" reader may first look. The opinion expressed by a fictional character or a narrator – even a first-person narrator – is not necessarily the author's own. "What the author thinks" is not so much to be found in a strand of dialogue or in a statement made by a narrator, as in the coming together of elements, of points of view, in the relationship, the delicate balance – or perhaps the imbalance – between them all.

Now, Jacques Ferron was a great polemicist. Not only did he give interviews, he wrote letters to newspapers, articles in magazines, and essays, where there may be an element of "pose" or "persona," but there is no significant fictional disguise. In 1975, for example, he published *Escarmouches*, a collection of short essays that had previously appeared in periodicals. "*Escarmouches*," or "skirmishes," is Ferron's term for "polemical texts." The "skirmishes" are identified here as taking place on three fronts: literary, political and medical. The medical skirmishes – forty-seven of them – make up the second section of the book.[5] Then, there are his collected "letters to the editor" – many of them signed "Jacques Ferron, m.d."[6] These were published only months after he died, in 1985. *Les Lettres aux journaux* is a five hundred and eighty-six page volume. The letters themselves run to four hundred and seventy pages.[7] More recently, in 1997, the transcript of over thirty hours of taped interview has been made available in book form. Conducted with Ferron over a period of several weeks in 1982, this interview has produced over three hundred pages of text, and some forty of these pages are on the subject of medicine.[8] It is from sources such as these that "opinion" is most easily extracted, though it can also be identified in short stories or novels where, in spite of all the subtleties I have alluded to, there are still bold authorial intrusions, clearly recognizable as such, and Ferron comes as close as one can in fiction to speaking in his own name. (In fact, as an author of fiction he sometimes finds it very difficult not to "upstage" his narrators or characters and have his own say. He has often been reproached, and often reproached himself for this.) It is on what he "says" in this particular type of text or passage that I will base my second part.

My third and final approach is to examine the incorporation of medical material into Ferron's fictional works. I will ask first: What are the situations, the experiences, that have found their way from medicine into literature? There is much that medical professionals will recognize here. But since these are not case histories transcribed from medical files, since they are literature and, as such, experience transformed, I will also ask: What has been done here with medicine – and for medicine? What is the nature of the literary transformation that has taken place? What is there in this transformation that I would most want to draw a doctor's attention to? And I will touch on the notions of "context," "voice" and "story," as well as on the question of "points of view."

In this last part in particular, but to a greater or lesser extent throughout, I will be concerned not only with the writing itself, but with its reception. I will make reference to the challenge I myself face as a reader in turn called upon to "make sense" of Ferron's "making sense." That challenge is great when it comes to interpreting the complex works of fiction, but even Ferron's explicit commentary on medicine is not always straightforward to read, particularly for a lay reader like myself. I will be reading reflexively, conscious of being outside the medical profession looking in, but keeping at all times in the back of my mind another reader, a medical reader, imagined by me. It was for just such an imagined reader that I first undertook to sift out the medical content of Ferron's writing, foregrounding that content in literary studies of his work.[9] Implicit, but undeveloped in this paper, are questions like: What could be the significance of Ferron's texts for the medical profession? What might occur when a medical professional takes on the role of active reader of these texts? Curious about the function of literature in a medical context, I am endeavouring to read not only through my own but through someone else's eyes. And underlying my "double" reading is the intuition that there are parallels between the role played by the active reader in the presence of the literary text, and the "making sense" that takes place in the face of illness – and in particular during the physician-patient encounter – in the physician's mind. I will be reflecting not only on the doctor as writer, but on the doctor as reader, not only on medicine and writing, but on the relationship between medicine and reading as well.

Finally, as I move through these three sections, it will be important to bear in mind my title. In Ferron's case, literature and medicine have come together in a most critical and self-conscious way. The doctor in him is constantly being subjected to the writer's gaze. In more senses than one, literature can be seen to be "putting medicine in its place."

2. The Physician-Writer

Ferron was – or so he would have us believe – something of a "doctor in spite of himself," in the sense that this was not his calling, not what he "wanted" to be. On the other hand, he seems to have known by the age of twenty that he would be a writer. That was the authentic choice. For the rest, it was simply a matter of earning a living. "I needed a backer," he said. "Thanks to medicine, I wasn't at the mercy of literature. I was able to choose it."[10] Literature, he felt, should not have to pay for itself. He wanted to free it from the strings of economic dependency.

Writing for Ferron was above all a freedom and a right, something as inalienable as the right to speak (he often tried to persuade others to write, to avail themselves of that freedom, that right). "It's not a profession," he wrote, "it's a freedom. When our material is the words used by everybody, the wisdom of nations, then the least I can say is that we should do it at our own risk and expense."[11] And he insists again: "Writing is not a profession. The proof is that there aren't any degrees in writing. If there were, it would be the end of literature."[12] Besides being a right and a freedom, there is also a suggestion that writing was for Ferron a kind of duty, performed in the name of others – on behalf of one's collectivity, for example. This, however, was an idea he developed as time went on and he became aware that he was writing for a francophone readership whose very survival was threatened. If it was a duty as well as a freedom, it was because he found himself in a situation where that freedom was threatened.[13]

These principles aside, there is no question that in the Quebec of the 1940s it would have been almost unheard of to make one's living as a writer. There was already a literary institution in place. There was a long tradition of doctors and lawyers and some clerics engaging to a greater or lesser degree in writing, and of writers with private means. But there were few – very few – figures sustaining themselves solely from the sale of their words. So Ferron had to pick himself a "backer." Because he came from a middle-class family, the choice open to him at that time in Quebec was law or medicine. His father was a notary and apparently considered it a foregone conclusion that his son would follow in his footsteps. It is a familiar story, and this "doctor in spite of himself" was perhaps also a "doctor out of spite," choosing the medical profession to spite his father, or at least to assert himself vis-à-vis this rather domineering man.[14]

Ferron made the decision early on, then, that income and writing would be kept separate. While he never went back on that decision, he did admit that the money he earned from his books gave him real pleasure, that he was proud of it, and that he could not say the same thing for the money medicine paid.[15] He also made no secret of the fact that he felt tremendous admiration for the one or two Quebec writers of his generation – writers like Yves Thériault – who did manage to earn a decent living from their books.

And so, for forty years medicine supported Jacques Ferron, gave him the independence to write what he wanted to write. But he owed more to his practice than financial security. Medicine was conducive to writing in ways another profession might not have been. "If I'd become a notary," he said in retrospect, "and had to draw up legal documents, I'd probably not have written books."[16] He was also conscious of having been transformed by medicine, and was careful to give it its due, albeit at times in a somewhat backhanded way: "I don't believe in what they call a vocation," he said in 1982. "You choose a profession and you adapt to it; it transforms you. … It's the profession that shapes you. … You're not necessarily called to it. You adapt."[17]

If he felt a certain gratitude to medicine, his attitude to it was nevertheless ambivalent. "I write in a medical context," he said around 1970, "which I like very much, because it keeps me in touch with reality, and which I dislike because it distracts me."[18] On the one hand, the writer recognizes that the medical context is vital to him. He "like[s it] very much." It keeps him in contact with people, and in particular with the lower classes (first the rural population of the Gaspé, then his working class patients in Montreal). This contact was healthy in a society where writers and intellectuals of his class were in some danger of cutting themselves off from the masses, and he knew that it nourished his writing. His experiences in the Gaspé had given him the sense of a rich and vigorous linguistic heritage and a robust oral tradition, both of which he would try to preserve in his writing. They furnished many of the situations and characters in his fiction, as would the long years spent making house calls in the suburbs or receiving patients in the little basement office, under a pharmacy, on Longueuil's sprawling Chemin de Chambly. House calls in particular gave him an entry, privileged access to what he called "life through the back door" – "*la vie par la porte d'en arrière*."[19] There is, then, on the one hand, an admission of writing's indebtedness to medical practice. But there is also in that same statement a hint of frustration and resentment, because medicine took up so very much of his time. Time he would have preferred to spend writing. One wonders when he did write. Often between patients, it seems, or at night, or early in the morning, before the calls began. This might be one explanation for his apparent predilection for shorter pieces – smaller forms like the *conte* (a short story, or "tale"), the *historiette* (a brief, often polemical humorous sketch), or the very short novel, or novella. He certainly stressed the connection between leisure and literature; he had enjoyed the luxury of long periods of uninterrupted time during his year as an army doctor, and credited this early leisure with helping to launch him on his literary career.[20] Later, once established in his practice, he did complain, as many women writers have, about the difficulty of "getting into" longer works, because of the fragmentation of his nights and days.[21]

But the resentment towards medicine – because more and more that is what it was – was based less on this kind of frustration than on the growing sense that there was something "unworthy" in the solution he had found. As time went on, he seems to have become more and more conscious of the difference between himself and certain other Quebec writers, who had staked all on their work, for whom writing was everything, and who refused to do anything else, even at the risk of having to live like beggars. One of them was poet Claude Gauvreau. Gauvreau's bouts of insanity and the death or internment of other writers he knew, caused Ferron to call into question his own compromise. Should he perhaps have declared himself to be a writer, unequivocally, unambiguously?

In an autobiographical text entitled "Purple Loosestrife" ("*Les salicaires*"[22]), dating from the early 1970s (by now Ferron had spent nearly thirty years as a doctor), he speaks to himself in the second person, with a kind of melancholy detachment:

> As a doctor it wasn't very often you did any good, and when you did, it was with cases that probably would have worked out on their own. You hadn't been spectacularly useful to anyone but yourself, salving your conscience a little.[23]

And he reflects on the value of his writing:

> You write in the common tongue, straight [out of] the wisdom of the nations, without inventing one single word, taking no risks, like a scribe or a notary. And you'd just seen two colleagues who risked all, the one dead, the other mad. … If they were dead, if they were mad, what were you? Nothing at all.[24]

He is filled with a sense of his own unworthiness. "What right have you to write? … [O]fficially you're a medical doctor, not a writer." "Who should commit suicide," he asks finally, "Sauvageau [a writer whose death he had just heard about], or yourself?"[25]

A few years later, Ferron was to give startling expression to the uneasy partnership between doctor and writer. During a period of weariness and depression (no doubt due in part to the exhaustion brought on by his intense activity on two fronts) he attempted suicide, and in an extraordinarily moving text entitled "The Execution of Maski," (*L'Exécution de Maski*[26]), which was written some time after (and which is neither fiction nor autobiography, but a kind of autobiographical fantasy), he came up with a fictional device to account for what he now saw as the split within him between conflicting selves. Each self becomes a character: one, he calls "Notary," and identifies as being the writer, or scribe; the other, a doctor, called "Maski," is the overpowering, shamelessly invasive man, whose life has inspired but also taken over the literary work. The two selves have collaborated as one, and in the text are tenuously held together by the pronoun "we" ("In the ten years between 1963 and 1973 we wrote a lot, maybe too much").[27] Notary, who is the narrator, longs to be free of Maski, to be at last "only a writer" (perhaps also "the only writer"?) – "*enfin seul écrivain.*"[28] While it is tempting to interpret the Maski/Notary split as a simple division between doctor and writer, nothing is quite that clear-cut. The self that is called "Maski" contains but is much greater than the doctor-self. The relationship between Maski and Notary includes but cannot be reduced to that between doctor and writer. It is nevertheless revealing of the doctor-writer relationship.[29]

Dissatisfied, unfulfilled, Notary conspires to get rid of his "other," whom he looks on as an embarrassment and an encumbrance, and on whom he realizes he has become overly dependent:

> If it hadn't been for Maski I never would have found the time to write. He not only supported me but took a vital interest in what I was doing. He beat the bushes to find me subjects to write about whenever I sat dazzled by the white page. He stood behind me, pretending to be watching me work, while I focused all my attention on my precious pen and never noticed [it was he] who was dictating everything I wrote.[30]

Further on he reflects:

> Perhaps Maski saw his role that way, hidden behind my shoulder, dictating the work I was counting on to make me famous, as if I were nothing but his scribe … and he the true author. … I'd already decided to get rid of him. I didn't want to think too much about what it might cost me.[31]

But of course he cannot live – or write – without Maski. "Maski's execution announced my own."[32]

L'Exécution de Maski was published in 1981. After this point, Ferron did not write very much at all. In some ways, quite objectively speaking, we might say that the "partnership" had been a huge success, given the number of fine texts that had grown out of it (and it is on these that his reputation rests). But in the end, Ferron himself seemed only to be aware of its failure. This is partly because in the last decade of his life there was one specific failure that he was unable to forget.

Although Ferron's work draws heavily on his experiences as a country doctor and as a general practitioner in suburban Montreal, it was his intense involvement with mental patients, particularly women and children, that was to provide the most powerful inspiration in later years. After leaving his post at St. Jean-de-Dieu psychiatric hospital in 1971, he attempted for more than a decade to write what he called his "great book on madness," his "*grand livre sur la folie*". "*C'est le premier livre que j'ai raté*," he said in 1982 – "the first book I've failed to bring off".[33] He would publish fragments of this vast work – among them, *L'Exécution de Maski* – and managed to complete other, smaller, quite different projects, like *Rosaire* (an account, reworked from his own doctor's diary, of the case of a patient he had fought to keep from being committed, a work "so mediocre I find it reassuring … [with] no other merits than accuracy and simplicity … a kind of document composed from notes taken in 1961"),[34] which he published alongside *L'Exécution de Maski*, in 1981;[35] and "*Le pas de Gamelin*" (a seventy-page text bearing the title of the "failed" book, and containing his reflections on the cases of half a dozen women patients he had known), which was published after his death, in 1987.[36] But in 1982, he announced that he had failed.

On a number of occasions Ferron tried to explain – to himself, to others – why it was so difficult to write a book about the insane. You have to share a little in their madness to write about it, he said. You have to be able to get inside it, so to speak. Otherwise you risk adopting the arrogant outside stance of the doctor-psychiatrist. The other excess to be avoided, and all too easy to succumb to, is the desire to achieve release. The insane he would be writing about were patients, and confined. Confinement is unbearable. Release from confinement is one of the great motivating forces in literature. The reader longs for the freedom of the captive. And the writer longs to bring it about. It was all too easy to fall into the trap of the facile, of the literary cliché.[37]

The reasons for this failure have a lot to do with Ferron's perception of the nature of mental illness and of the relationship between writing and "madness."[38] They also have to do with the fact that in Ferron's own experience of mental illness there was a blurring of the boundary between doctor and patient. It is not possible to go into all that here. Suffice it to say that in Ferron's eyes writing had failed in its attempt to "make sense" of "madness." His book itself was "crazy," he insisted, "unpublishable" – " [*un livre*] *fou*."[39] He saw this as a personal failure, not as the failure of writing itself – he claimed that writers like Shakespeare, Dostoyevsky, or Proust had come closer to the "truth" of madness than psychiatry ever would.[40] The failure to "bring off" this ambitious book sealed for him the failure of the uneasy partnership between writer and physician. There is no question that by the time he came to write it, the doctor and the writer could no longer collaborate the way they had in the past. The writer had struck a deal with medicine. Or so he thought. In the end, it had proved impossible to keep medicine "in its place." The relation was one of constant shifting, constant renegotiation – unsettled, unsettling – like the relation of self to other, self to self.

Ferron's own interpretation of the relationship between medicine and writing is marked, then, by the unequal value he placed on the two activities, by his perception of a split within him between two selves (corresponding in part to those two distinct but interconnected activities), and by the sense of the unworthiness and, ultimately, of the failure of the collaboration between the two. To adequately interpret Ferron's interpretation one would need to move beyond the limits of the terms he himself devised. In this brief summary of mine, I am conscious not only of having left out much rich detail, but above all of having allowed myself to re-apply – and in so doing, risk over-simplifying – Ferron's own terms. In this sense, the greatest challenge to reading these troubled and troubling texts has not been taken up.[41]

3. Ferron on Medicine: A Doctor's Views

"When it comes to medicine," Ferron once said, "I'm something of an atheist."[42] One of the most striking things about this doctor's attitude to his profession is his doubting of its claims. It is a doubting that borders at times on cynicism, but at others seems like just good healthy (and typically Ferronien) disrespect. Humility too. He once remarked that there were only two kinds of doctor: the arrogant ones, and the humble ones, whose only consolation was their lucidity.[43] He often suggested that in the end the only true healer, the only true cure, was death. "Death," he wrote, "is the one great remedy, the principle of regeneration."[44] He liked to point out that doctors were no longer indispensable, that the human race did not depend for its survival on them.[45]

For Ferron, one of the hardest things was knowing that he had perhaps not been particularly useful. Like the autobiographical doctor-self in "Purple Loosestrife," of whom the narrator comments that when he appeared to have done any good it was probably in cases that would have worked out by themselves anyway, Ferron often suggested that his greatest successes were cases where the patients had simply got better of their own accord. There was some satisfaction for him in performing specific tasks that required manual dexterity. (In relation to this notion of manual dexterity, I am reminded of a comment by another disabused doctor-narrator, who of course should not be identified in any absolute way with Ferron himself, but whose story incorporates a number of autobiographical details and reads like a confession: "I'd have been happier as a vet or a puller of teeth.")[46] Skeptical about his own usefulness as a doctor, Ferron did take considerable pride in having helped to bring babies into the world. He loved obstetrics and delivered all four of his own children. In his writing on childbirth, there are passages that are truly celebratory. However, the doctor in attendance is never glorified. More often than not he is humbled. Traditional midwives command considerably more respect than doctors, and it is generally birth itself, not obstetrical art, that is being celebrated.[47]

Given his skepticism towards medicine and his ambivalence towards his doctor-writer partnership, it is hardly surprising that Ferron should have had harsh words for individual doctors and for the medical profession as a whole. The twentieth century's glorification – and disproportionate remuneration – of doctors was, he felt, a disturbing – and unhealthy – sign . "When doctors are too well off, perhaps it's civilisation itself that's sick."[48] He was concerned above all with structures of power. His work is full of references to the dictatorship of medicine – a quasi-religious dictatorship, he maintained. In an article called "*La difficulté d'être médecin*" ("The Difficulty of Being a Doctor"), published in 1970 in a bi-weekly journal for doctors, called *L'Information médicale et para-médicale*, to which he contributed several hundred pieces between 1951 and 1980,[49] Ferron writes that medicine is no longer a calling. If it had once been possible to compare priests and doctors, both of whom had chosen a kind of ministry, if it was true that there had indeed been something like a calling in the days when payment had been made in cords of wood and sacks of potatoes (and sometimes a meagre sum of money to top that up) and intolerable conditions had driven underpaid, sleep-starved doctors to alcoholism or drugs, there were now no longer in the profession any "priests" or "curates," only – because of the high incomes – archbishops. "*Tous les médecins sont archevêques*" ("All doctors are archbishops"). The specialists, he said, were the "cardinals" and the "popes." Without any solid structure to support it, without contact with any grass-roots beneath, the profession floated on high, infatuated with its own importance. And only the state of generalized hypochondria that prevails in the western world allowed it to remain there unchallenged. On the subject of hypochondria, he felt that the whole concept of what constituted "good health" had undergone a profound change. For a kind of naïve and innocent confidence, a sense of well-being or euphoria, we have substituted a more or less permanent state of accusation. We have become the accused, answering to medicine's "Holy Inquisition."[50] While he does not name it specifically in this article, it is clear that Ferron is alluding, among other things, to the influence of preventive medicine, which he condemned quite explicitly elsewhere. Because of the emphasis on prevention, doctors, he claimed, now "treat[ed] the well" as a matter of course, and, as a result, "neglect[ed] or ignor[ed] the suffering and the dying."[51]

In "*La difficulté d'être médecin*," and in many other contexts, Ferron refers to the doctors of Molière's plays, insisting that today, as in the 17th century, the profession is guilty of the same mighty deceit. The doctor, whose science is fallible, refutable, incomplete, is always in a position of knowing more than the patient. This superior knowledge gives him his edge, and establishes the patient-doctor relation as one between powerful and powerless, rendering communication all but impossible. Ferron also points out another major difference that separates the doctor from the patient: for the patient, illness is always lived, always in the realm of "*le vécu*," whereas for the doctor it tends to be learned about, "*appris*." There is no comparison between "*l'appris*" and "*le vécu*." and this enlarges the gulf between the two. "You have to have seen a doctor who has crossed the border and suddenly become sick himself, to know what I mean. He loses his head, completely, and in his fright is little better than a hunted animal."[52]

Ferron was aware that this gulf is perhaps never wider than between male doctor and female patient, and that because medicine has been a largely male profession, male arrogance and professional arrogance can combine, not only to intimidate women but to dispossess them of their bodies and their minds. "*Le pas de Gamelin*," the posthumous text in which he writes about his women patients at Saint-Jean-de-Dieu, is particularly eloquent in this regard. Of the treatments prescribed for Mariette, a patient in her twenties, who between 1946 and 1951 underwent in rapid succession electro-shock therapy, hysterectomy, ovariectomy, lobotomy, he has this to say: " It's a man's medicine, at the very least ambiguous, possibly perverse. … A man's medicine. I've already said it, and I say it again, to my own shame."[53]

One of the areas where male dominance sought to assert itself most was, he felt, in childbirth – a striking instance, if ever there was one, of the gulf between "*l'appris*" and "*le vécu*". In an article entitled "*L'impérialisme masculin*" ("Male Imperialism"), published in the Montréal newspaper *Le Devoir* in 1975, he denounces the industrialisation of birth, in terms that reflect a decidedly feminist stance. He speaks of the doctor as the arch usurper, who sets out to displace and dispossess. "Male imperialism," he writes, "uses every means at its disposal to dispossess woman of herself." He describes how it happens – the "industrial" setting, the elaborate preparation by the nurses. Then, finally, the "usurper" arrives. He comes, Ferron writes, to make the ritual sign – the sign, not of the cross, but of the episiotomy. "Maybe there'll be time for a chat with the nurses. Under the sheet there's a nuisance who's making conversation difficult. They do their best to keep her quiet and to let her know she's in the way."[54]

If medicine draws its arrogance from a false sense of its own superiority, it also bases many of its suppositions on a mistaken premise – that of the "pathological lesion," on which Ferron maintains the teaching of medicine is still founded, and which for him constitutes the supreme illusion. The concept has been responsible for doctors' focus on "*la maladie*" as opposed to "*le malade*" – on sickness as opposed to the sick person. The term he uses in referring to it is "*la lésion cadavérique*." Since most patients have not yet reached the stage of being corpses, he says, in the days before exploratory surgery diagnosis based on what was known about cadavers was approximate, to say the least. Modern exploratory surgery merely perpetuates the illusion of the preeminence of the physical. Ferron sees a dangerous tendency for this "pathological" or physical premise to become an obsession –"*une hantise*" – and for it to "haunt" the minds of doctors, even in those areas of medicine – like psychiatry – that are the least physical, the least material, and where it should, by rights, have taken least hold. He sees psychiatry's use of lobotomy, electro-shocks and mega-dose drug therapy as an attempt to reassert its dominion over illnesses that escape it, by reassigning them a place in the physical realm and even (in the case of surgical intervention, for example) providing the doctor at last with his missing "lesion," his "scar."[55] I have said Ferron was a great polemicist. His polemics against certain psychiatric practices were famous, and every bit as vehement as those he waged in the political arena against federal politicians or corrupt provincial ones.

Against the obsession with the physical Ferron set other notions, like that of the "biographical" or the "social," which he felt had been far too often ignored. In the case of mental illness, the implication of these notions is obvious. More important than anything else, he felt, was the patient's story, which, in their hurry to classify and diagnose, psychiatrists tended to ignore. Biography, was worth more than a diagnosis any day.[56] Inseparable from the biographical dimension is the social one. Ferron stressed the importance of the wider social fabric of which any individual is a part. And he insisted that no diagnosis should be attempted before the ties are unraveled that bind a patient to a group.[57] For this reason he was concerned, too, about the confinement and isolation of patients. He refers quite often to doctors as "jailers" and is unforgiving of families who "imprison" undesirable "loved ones" behind institution walls. Here is one of his doctor-narrators, whose voice has a very authorial tone:

> The fact is, Doctor, my Aunt has been behaving very strangely." And he had come to ask for my help in getting her into a mental hospital. I was not surprised: it's the fashion now to shut people up. Faced with an undesirable who's not a criminal, we simply say he's sick, and he can be imprisoned without trial. In this

> respect medicine is a most useful institution, a branch of the law. Doctors themselves are generally well fitted for their role; they make excellent jailers. All they have to learn now is the executioner's trade.[58]

The relevance of notions like the social and the biographical would, one suspects, be readily accepted in the case of mental illness, although opinion as to their precise significance could be expected to vary. What to the lay reader is a little more surprising is the way in which these notions are extended by Ferron to include some other illnesses – leprosy, for example.[59] Or tuberculosis.

Ferron wrote quite often about tuberculosis. The illness had claimed the life of his mother (she died when he was only ten), his mother's two sisters, and several cousins. He himself developed it in his late twenties and spent some time in a sanatorium in the Laurentians.[60] He loved to tell the story of his maternal cousin, Annette. Annette was brave and impulsive. As a young woman she had fled the stifling atmosphere of her Quebec small town for Toronto, where she had achieved a kind of dramatic liberation. Soon after her arrival in the big city she had flung herself, in a fit of depression, in front of a passing car. Not only did Annette survive her suicide attempt, it seems she became the mistress of the driver of the car, and went on to become the only female cousin on Ferron's mother's side not to have succumbed to tuberculosis.[61]

When Ferron is discussing tuberculosis, the authority he most readily cites is, significantly, André Gide, in whose novel, *L'Immoraliste,* cure takes place outside the sanatorium.[62] Here, then, as in the case of "madness," he credits the literary mind with having achieved the most valuable perceptions of illness. Ferron wrote again and again that tuberculosis was a social illness, an illness of confinement, an illness of societies turned in upon themselves. The proof, he said, was that monkeys in cages contract it, whereas monkeys in the wild do not.[63] In human societies, mentalities change, and although doctors seldom recognize it, the change itself (as much as the discovery of any new substance or medication) is the cure. Victory over tuberculosis, he noted, had coincided with the early euphoria of consumer society (had he lived to see it, he might have associated the return of the disease with that society's decline).[64] Commenting on his own recovery, he often declared that he had cured himself of tuberculosis by "contracting" communism.[65]

The scholar of literature will be aware of an element of style – or rhetoric – in all this. I am very conscious, for example, when reading Ferron, that he hammers away relentlessly at single ideas that go against the mainstream, seeming to "exaggerate" this, and therefore, to "deny" that. A statement like "Tuberculosis is a social illness" should not be taken to mean that the bacillus does not exist, that contagion does not exist. Looking at Ferron's assertions, it is possible for the conscientious lay reader to understand something like this: Living together in large numbers in confined conditions favours the spreading of this disease. Societies who live like this are often claustrophobic, repressive – or at least restrictive. There is a lack of air and light that is psychic as well as physical. To escape from the psychic confinement can favour the elimination of the disease. It can be enough to escape the prison walls for a healing to take place. That is how I, as a lay reader, have interpreted Ferron in this particular instance – temporarily.

Ferron reflected – and spoke or wrote provocatively – on many other aspects of medicine: for example, the introduction of state medicare (which in Quebec saw the displacement of the religious as health-care givers), or the prevalence of psychosomatic illness in western society.[66] As I attempt to convey his views, I am acutely aware of the limits of my own knowledge. How do statements by Ferron fit into a larger controversy? With whom is he agreeing? More often than not one has the impression that he is a solitary polemicist not speaking for any group, just speaking out in the name of humanity. When he gives references, they are, as we have seen, very frequently literary. It is clear, however, that he has read widely on the subject of medicine, as on almost everything else. But what exactly? Lacan, he knows; he refers to him once or twice.[67] Foucault too.[68] He is conscious of having anticipated Illich.[69] And his language, when he speaks of medicine – and psychiatry in particular – bears a striking resemblance to that of Thomas Szasz.[70] But my own sense of the context is at best fragmentary. It is here that my position as a reader outside the profession becomes most problematic. In order to adequately interpret Ferron's interpretations (interpretations of tuberculosis, for example, or of mental illness, of obstetrical practice, or of the psychosomatic), the conscientious reader will want to situate them in relation to particular issues, controversies or debates in the history of medicine, and place them in the context of current critical reflection on these issues. It is a task that, with a few notable exceptions, scholars have yet to undertake, and that I cannot undertake here.[71] Without recourse to the medical context, indeed, to the medical intertext, this reading of Ferron is incomplete.

4. Medicine in Literature

The reader of Ferron's work – and I will concentrate now on his fiction (and autobiographical fictions) – is confronted with a whole array of medical situations – some of them narrowly, clinically medical, others broadly so. There is heart attack, tuberculosis, cancer. There are vague gastric or intestinal disturbances, variously designated as "colic" or "diarrhea." There is an automobile accident. There is venereal disease. There is drug and alcohol abuse and a wide range of mental conditions – from simple-mindedness or retardation to colourful eccentricity, from post-partum depression to the traumas of bereavement and old-age.

In the case of old age, the "empty nest" is a recurring theme. The departure of the children is particularly hard for the wife:

> Mélie Caron had only thirteen children. She expected to have more, one a year until she died; but after the thirteenth, Jean-Baptiste Caron, her husband, said to her, "Stop, Mélie!"
> So the poor woman stopped, not yet fifty years old. She remained unsatisfied, deprived of her due, all warm and trembling like an animal checked in full career. However, her trouble was not without remedy: did she not have her thirteen children? Thirteen children is not much; but it is a family. Alas! the consolation was shortlived. One by one her children left her. She had fed them too well: full of ardour were the boys, ripe and tender the girls; once full grown there was no holding them back. In the end Mélie lost them all. She remained alone with her old man.[72]

In this story, called "Mélie and the Bull" ("*Mélie et le bœuf*"), a fantastical narrative unfolds when, seeming to "take leave of her senses," Mélie transfers her affections to a newborn calf. Another story, "The Parakeet," ("*La perruche*") begins like this:

> The departure of her eldest had never upset her, for she had always managed to replace them as she went along. But there came a year when she was no longer able, having, as it turned out, produced her lastborn the year before. This was the end of her family. The lastborn grew and, growing, nudged the rest, who one after another went their way.
> "Soon they'll all have left."
> "I hope so," said the old man.[73]

In "The Grey Dog" ("*Le chien gris*"), there is old age and gradual decline – physical and mental – , this time in a man.

> Peter Bezeau, Seigneur of Grand-Etang, had become a widower soon after his marriage, and had replaced his wife with the bottle of rum he drank each night. As the years went by he drained his bottle faster and got to bed earlier, and in this way, little by little, went into his decline.[74]

In "Black Cargo Ships of War" ("*Les cargos noirs de la guerre*"), we see bereavement, denial of the loved one's death and a wait that prolongs life indefinitely:

> A widow loved her son too much. One day he left her. She began to wait for him. The years passed. Even after he had died she went on waiting. Because of this he remained in Purgatory. Saint Peter had said to him: "My poor boy, I cannot take you: your mother is waiting for you." So he too had begun to wait. And the years had passed. He wandered in Flanders, held back by his grave. On foggy nights he was able to go as far as the sea. On the other shore, in the land of his birth, an old woman never lost faith. Her son was her whole life. Of her own accord she would never have died. And the wide ocean lay between them.[75]

Here, in a story called "The Parrot" ("*Le perroquet*"), is one of the many shades of "madness":

> If she had been vulgar, coarse, fleshy, it might not have been so surprising, but she was, on the contrary, a very prim and proper lady, bony to say the least. What, then, could have possessed her to show her behind?[76]

Finally, there is life at its very beginnings, in scenes of childbirth, or in its last throes, in scenes of dying and death. Childbirth is one of the most important themes in Ferron's work. He returned to it again and again (and in an intensely emotional autobiographical evocation entitled "Credit Due" ["*La créance*"][77] even undertook to describe his own birth). In the short story "Little William" ("*Le petit William*"), the obstetrical issue is maternal posture in labour and delivery.

> The young woman [refused] to stay on her back. No matter how many times we turned her [over] she would look [up] at us through blurred eyes and then roll onto her side again, tucking her knees up to her stomach, hiding her face in the pillow, sulking her way through labour. I stood near the bed, gloved to the elbows, looking like a priest stalled in the middle of his *Dominus vobiscum*.[78]

This is happening somewhere along the Gaspé Shore, sometime in the 1940s. The narrator, fresh from medical school and the hospitals, is being introduced to the mysteries of the left lateral semi-prone position (known here as "the English position" because it has been introduced to the region by "*un Anglais*," and because it accommodates female modesty so nicely). He is disconcerted – *il perd son latin.* Fortunately there is a midwife present. She is in command of the situation and sits the helpless doctor down for a cup of tea and a lesson in humility.[79]

As for death, Ferron deals with the subject in a tone that is often familiar, joking, cynical. There is little sense of awe or mystery. Although he is occasionally quite lyrical, he seems to delight in mocking the solemnity surrounding the event. "How the Old Man Died" ("*La mort du bonhomme*") is a light-hearted look at a fatal illness, seen through the eyes of the medically naïve:

> There was a bone askew above his stomach; he was not sick, but the bone made him uncomfortable, stabbing him with every breath he took. He would have to stay quiet until the bone reset. After three or four weeks the wretched bone had not moved, the old man was going from bad to worse; they sent for the manipulator, but the manipulator, having felt him, refused to manipulate him, since in shifting the bone he would at the same time have dislocated the nerve of the heart. The old man was done for. They sent for the priest.[80]

In the scenes of death and dying, it is usually the fact of dying itself that is important, and it is often almost impossible to deduce the causes of death. Here are the opening lines of "The Child" ("*L'enfant*"):

> A husband was on his deathbed; his beard was long, he looked like a seal. However, he was in no hurry to die. His wife had been sitting up for a week; she was beginning to lose patience. It would have been different had there been a steady decline, but no: he had ups and downs; he was playing games with death – he was not taking dying seriously.[81]

The husband not only looks like a seal, he behaves like one, diving in and out of consciousness, disappearing for a time beneath the surface, then bobbing up again. The wife is exhausted by her long wait, and with a slight increase in the medication she nudges the husband into the final plunge. As he goes under, we learn more about the wife. Then, her life and his are reduced to their essence in the moment of hyper-consciousness they share before he dies.

> She was a good woman, and had been a good wife as long as the husband had seemed a good man. Together they had built a house, put money aside, and in comfort

> had nourished fond hopes of having children. They had had none. Whose fault was it? She had taken the blame; it is always the innocent who admit guilt. This had given her the strength to endure, for ten years and more, the pecking of a useless cock.
> The potion had its effect, the priest had to be called in to administer the last rites to the dying man. When the ceremony was over, the priest lit a candle and went away. The wife remained alone with her husband; she fell asleep and dreamed she held a child in her arms. While she was sleeping, the poor man came up again – he was a hard one to kill. A bubble burst on the surface of the water; he saw his wife, the child, and the candle: his wife happy, the child looking at him in terror, and the candle half burned away. He did not know what to think. Who was he? A seal? A wet cock? He was certainly no longer the husband. Then he found the strength to raise himself up, put out the candle, and die.[82]

This small sampling of "situations" – all taken from Ferron's short stories, or *contes* – will have indicated at least some of the recurrent themes around which one could organize a study of the doctor-writer's work.[83] It will also have served to direct attention to the patient figure. I would hesitate, however, to call all the characters I have evoked "patients." If they are that, it is often only "by the way." To label them as such is to limit them to their medical status. And for the human beings they present, Ferron's stories – like his other works of fiction – are anything but limiting. Beyond the clinical facts, some other truth is being revealed. Diagnosis is rarely the point. Often there is a doctor in attendance, but not always. And if there is, it is rarely through any action of his that resolution is brought about.

Yet Ferron's fiction is full of doctors. It would be possible to foreground the doctor figure as well as the patient figure, to cite passages where the doctor sees himself or is seen. One could construct a kind of composite portrait of him, show him interacting with his patients, expressing bewilderment, uneasiness, resentment, anger, mirth. This is no "ideal" doctor preaching an ideal of patient-doctor relations. He is conscious of playing a role, and he is far from being a "saint." Ferron's doctor is capable of being compassionate, but there is no "holier-than-thou" attitude, no preachiness. He is flawed. He admits to a kind of callousness, a heartlessness. He is uncomfortable with the power bestowed on him, but at times he admits, regretfully, to having enjoyed the authority his position confers. He is often disillusioned. Sometimes he is positively abject. He judges himself harshly and is in turn judged by those he treats.

In considering the representation of medicine in Ferron's writing, one might concentrate, then, on the treatment of individual themes, or on the portrayal of doctors and patients. But I prefer now to shift the focus somewhat. I would like to leave the specific content of the works aside, or at least to see beyond it, to what I have already referred to as "the literary transformation that has taken place." I would like to ask what literature has done here for medicine, and try to define just what it is in the process that I would most want to draw the medical profession's attention to.

Fictions like Ferron's contain the essence of situations life presents us with – sometimes over-whelmingly, shapelessly. Medical training gives its own set of rules and guidelines for making sense of things and shaping into meaningful patterns that profession's raw encounters with reality. In literature, a process of selection, shaping, highlighting, has already occurred. In a sense "once removed" from reality, a literary text can, paradoxically, bring us closer to it. It seems to me that through contact with this "shaped" reality, doctors or medical students could not help but gain insight into situations in which at one time or another they may be called on to intervene. They may be forced to take notice of things whose significance they might not otherwise have seen.

But there is not only the question of "essence" and pinpointed significance. I have already implied that in Ferron's work the narrowly, clinically medical opens out onto broader, medicine-related concerns. But it is also true that these situations I have called "broadly" medical in turn connect with political, social, moral or existential concerns. A Ferron story is never just about a heart attack, a stomach cancer, a car accident, senility. An obstetrical issue can connect with issues of cultural and political survival, individual "madness" with the alienation of a whole society. Specific situations or symptoms that inevitably draw the medical gaze are in fact small pieces only, fitting into a much bigger picture, which is a literary vision or "version" of a "scheme of things." Ferron gives them a context. The medical is integrated into something much vaster, put revealingly – one could almost say "holistically" – "in its place."

I would like to say a word now about the importance of listening, and about story, presenting the writer as listener but stressing at the same time the significance of listening in the doctor-patient encounter, and positing something like a transferability of listening and reading skills. As I think further about Ferron's stories and their possible function in a medical context, it occurs to me that exposure to literary texts hones reading skills and that there are parallels between reading and listening – the kind of active listening that interprets and makes sense of things. Doctors are called upon to listen. Ferron maintained that in many cases they simply do not know how. I do not think it would be presumptuous to suggest that most doctors could probably become better listeners, could do better at the kind of listening a writer constantly does and that an attentive reader does in the presence of the writer's text.

One of Ferron's doctors, the first-person narrator of the novel *The Cart (La Charrette)*, is a reader and a listener both. He loses the ability – and the will – to treat his patients in the weeks that precede his death (doctors die too in Ferron's universe, and this also helps to put them "in their place"). This doctor does not know he is going to die, but in the end, weary and disillusioned, he is reduced to the simple and primordial function of listening. In the presence of his patients, he can do nothing else.

> My patients introduced themselves humbly and I listened to them in the same way. ... There was no need to play super-healer, but I knew they'd have liked me to listen with just a little more assurance and serenity. Yet for me assurance and serenity would have been a cheap trick, and I could never have fooled myself. So I listened as best I could. They said they were sick and I believed them, thinking it was a wonder they weren't a lot sicker, considering the lives they led and the society they lived in. If I [had no] remedy, I could at least tell them that. But they looked at me suspiciously. It's normal to be suspicious of a doctor who doesn't want to treat people any more. I'd have liked to; I just couldn't. The whole species seemed so rotten, I couldn't promise to keep any one individual afloat. The best I could do was listen, very humbly, never being quite sure I understood.[84]

To all intents and purposes this doctor is a failure. But he is interesting to us. Even though he speaks with the voice of disillusionment, in a strange way he is exemplary. Ferron has isolated this essential function, the listening function. It is the one the fictional doctor clings to, the one he cannot let go. It can be no coincidence that in his lifetime he has been a lover of literature, a reader of books.[85] This character is also not unlike Ferron the writer, it seems to me. "The best I could do was listen, very humbly, never being quite sure I understood." Literature such as Ferron's is not strong on "prescription." It is an exercise in listening, a coming to terms with uncertainty.

Ferron has listened. Behind every one of the situations I have referred to – embedded in it, or growing out of it – there is a story. Someone's story, that has been heard. I have already conveyed to you something of Ferron's view of the importance of story (not story in the sense of something to entertain, but story as biography, as meaningful events), so it should be clear that just by hearing these stories and letting them be heard again, he is reasserting their significance in human life. Psychiatrist Julien Bigras, one of Ferron's most attentive readers, has paid tribute to the particular quality of listening ("*écoute*") that can be detected in Ferron's approach to psychiatric patients, an approach, Bigras says, that respects the integrity and "wholeness" of the patient's biography, and acknowledges imagination as an adjunct, a vital accompaniment to the listening act.[86] Something of that same listening quality no doubt characterized Ferron's approach to all patients – all characters – and carries over into the stories that he writes.

By telling these stories Ferron is also reasserting the importance of voice, reassigning, legitimizing voice. In relation to his physician-authored fiction, where it goes almost without saying that there is a predominance of doctor's story, of doctor's voice, I am thinking particularly of access to the patient's story and the patient's voice. The following is a passage from Ferron's author's preface to a "Love Letter," a short text that he himself rewrote from the almost incoherent scribblings of a schizophrenic patient, making them into a "readable" text, allowing that voice to be heard.

> The insane are witnesses. Their language is hermetic. No one knows what cause they plead nor what the charges are. And no one listens to them. We shut them up together in places where time stands still and nothing happens, only what has already happened somewhere else, only what they insist on bearing witness to, shouting to make themselves heard above the senseless clamour of voices, drowning each other out. They all talk at once and no one listens, except for those who pretend, those whose job it is to be kind and patient, those authorized to listen, who are around less than anyone else. While time in the asylum stands still, outside the walls real time marches on. Before long the trial is suspended for want of all the parties. The case cannot be heard, and the evidence of the insane becomes meaningless, proof that they have not been locked up for nothing, that they really were mad.[87]

In another work, a short story narrated by a disenchanted and seemingly heartless doctor, the voice of a dying woman patient is allowed to come through the text, is heard along with his unfeeling, cold and cynical narrator's voice. And when we realize that this narrator is also a writer, it becomes clear that he is consciously the medium through which her truth is being expressed. There are passages of poetry that erupt in the prose text. The woman speaks through them. And we realize that the doctor-narrator is the author of these. He comments on the words he has put in her mouth. In this story, called "The Lady from Ferme-Neuve" ("*La dame de Ferme-Neuve*"),[88] we have a glimpse into authorial consciousness and into a crucial process I will call simply "exploration of narrative points of view." This process is one of the most important ways in which literature can act on reality. In Ferron's work medical reality is recounted from a whole range of points of view: he has created outside omniscient narrators relating things successively from the patient's and from the doctor's point of view; doctor-narrators giving an account of their own experience; first-person patient-narrators telling the story from their point of view. The mere accumulation and juxtaposition of these points of view is significant. Sometimes there is an interconnectedness which is even more remarkable. The notion, for example, of an author-physician creating a physician-narrator holding in his consciousness a patient as well as himself, and merging their two consciousnesses in the poetry he writes – that notion fascinates me. As does that of the author-physician creating a patient-narrator who in turn holds in his or her consciousness a doctor as well as his or her own self.

For me to tell someone's story, either by letting them speak through me in their own words, or by using my words to tell it from their point of view, requires that I become like the other person, reaffirms a kind of bond. One takes into oneself and gives new existence to another. One does what I am told doctors are discouraged from doing. It is a form of empathizing. What in everyday life we cannot do beyond a certain point without seriously compromising our own identity – and no doubt in many instances our professional efficacy. It is an instance of being at once oneself – the same – and someone else – other. It is a state – momentary, fleeting, elusive at best – which we pass through dozens of times in our day to day existence, but which writing and reading both allow us to sustain. Along with the openness to another's story, the listening to another's voice, there is, then, the ability to actively sustain in one single mind a diversity of interconnecting points of view. It is this ability – this agility – that literature such as Ferron's demonstrates and at the same time invites us as readers to share.

5. Conclusion

I have indicated some of the ways in which literature like Ferron's "puts medicine in its place," creating for it perspectives, contexts, meanings, that both elevate and humble it. Let me now, in conclusion, play with my title a little, turn it round, asking the question: What place is there for literature in medicine? What would it be for medicine to put literature in its (rightful) place?

Medicine fills the lives of those who practise it with powerful experiences that need response. I am referring, of course, to something beyond professional response: the deep response of one's whole being that literature allows – and requires. Medicine needs literature. We cannot ask of all doctors that they be writers. In spite of the agonies of his own "uneasy partnership," Ferron would no doubt have encouraged them to exercise that privilege, that "right." Medical practice might seem to work against writing. Certainly the demands on a writer's time and a physician's time could appear irreconcilable. It is also tempting to invoke the difficulty of reconciling the very different emotional strategies the two employ, though on the latter point I would ask you to consider whether the difference has not been overstated. Is the much-vaunted writer's empathy not of little use if it is not combined with the ability to achieve distance and to curiously observe? For the medical practitioner, can professional detachment on its own, without some degree of empathy, really suffice? To reconcile writing and medicine in the sense that one has two complete professions is something not many can do. But if we cannot ask of all doctors that they be professional writers, we might at least suggest to future physicians that they explore the benefits of writing for themselves – diary writing, for example. And we can, most assuredly, as more and more medical educators now do, stress the value of reading works of literature, like those by Jacques Ferron. That is the invitation – at once very general and quite specific – that I would leave you with.

To reflect on Ferron's work is to reflect on the place of literature in the lives of health professionals. In *The Cart*, as we have already seen, there is a doctor-listener who has been a reader of books. There are also, throughout Ferron's work, doctors who themselves write – like the narrator of "The Lady from Ferme-Neuve," who does so "between nights, … to bring [him]self back in touch with day;"[89] like Mithridates III in *Le Saint-Élias*, who "remake[s] the reality of [his] country according to [his] own desires;"[90] or like the narrator and Maski, whom we see, this time in *Gaspé-Mattempa*, delivering babies at the start of their career, and whose aspirations are summarized in retrospect thus: "to go back to the beginning, one's own beginning, the beginning of everything, in the middle of the Alleghanies and the Shickshocks, … to steep oneself in [the event of childbirth], to live it, and then write it, in order to understand it, because that was the only way there was to understand."[91] By creating fictional doctors and exploring their relationship to reading or writing – or both – Ferron has achieved a kind of meta-commentary on the relationship between literature and medicine.

I would like now to consider one of the most famous of these fictional doctors. He is called Cotnoir. In the novel of this name there is a character who writes – not books, but a humble diary. This character is not the doctor of the title, but the doctor's wife, and in the eyes of her doctor husband she is creating a kind of ark. This doctor talks to his wife at the end of each day, offering up his experiences to her for safekeeping, and he tells us: "I've gotten a good many people aboard that ark of hers – and all the animals I've met over the past twenty years around every corner of the suburb."[92] Had the doctor written, he would, of course, have listened to himself. As it is, she fulfills that function for him. She listens to him, and then she writes. The two are in partnership. Writing is occurring on his behalf. What is important is that the doctor takes for granted that he, like his patients, will have found a place aboard the writer's ark. He has never looked inside his wife's diary, but he knows one day he will, and he wonders if he will recognize himself when he comes to read what she has written over the years. Transformed he will most likely be, but saved in some miraculous sense, too, he is sure. By creating those two distinct characters of husband and wife, Ferron has separated the writing and the reading functions out and held them up to view. What is clear is that writing and reading "accompany" this doctor's practice. The doctor needs them both. He may have delegated the writing to his wife and put off the reading to some future time. But he knows he needs them both.

Notes

[1] Yves Taschereau, *Le Portuna: la médecine dans l'œuvre de Jacques Ferron* (Montréal: l'Aurore, 1975) is an early attempt to examine the medical content of Ferron's writing – in particular his treatment of the figures of the doctor and the patient – and to identify points of contact between medicine and literature. It provides a useful overview of material in works published prior to 1975, and to this day stands alone. The first introduction to Ferron as a doctor-writer to be written in English was a brief homage by one of Ferron's translators, a professor of literature, published in 1985: Ray Ellenwood, "Homage to Jacques," *MD's Companion,* December 1985, 38-39. Other studies (e.g. Bednarski and McAlister, Kègle [1992,1993], Viau, Olscamp [2002]) focus more closely on particular themes or conditions, or on individual works.

[2] The most notable of Ferron's medical readers (and explicit interlocutors) have to date been psychiatrists. See Julien Bigras et Jacques Ferron, *Le Désarroi: correspondance* (Montréal: VLB éditeur, 1988), and Pierre Migneault, "Je vais essayer de m'expliquer," *Spirale*, mai-juin 2000, 16.

[3] Elements of the present study have been developed in the course of my on-going conversation with students and teachers in the Dalhousie Faculty of Medicine, in particular in the context of the "Medicine and the Humanities" conference, Dalhousie University, February 7-9, 1991, and during the fall term of 2001, when I was the Hannah Millennium Visitor in the Dalhousie Medical Humanities Programme. The broad lines of this study are those set out in the paper "Making Sense of Medicine Through Writing," presented at the Oxford "Probing the Boundaries" conference, in June 2002. I have also incorporated ideas since developed for the November 2002 Hannah Lecture on the History of Medicine, titled "Putting Medicine in its Place," and delivered in Montreal, at the Family Medicine Forum of the College of Family Physicians of Canada and the Collège québécois des médecins de famille.

[4] The reader may wish to consult the one completed volume of Ferron's biography: Marcel Olscamp, *Le fils du notaire: Jacques Ferron 1921-1949* (Montréal: Fides, 1997).
[5] Jacques Ferron, *Escarmouches: la longue passe*, tome 1 (Montréal: Leméac, 1975), 247-391.
[6] He also occasionally signs "Dr. Jacques Ferron" or "Jacques Ferron, écrivain et médecin". Most letters, however, are signed simply "Jacques Ferron."
[7] Jacques Ferron, *Les Lettres aux journaux*, ed. Pierre Cantin, Marie Ferron and Paul Lewis (Montréal: VLB éditeur, 1985).
[8] Jacques Ferron et Pierre L'Hérault, *Par la porte d'en arrière: entretiens* (Montréal: Lanctôt éditeur, 1997). Two shorter published interviews are also useful: Taschereau, 107-114; and Pierre L'Hérault et Jacques Pelletier, "L'écrivain est un cénobite, entrevue avec Jacques Ferron," *Voix et images,* 8, 3 (1983): 397-405.
[9] See, for example, the article I have written in collaboration with a physician-reader (a professor of surgery). Betty Bednarski and Vivian McAlister, "Literature and Obstetrics: Reading Maternal Posture in Jacques Ferron's 'Little William'," *Literature and Medicine*, 21, 2 (2002): 216-241.
[10] Quoted in Jean Marcel, *Jacques Ferron malgré lui* (Montréal: Éditions du jour, 1970), 18. My translation.
[11] Jacques Ferron, "Alain Grandbois, les écrivains crétins et le Zigoteau," in *Escarmouches: la longue passe*, tome 2 (Montréal: Leméac, 1975), 143. This quotation is translated by Ray Ellenwood in *Brick* 16 (1982): 18.
[12] L'Hérault et Pelletier, 404. My translation.
[13] Like many *québécois* writers of his generation, Ferron came to political consciousness through literature, and he came to envisage writing as a means of bringing his troubled and uncertain Quebec to some kind of certainty. Politics was nevertheless for him a burden, and he dreamed of one day writing in peace, "as [writers do] in normal countries." See Marcel, 19-20, 34.
[14] Ferron et L'Hérault, 78.
[15] L'Hérault et Pelletier, 404-405.
[16] Ferron et L'Hérault, 78.
[17] Ibid.
[18] Quoted in Jean Marcel, 23. My translation.
[19] Ferron et L'Hérault, 109.
[20] Taschereau, 111.
[21] L'Hérault et Pelletier, 405.
[22] Jacques Ferron, "Les salicaires," in *Du fond de mon arrière-cuisine* (Montréal: Éditions du jour, 1973), 267-288. Translated by Ray Ellenwood as "Purple Loosestrife," in *Brick* 16, Fall 1982: 25-30.
[23] *Brick*, 28.

[24] Ibid., 27.
[25] Ibid., 29.
[26] In Jacques Ferron, *Rosaire*, précédé de *L'Exécution de Maski* (Montréal: VLB éditeur, 1981), 11-36. Translated by Ray Ellenwood as "The Execution of Maski," in *Brick* 16, Fall 1982, 41-46.
[27] *Brick*, 42.
[28] Ibid.
[29] The two selves also appear in a short lyrical (and autobiographical) evocation of the Gaspé, called *Gaspé-Mattempa*, first published in 1980. Maski is remembered here as a young doctor-writer in practice in the Gaspé. The narrator, Maski's friend and correspondent, and himself a doctor and aspiring writer, has practised in a more prosperous region further inland. Critic Marcel Olscamp sees in the exchange between the two a dialogue between two doctor-selves – the modest Gaspé country doctor Ferron had in fact been, and the hypothetical prosperous bourgeois "other" he might have become. See Jacques Ferron, *Gaspé-Mattempa* (Montréal: Lanctôt éditeur, 1997), 11.
[30] *Brick*, 41.
[31] Ibid., 42.
[32] Ibid., 46.
[33] L'Hérault et Pelletier, 397-398; Ferron et L'Hérault, 278.
[34] *Brick*, 46.
[35] *Rosaire* précédé de *L'Exécution de Maski,* 39-197.
[36] Jacques Ferron, "Le pas de Gamelin," in *La Conférence inachevée* (Montréal: VLB éditeur, 1987), 21-94.
[37] L'Hérault et Pelletier, 405.
[38] In one of Ferron's novels, a young woman reads her dead father's letters, finds them "beautiful, [...] almost literary," and wonders whether writing is not "madness that has been transcended and seeks its own cure." Jacques Ferron, *Les roses sauvages, petit roman suivi d'une lettre d'amour soigneusement présentée* (Montréal:Éditions du jour, 1971), 117.Translated by Betty Bednarski as *Wild Roses* (Toronto: McClelland and Stewart, 1976), 79.
[39] *Brick*, 46. The manuscript of this "failed" book is in the Fonds Jacques Ferron of the *Bibliothèque nationale du Québec.*
[40] Ferron, "Shakespeare et l'entomologie psychiatrique," in *Escarmouches: la longue passe*, tome 1, 368-372.
[41] One way of taking up the extraordinary challenge these texts pose is to make use, as some scholars have done, of the insight psychoanalysis can provide. See, for example, Christiane Kègle, "D'une position idéologique à une solution éthique: la traversée des discours de la folie dans l'œuvre de Jacques Ferron," in *Littératures* 9-10 (1992): 55-80, and, by the same author, "Truchement, transfert, figures de la folie chez Jacques Ferron," in *Voix et images* 54 (1993): 495-506.

[42] L'Hérault et Pelletier, 405. My translation.
[43] Ferron, "La difficulté d'être médecin," in *Escarmouches: la longue passe*, tome 1, 250.
[44] Ferron, "Adacanabran," in *La Conférence inachevée* (Montréal: VLB éditeur, 1987), 211. My translation.
[45] Taschereau, 109.
[46] *La Conférence inachevée*, 211. My translation.
[47] See Bednarski and McAlister.
[48] Ferron et L'Hérault, 83; Taschereau, 108.
[49] This tabloid-style journal was predominantly physician-subscribed. Besides essays and opinion pieces on medical and other topics, Ferron first published in its pages many of his short stories and first drafts of passages later to be incorporated into his novels. For close to thirty years, physicians were thus among the very first readers of many of his texts.
[50] *Escarmouches: la longue passe*, tome 1, 247-250.
[51] *Gaspé-Mattempa*, 42. My translation.
[52] Ibid., 248.
[53] *La Conférence inachevée*, 59. My translation.
[54] *Les Lettres aux journaux*, 415-416.
[55] *La Conférence inachevée*, 54.
[56] Ibid., 77.
[57] Ibid., 79.
[58] Jacques Ferron, "Le perroquet," *Contes*, édition intégrale (Montréal: Éditions HMH, 1968), 51. Translated by Betty Bednarski as "The Parrot," in *Selected Tales of Jacques Ferron* (Toronto: House of Anansi, 1984), 72.
[59] Ferron et L'Hérault, 86.
[60] For a first-hand account of Ferron the doctor-patient, see Ronald Bayne, "Ascending the Magic Mountain," *Canadian Medical Association Journal* 159 (1998): 517-518.
[61] For one version of the story, see Jacques Ferron, *Les Confitures de coings et autres textes* (Montréal: Parti Pris, 1972), 290. Translated by Ray Ellenwood, in *Quince Jam* (Toronto: Exile Editions, 1977), 232.
[62] *Les Confitures de coings*, 285; *Quince Jam*, 228; Ferron et L'Hérault, 85. On Ferron, Gide and tuberculosis, see Marcel Olscamp, "A la recherche de Lafcadio: Jacques Ferron, lecteur d'André Gide," in *Jacques Ferron; le palimpseste infini*, ed. Brigitte Faivre-Duboz et Patrick Poirier, Montréal: Lanctôt éditeur, 2002, 235-247.
[63] *Les Confitures de coings*, 284; *Quince Jam*, 227.
[64] Ferron et L'Hérault, 86.
[65] *Les Confitures de coings*, 285; *Quince Jam*, 228; Ferron et L'Hérault, 85.
[66] Ferron et L'Hérault, 81.
[67] *Escarmouches: la longue passe,* tome 1, 249.

[68] "L'Alceste à la Fernandez," in *Du fond de mon arrière-cuisine,* 24; "Le forgeron et le goglu," in *Escarmouches: la longue passe,* tome 1, 309.
[69] L'Hérault et Ferron, 97.
[70] Thomas Sasz, *The Manufacture of Madness: A Comparative Study of the Inquisition and the Mental Health Movement* (New York: Harper & Row, 1970).
[71] Both Robert Viau and Christiane Kègle have written very useful studies that situate Ferron's ideas on the care of the mentally ill in their historical context. See Robert Viau, *Les Fous de papier* (Montréal: Éditions du Méridien, 1989), 197-296, and Kègle (1992). For his part, Marcel Olscamp has indicated some of the connections to be made between Ferron's ideas on tuberculosis and certain social and psychological theories of the disease. See Olscamp (2002).
[72] *Contes*, 25; *Selected Tales*, 37.
[73] *Contes*, 113; *Selected Tales*, 154.
[74] *Contes*, 70; *Selected Tales*, 96.
[75] *Contes*, 57; *Selected Tales*, 205.
[76] *Contes*, 51; *Selected Tales*, 72
[77] *Les Confitures de coings*, 233-260; *Quince Jam*, 186-208.
[78] *Contes*, 144. Translated by Ray Ellenwood in *Impulse* 3, 2 (1974): 11.
[79] See Bednarski and McAlister.
[80] *Contes*, 23; *Selected Tales*, 34.
[81] *Contes*, 56; *Selected Tales*, 78.
[82] *Contes*, 57; *Selected Tales*, 79.
[83] For a summary of some of Ferron's most important themes see Betty Bednarski, "Jacques Ferron," in *Profiles in Canadian Literature* 5, ed. Jeffrey M.Heath (Toronto: Dundurn Press, 1986), 121-128.
[84] Jacques Ferron, *La Charrette* (Montréal: Éditions HMH, 1968), 47-48. Translated by Ray Ellenwood in *The Cart* (Toronto: Exile Editions, 1980), 32.
[85] *La Charrette*, 82-84; *The Cart*, 54-55.
[86] Bigras et Ferron, 11-12.
[87] *Les Roses sauvages*, 127; *Wild Roses*, 87.
[88] *Contes*, 179-186; *Selected Tales*, 220-230.
[89] *Contes*, 179; *Selected Tales*, 220.
[90] Jacques Ferron, *Le Saint Élias* (Montréal: Éditions du jour, 1972), 185. My translation.
[91] *Gaspé-Mattempa*, 39-40. My translation.
[92] Jacques Ferron, *Cotnoir* (Montréal: Éditions d'Orphée, 1962), 83. My translation.

Bibliography

Bayne, Ronald. "Ascending the Magic Mountain." *Canadian Medical Association Journal* 159: 517-518.

Bednarski, Betty. "Jacques Ferron." In *Profiles in Canadian Literature* 5, edited by Jeffrey Heath, 121-128. Toronto: Dundurn Press, 1986.

---------- and Vivian McAlister. "Literature and Obstetrics: Reading Maternal Posture in Jacques Ferron's 'Little William'." *Literature and Medicine* 21, 2 (2002): 216-241.

Bigras, Julien et Jacques Ferron. *Le Désarroi: correspondance.* Montréal: VLB éditeur, 1988.

Ellenwood, Ray. "Homage to Jacques." In *MD's Companion*, December 1985, 38-39.

Ferron, Jacques. *Gaspé-Mattempa.* Montreal: Lanctôt éditeur, 1997.

----------. "Adacanabran." In *La Conférence inachevée*: *Le pas de Gamelin et autres récits*, 199-217. Montréal: VLB éditeur, 1987.

----------. "Le pas de Gamelin." In *La Conférence inachevée*, 21-94.

----------. "L'Impérialisme masculin." In *Les Lettres aux journaux*, colligées et annotées par Pierre Cantin, Marie Ferron et Paul Lewis, 415-416. Montréal: VLB éditeur, 1985.

----------. *Rosaire.* In *Rosaire* précédé de *L'Exécution de Maski*, 39-197. Montréal: VLB éditeur, 1981.

----------. *L'Exécution de Maski. In Rosaire* précédé de *L'Exécution de Maski*, 11-36. Translated by Ray Ellenwood as "The Execution of Maski." In *Brick* 16 (1982): 41-46.

----------. "La difficulté d'être médecin." In *Escarmouches: la longue passe*, tome 1, 247-250.

----------. "Le forgeron et le goglu." In *Escarmouches: la longue passe*, tome 1, 308-311.

----------. "Shakespeare et l'entomologie psychiatrique." In *Escarmouches: la longue passe*, tome 1, 368-372. ----------. "Alain Grandbois, les écrivains crétins et le Zigoteau." In *Escarmouches: la longue passe*, tome 2, 142-144.

----------. "L'Alceste à la Fernandez." In *Du fond de mon arrière-cuisine.*, 23-31. Montréal: Éditions du jour, 1973.

----------. "Les salicaires." In *Du fond de mon arrière-cuisine*, 267-288. Translated by Ray Ellenwood as "Purple Loosestrife." In *Brick* 16 (1982): 25-30.

----------. *Le Saint-Élias.* Montréal: Éditions du jour, 1972. Translated as *The Saint Elias* by Pierre Cloutier. Montreal: Harvest House, 1975.

---------- *Les Confitures de coings et autres textes.* Montréal: Éditions Parti-pris, 1972. Translated by Ray Ellenwood as *Quince Jam.* Toronto: Exile Editions, 1977.

----------. *Les Roses sauvages, petit roman suivi d'une lettre d'amour soigneusement présentée.* Montréal: Éditions du jour, 1971. Translated by Betty Bednarski as *Wild Roses.* Toronto: McClelland and Stewart, 1976.

----------. "Le Petit William." In *Contes,* édition intégrale, 144-146. Montréal: Editions HMH, 1968. Translated by Ray Ellenwood as "Little William." In *Impulse* 3, 2 (1974): 11-12.

----------. "La mort du bonhomme;" "Mélie et le boeuf;" "Le perroquet;" "L'enfant;" "Le chien gris;" "La perruche;" "Les cargos noirs de la guerre;" "La dame de Ferme-Neuve." In *Contes*, édition intégrale, 23-24; 25-38; 51-55; 56-57; 70-73; 113-114; 157-161; 179-186. Montréal: Éditions HMH, 1968. Translated by Betty Bednarski as "How the Old Man Died;" "Mélie and the Bull;" "The Parrot;" "The Child;" "The Grey Dog;" "The Parakeet;" "Black Cargo Ships of War;" "The Lady from Ferme-Neuve." In *Selected Tales of Jacques Ferron*, 34-36; 37-55; 72-77; 78-79; 96-101; 154-156; 205-210; 220-230. Toronto: House of Anansi, 1984.

----------. *La Charrette.* Montréal: Éditions HMH, 1968. Translated by Ray Ellenwood as *The Cart.* Toronto: Exile Editions, 1982.

----------. *Cotnoir.* Montréal: Éditions d'Orphée, 1962. Translated by Pierre Cloutier as *Dr. Cotnoir.* Montréal: Harvest House, 1973.

---------- et Pierre L'Hérault. *Par la porte d'en arrière: entretiens.* Montréal: Lanctôt éditeur, 1997.

Kègle, Christiane. “Truchement, transfert, figures de la folie chez Jacques Ferron.” *Voix et images* 54 (1993): 495-506.

----------. “D’une position idéologique à une solution éthique: la traversée des discours sur la folie dans l’oeuvre de Jacques Ferron.” *Littératures*, 9-10 (1992): 55-80.

L’Hérault, Pierre et Jacques Pelletier. “L’écrivain est un cénobite, entrevue avec Jacques Ferron.” In *Voix et images* 8, 3 (1983): 397-405.

Marcel, Jean. *Jacques Ferron malgré lui*. Montréal: Éditions du jour, 1970.

Migneault, Pierre. “Je vais essayer de m’expliquer.” *Spirale*, mai-juin 2000, 16.

Olscamp, Marcel. “À la recherche de Lafcadio: Jacques Ferron, lecteur d’André Gide.” In *Jacques Ferron: le palimpseste infini*, sous la direction de Brigitte Faivre-Duboz et Patrick Poirier, 235-247. Montréal: Lanctôt éditeur, 2002.

----------. *Le Fils du notaire: Jacques Ferron 1921-1949*. Montréal: Fides, 1997.

---------- “Préface.” Jacques Ferron, *Gaspé-Mattempa*, 7-11. Montréal: Lanctôt éditeur, 1997.

Sasz, Thomas. *The Manufacture of Madness: A Comparative Study of the Inquisition and the Mental Health Movement.* New York: Harper & Row, 1970.

Taschereau, Yves. *Le Portuna: la médecine dans l’œuvre de Jacques Ferron*. Montréal: L’Aurore, 1975.

Viau, Robert. *Les Fous de papier*. Montréal: Éditions du Méridien, 1989.

Note on Contributor

Betty Bednarski is a Professor of French and the Coordinator of Canadian Studies at Dalhousie University, Halifax, Nova Scotia. She has published widely in the field of Quebec literature and is well known for her translations of physician-writer Jacques Ferron.

Florence Nightingale's Sensational Narratives of Contagion and Contamination

Louise Penner

Throughout her career as a nurse, and later as an influential figure in English politics, Florence Nightingale was deeply committed to the field of medical statistics. Through statistical study, she claimed, one could prove the correlation between the poor hygiene and sanitation laws of various regions including England, and the presence of disease. While we associate "hygiene" and "sanitation" with the environment, we probably do not do so to the extent that Nightingale did in her writings addressed to government officials and others involved in public health movements of the nineteenth century. For Nightingale associated hygiene and sanitation *exclusively* with long-term exposure to the environment – and to the exclusion of what she called "contagion." Contagion was understood to be transmission of disease by unobservable agents called "germs" via the clothing, breath, and effluvia of infected persons possibly even by a single such contact.

Throughout this essay, I use the term "contamination" when referring to disease transmission explained as resulting exclusively from long-term exposure to environmental or miasmatic causes, while I reserve the word "contagion" for referring to disease transmission explained as occurring possible through a single contact between bodies.

We now know that Nightingale's view – that disease origins and means of transmission were explicable entirely as the result of environmental contaminants or miasma, and not the result of contagion between bodies – was wrong. We know, in fact, that within hospitals the majority of hazards involve contagion from agents previously unobservable, now observable with powerful microscopes. However, until very recently historians have agreed that Nightingale was, up to the end of her life, a virulent anticontagionist.

Hugh Small's recent book *Florence Nightingale: Avenging Angel*, however, claims in passing that hitherto unnoticed evidence from a short essay privately circulated, "Notes on Contagion and Infection" (1858), prove that Nightingale actually privately accepted the notion that unobservable germs might cause disease.[1] "On careful examination," he claims, "the widespread allegation that she refused to accept germ theory turns out to be false."[2] He justifies this claim on the basis of a passage from "Notes on Contagion and Infection" where Nightingale says, "There are two or three diseases in which there is a specific virus which can be seen, tasted, smelt, and analysed, and which, in certain constitutions, propagates the original disease by inoculation, such as small pox, cow pox, and syphilis, but these are not 'contagions' in the sense supposed."[3] The passage certainly does show Nightingale accepting that there is such a thing as contagion via observable viruses, those "which can be seen, tasted, smelt, and analysed," and via actual inoculation. But she regards this sense of contagion as irrelevant to contagion theory as she sees it, whereas Small's thinks this shows Nightingale should therefore accept any version of contagion theory. He does not distinguish adequately between the two kinds of contagion Nightingale clearly distinguishes, both opposed to the notion of environmental contamination: 1) contagion via observable viruses or via actual inoculation (this she grants as possible), and 2) single exposure contagion via unobservable agents, transmitted via the clothing, air, and effluvia of the infected.

Small's theory that Nightingale actually privately endorsed germ theory, if true, would initiate a radical change in the perception of Nightingale, as his theory would surely leave her open to accusations that she was willing to put patients at terrible risk of catching contagious disease when she wasn't willing to admit she was wrong about contagion. For example, she insisted as late as 1860 that, "With proper sanitary precautions, diseases reputed to be the most 'infectious' may be treated in wards among other sick without any danger."[4] Thus, I suppose, she would have claimed that even cholera or scarlet fever patients might have been kept without danger in the same room with other patients.

While I am not willing to accept that with her extensive anti-contagionist campaign Nightingale actually had no qualms about granting *any* form of contagionism whatever, I do find his observation that there is some evidence to suggest inconsistency within her anti-contagionist rhetoric provocative. But what that evidence showed me was not so much an inconsistent embrace of contagionism as an appearance of inconsistency brought on by certain rhetorical strategies Nightingale engages in, particularly in the rhetoric of her major post-Scutari writings, *Notes on Nursing: What it is* and *What it is Not* and *Notes on Hospitals*.[5] The inconsistencies Small observes may be taken as an indication of Nightingale's fearing that the germ theory hypothesis could be true. As a rational thinker she could hardly fail to entertain this possibility. Even if that possibility were realized, the greater worry for Nightingale would still be that belief in contagion theory would allow people to ignore the importance of proper hygiene. This is as far in the direction of Small's thesis as I would be willing to go. On the other hand, Nightingale may also have been deliberately using fear of contagion strategically to influence others into acting on the hygiene and sanitation issues she held so dear.

I find this possibility to be the most convincing one, in part because I see her treatment of the disease origins issue as the place where Nightingale seems most to dramatize her explanations, drawing from the language of sensationalism to reach a popular audience. She makes use of this sensational rhetoric particularly in writings addressed to middle- and working-class women.

By sensationalizing fear of contagion, Nightingale finds herself emphasizing almost excessively the dangers of body products for sick patients. With its apparent phobia of the body and body products, her language imitates that of the sensation fiction novels written at just the time that she was writing *Notes on Nursing* (1860 – addressed to middle-class women) and publishing a new edition of *Notes on Hospitals* (addressed to government officials). My reading of her willingness to engage in sensational language when addressing middle-class women helps to counter Small's claim about Nightingale's private acceptance of contagion theory. The language in *Notes on Nursing* especially might at first appear to support Small's view. When Nightingale addresses middle-class women, insisting on the need for hygiene in the home in *Notes on Nursing*, the narrative she creates of the infiltration of contaminants both from within and outside of the home, shows her applying a clinical eye to diagnose the places of environmental contamination in the home, the curtains, sheets, etc. What is confusing for readers, and perhaps for Nightingale herself, is that the contaminants she focuses on are products of human bodies. For the question surely arises whether the products of human bodies affect humans via a single contact with another human body, or whether a single contact infection of the environment could also effect humans living in that environment. In either case, we would have an appeal to contagion.

Nightingale's narrative itself thus raises scientific and narratological questions about the status of the body in narratives of contagion and contamination. Does the body or do the products of the body infect the environment? Does disease originate in the environment? Is it the case that, as Nightingale argues in *Notes on Hospitals* and elsewhere, the environment is the only force that influences disease? Do these narratives thus invite or eschew discussion of the body? In her own insistence on the need for the clean home and body, Nightingale provides a description of the relationship between the body and the environment that seems clearly body phobic. Her phobia would appear to challenge the belief that she was convinced of the anticontagionist argument described earlier. Why would she not admit publicly, something that, if Small is right, she appears to have feared privately? Though I doubt she believed in contagion between bodies, because it could not be observed empirically, I do see her as willing to exploit fear of contagion to its fullest, and allow the language of sensation fiction to help her make her case as dramatically as possible.

There are two beliefs she confirms over and over, both of which convince me that she had not privately accepted contagion theories. First, she believed one could use statistical analyses to "observe" facts about sanitation and hygiene, facts that she thought clearly revealed natural laws about hygiene. And second, she rejects any belief in "natural" nursing abilities that would by themselves give sufficient indication of the need for hygiene. The nurse must think scientifically, and according to these so-called natural laws.

The view of Nightingale as a staunch anticontagionist and avid supporter of statistics seems well-supported as late as 1860 by her disturbing conclusion in *Notes on Hospitals* that the theory of contagion was a fiction created for social and political ends. She writes:

> The idea of "contagion," as explaining the spread of disease, appears to have been adopted at a time when, from the neglect of sanitary arrangements, epidemics attacked whole masses of people, and when men had ceased to consider that nature had any laws for her guidance. Beginning with the poets and historians, the word finally made its way into medical nomenclature where it has remained ever since, affording to certain classes of minds, chiefly in the Southern and less educated parts of Europe, a satisfactory reason for pestilence, and an adequate excuse for non-exertion to prevent its recurrence. [6]

Leaving aside for a moment the ideological problems evident in Nightingale's derogatory remarks on "the Southern and less educated parts of Europe," I want to focus on the impression Nightingale gives here of rejecting contagion theory on two grounds: First, according to the logic she invokes here, only those who rely on observation and statistical analysis to verify the laws of nature, can perceive the so-called "facts" of disease. In other words, by observing what David Hume would call, the "constant conjunction" of particular environmental factors and disease, one can establish laws to explain the causes and spread of disease.[7] Our willful ignorance of those laws, she argues, makes us responsible for the diseases and ill health that result from it. In her words:

> God lays down certain physical laws. Upon His carrying out such laws depends our responsibility (that much abused word), for how could we have any responsibility for actions, the results of which we could not foresee – which would be the case if the carrying out of His laws were not certain. Yet we seem to be continually expecting that He will work a miracle – i.e. break His own laws expressly to relieve us of responsibility.[8]

The reference to the impossibility of God "breaking his own laws," indicates her rejection of the idea that God strikes down individuals or communities by introducing contagious diseases as divine punishment for misdeeds. Instead, God sets up nature according to laws, which can be revealed through observation, and the clever nurse will act according to them.

The second ground on which she bases her rejection of contagion in the passage above is her claim that belief in contagion itself derives from storytelling. Thus the language of contagion has itself infected both the medical and popular perceptions of disease, misleading the general public about the causes of disease and allowing for their indifference to issues of sanitation and hygiene. She places the onus for such neglect on "the Southern and less educated parts of Europe." Is this accusation just radical empiricist rejection of anything departing from Humean canons, or does it involve also in an attempt to manipulate the disease question into one that could be swayed by the language of national pride and the government's benevolent paternalism?

Nightingale's anxiety about the language of contagion in *Notes on Hospitals* and other writings is matched only by the near-paranoid narrative voice of *Notes on Nursing*. Nightingale appears to have wanted *Notes on Nursing* to be a means for her to transfer her own knowledge about hygiene to primarily middle-class women.[9] While she does not use the essay explicitly as a platform from which to make the anticontagionist argument she makes so strongly in *Notes on Hospitals*, written the same year, her advice is clearly geared toward promoting household management according to prevailing anticontagionist beliefs.

Her account of the average, dirty middle-class home presents a call for strict rules of hygiene and intolerance of laziness similar to that contained in her critique of the "Southern Europeans." Where this narrative differs substantially from *Notes on Hospitals*, however, is in her own obsession already noted above with the body's products and their effects on the environment. She often identifies the source of contamination within the home as the products of the sick patient's body, including the breath, sweat, and hair. She argues, for instance, against keeping the sickroom air warm by keeping windows closed and "making the sick repeatedly breathe their own hot, humid, putrescing [sic] atmosphere," an action that will serve only, she says, "to delay recovery or to destroy life."[10] Elsewhere, she claims that:

> Of all the methods of keeping patients warm the very worst is certainly to depend for heat on the breath and bodies of the sick. I have known a medical officer keep his ward windows hermetically closed, thus exposing the sick to all the dangers of infected atmospheres, because he was afraid that, by admitting fresh air the temperature of the ward would be too much lowered. This is a destructive fallacy.[11]

The logic of these claims may be evident to a twenty-first century reader, but her claims would have appeared to other anticontagionists as coming dangerously close to endorsing contagion theory. Her explanation of environmental contaminants even extends to rooms left closed up after the human inhabitants have left. She writes, "Old papered walls of years' standing, dirty carpets, uncleansed furniture, are just as ready sources of impurity to the air as if there were a dung-heap in the basement."[12] And the sink is even personified to add dramatic effect to her claim that "The ordinary sink is an abomination. That great surface of stone, which is always left wet, is always exhaling into the air."[13] Such passages may well seem to suggest that Nightingale is allowing for the possibility of single contact contagion (though environmental contamination may also be suggested by the talk of "repeatedly" breathing bad air, or the sink "always" exhaling into the air).

Because she comes so close to appearing to endorse contagion theory, Nightingale thus inserts a note to assure that her message is not misconstrued. In one of many explanatory footnotes throughout the text she writes,

> I was brought up, both by scientific men and ignorant women, distinctly to believe that small-pox, for instance, was a thing of which there was once a first specimen in the world, which went on propagating itself, in a perpetual chain of descent, just as much as that there was a first dog, (or a first pair of dogs,) and that small-pox would not begin itself any more than a new dog would begin without there having been a parent dog. Since then I have seen with my eyes and smelt with my nose small-pox growing up in first specimens, whether in closed rooms, or in overcrowded wards, where it could not by any possibility have been "caught," but must have begun.[14]

Small's insinuation of Nightingale's private endorsement of contagion theory seems almost impossible to imagine coexisting with this strident insistence that disease not only is transmitted, but also *originates* in the atmosphere. Her sensational language, the personified sink, and the "corrupt" air, seems to me much more strategically drawn from the language of novels, despite her complaint about the intersections between the language of medicine and literature in *Notes on Hospitals*. So, then the radical empiricist is here making maximum use of sensationalist rhetoric to move the empiricist program forward.

In her address to middle-class women in *Notes on Nursing*, her language takes on the quality of sensationalism, a sure indication that she was "pitching" this work so as to have the strongest effect possible. Here, instead of appealing to statistics and/or the language of science, she moves to language reminiscent of the sensational tabloid – at just the time when sensation fiction novels were beginning to be popular among the middle-class readership she clearly envisioned. In describing the workings of environmental contaminants, Nightingale employs metaphors of the silent and unobserved invasion of the middle class home. She interjects, for example, the following anecdote into her discussion of the kinds of inadequate hygiene that may cause disease and even death.

> A short time ago a man walked into a back-kitchen in Queen square, and cut the throat of a poor consumptive creature, sitting by the fire. The murderer did not deny the act, but simply said, "It's all right." Of course he was mad.
>
> But in our case [the case of inadequate hygiene], the extraordinary thing is that the victim says, "it's all right," and that we are not mad. Yet, although we "nose" the murderers, in the musty, unaired, unsunned room, the scarlet fever which is behind the door, or the fever and hospital gangrene which are stalking among the crowded beds of a hospital ward, we say, "It's alright."[15]

Of course, sensation fiction of the 1860s also often took its plots from current public scandals, bigamy trials, female murderers, etc. These popular novels stress vigilance and dispassionate observation as the only effective way of combating the insidious behavior of master criminals, such as Count Fosco in Wilkie Collins' *The Woman in White*.[16] Both the novel's hero, Walter Hartright, and its dark, heroine, Marian Halcombe write extensively in their journals about the need to observe rationally and without prejudgment to defeat Fosco. It seems no accident that the novel also features a hypochondriac who obsesses over the cleanliness of his home with a zeal reminiscent of Florence Nightingale herself. Marian's Uncle Fairlie also insists that people keep a comfortable distance from him, as he's sure that their noise will affect his constitution so dramatically as to make him ill. Fairlie, like Nightingale, uses fear of illness to conduct household management with an iron hand (though, of course, in her case, her effort is to scare others not herself!). Fairlie, and for that matter the novel's hero Walter Hartright would surely agree with Nightingale's assertion that "Apprehension, uncertainty, waiting, expectation, fear of surprise, do a patient more harm than any exertion."[17] Fairlie would appreciate too that Nightingale insists that nurses "value the patients 'fancies' as reliable indicators of what will make them well."[18] Both Fairlie, the fictional character, and Nightingale retired to their rooms, insisting on quiet, cleanliness, ventilation, and distance from other people.

Nightingale sets up the rather startling analogy between the sensational tabloid murder and the infection of the home through contaminants to shock her readers into complying with her prescriptions for household hygiene, but she insists also that the emphasis on strict observation must go further. She extends the discussion of the importance of vigilant empirical observation and detection into her later prescriptions for how a nurse (and, as Nightingale argues *every* woman is, at one time or another, a nurse[19]) might observe the symptoms of death correctly. She describes the different colors faces actually take in death's various stages, while observing that novel *de rigeur* always assume the coloring of the dying is white. Novels' coding of death, according to Nightingale, is not "true to life,"[20] or accurate in detail, something that the Pre-Raphaelite poets, artists, and the sensation fiction writers of the 1860s would have insisted that they be.[21]

But Nightingale later appears to abandon this need for rigid focus on the accuracy of representation, when she begins to mix the language of contamination (which she will have taken to be the only empirically sound language with which to discuss disease) with that of the moral imperatives incumbent on the nurse. Despite her wish to maintain a separation between the notions of contagion and morality – disease is *not* explicable through contagion between bodies introduced into the body as divine punishment from God – Nightingale nevertheless wishes in *Notes on Nursing* to establish in her readers' minds that there is a connection between hygiene and morality. As much as she would like to claim a strictly empiricist basis for the cause and transmission of disease, her instructions to middle class women insist that hygiene is a moral responsibility. She argues: "On women we must depend first and last for personal and household hygiene – for preventing the race from degenerating as far as these things are concerned."[22] The term she uses, "degeneration," is a loaded one, which suggests that the connection Nightingale perhaps inadvertently describes is fueled by her sense of English women's special role in preventing both immorality and disease. I find it impossible not to associate the term "degeneration" with Nightingale's lambasting of the "poor and less educated Southern Europeans." Her argument here seems one step away from the arguments of public health reformers, such as James Kay, that "other races" infiltrating England (and, in Kay's view, the Irish in particular are to blame) are responsible for the spread of poor moral hygiene, leading then to poor bodily health as well.[23] Her view does stop short of endorsing moral contagion, a step that would have led Nightingale away from her endorsement of the idea of contamination as expressing God's natural laws.

In *Notes on Nursing* Nightingale does not address the difficult scientific question of whether or not bodies or the products of bodies infect or indeed are part of the environment, something she is careful to do in *Notes on Hospitals*, clearly written for a different audience. Medical professionals with whom Nightingale corresponded struggled too with this question. Thomas Southwood Smith, for example, tried in 1829 to claim a middle ground between the contagion and environment positions by using the term "infection" to describe the transmission of disease through breathing air infected by the breath of a sick person. I have used the term above in describing Nightingale's view – which must make infection a matter of contagion. But Southwood Smith meant to use the term in a neutral way, rather than strictly attributing the spread of disease to either environmental pollutants or contagion through physical contact.[24] Nightingale, objecting to just such means of fence-sitting, responded with a clear statement denying that the term "infection" provided any room for belief in contagion. She argued, "The word 'infection,' which is often confounded with 'contagion,' expresses a fact, and does not involve a hypothesis. But just as there is no such thing as 'contagion,' there is no such thing as *inevitable* 'infection.' Infection acts through the air. Poison the air breathed by individuals, and there is infection".'[25] Small takes Nightingale's statement that "[T]he term infection ... expresses a fact and does not involve a hypothesis" as a ringing endorsement of the notion of germs causing disease,[26] in part because he leaves out the rest of the passage I cite here. While Nightingale certainly objects to the conflation of the terms infection and contagion, she offers no account of when or how body products become products of environmental contamination, rather than agents of contagion. As a means of coping with the difficulty of the question of infected air, sheets, curtains, etc., in *Notes on Nursing*, Nightingale herself allows the language of her medical advice to be infiltrated by the language of fictional narrative.

As I have already noted, Nightingale remains careful not to adopt the much more popular language of moral contagion, or disease as a form of divine punishment for bad conduct, that was present also in works by prominent fiction writers of the day. Charles Dickens, for example, indicates a belief in the mutual relation between moral and physical contagion through the narrator of his 1846 novel, *Dombey and Son*.[27] In this passage, for instance, the narrator explains the inseparability of poor physical and moral conditions among the poor in the most wretched of living conditions

> Those who study the physical sciences, and bring them to bear upon the health of Man, tell us that if the noxious particles that rise from vitiated air were palpable to the sight, we should see them lowering in a dense black cloud above such haunts, and rolling slowly on to corrupt the better portions of a town. But if the moral pestilence that rises with them, and in the eternal laws of outraged nature, is inseparable from them, could be made discernible too, how terrible the revelation![28]

In this passage, moral contagion appears in constant conjunction with environmental contaminants; it "rises with" and "is inseparable from" the presence of such "noxious particles." But Dickens goes even further to insist that the inseparability of environmental pollutants and moral contagion is an "eternal" law of "outraged nature." In other words, the claim goes beyond what an empiricist might observe about the habitual association of two things, beyond statistics and the observable, to create a law akin to the laws of nature. This is one step further than Nightingale is willing to allow in her own argument. There is no place for the language of moral contagion in her work, especially not when it is connected to a theory that assumes a relationship between morality and natural law though social reformers of her day wanted to make such claims.

Kay, for example, advocates the use of statistics in his treatise on the health of Manchester as the most "minutely accurate" form of investigation of disease origins,[29] but his "evidence" connected statistics about the numbers of Irish versus English in a region, to the numbers of taverns, the numbers of dissenters buried, and the numbers of churches in a region, all in order to connect such figures relating to morality to the presence of disease. Kay insists, in other words, that moral contagion is a readily observable entity through statistical analysis. He associates the spread of disease with the "[n]atural progress of barbarous habits" originating from the Irish.[30] He thus correlates the number of Irish with disease, as well as the number of drinking establishments and the numbers of faithful versus the numbers of dissenters. The source of the moral contagion, and hence the source of disease itself, is traceable in Kay's statistical analysis to the Irish.

In Nightingale's sensational story of the intruder – the intruder representing, of course, disease in general, and epidemic disease in particular – the culprit is ultimately the English middle-class woman who has allowed the disease into her midst through poor household management. While she avoids making any one race or religion the source of disease, she does manage to avoid slipping into the language of morality, which would clearly mark a falling away from the language of empiricism into metaphysics. In making her claim about the culpability of the unobservant middle-class woman early in her narrative, Nightingale seems to be setting up her later empiricist argument that women have no inborn ability to perform the necessary vigilant observation and detection of such intruders. Here, the metaphysical language of natural abilities to nurture, care and sympathize, have no place in Nightingale's narrative of good household management. Instead, she clearly would like nurses and women in general to be trained in empirical observation of the home.

As in *Notes on Hospitals*, she justifies her claim by emphasizing the natural laws of disease, which are confirmable through the observation of the constant conjunctions between poor hygiene and the presence of disease. Nurses, she worries, are

> not taught anything about those laws which God has assigned to the relations of our bodies with the world in which He has put them. In other words, the laws which make these bodies, into which he has put our minds, healthy or unhealthy organs of those minds, are all but unlearnt. [31]

She models the need for hygiene in the home on the similar need for it in hospitals. She writes:

> The everyday management of a large ward, let alone of a hospital – the knowing what are the laws of life and death for men, and what the laws of health for wards – and wards are healthy and unhealthy, mainly according to the knowledge or ignorance of the nurse) – are not these matters of sufficient importance and difficulty to require learning by experience and careful inquiry, just as much as any other art? They do not come by inspiration to the lady disappointed in love, nor to the poor workhouse drudge hard up for a livelihood.[32]

The problem she sees with nursing in the home, as in the hospital, is that novelists have created the expectation that the best nurse is the one that is "disappointed in love or fresh out of the drawing room."[33] These images of "heroines of nursing"[34] appear to be precisely the problem with nursing – the overemphasis on intangible qualities of affect and shared sympathy. But Nightingale's insistence on empirical truths here does not remain consistent.

Perhaps the passage that best exemplifies the confusion in Nightingale's essay between her call for strict empiricist observation and her desire to connect morality to both the presence of disease and "natural" law comes in her attempt finally to ascribe a superior "natural" capacity for good empiricist observation to the English woman. She writes:

> But I think in no country are women to be found so deficient in ready and sound observation as in England, while peculiarly capable of being trained for it. The French or Irish woman is too quick of perception to be so sound an observer – the Teuton is too slow to be so ready observer as an English woman might be. Yet women lay themselves open to the charge that is so often made

> against them by men that they are not to be trusted ... for want of a practiced and studied observation.[35]

In claiming an ability to measure "capability," which would seem to be like a person's capacity for love or imagination – impossible to observe empirically, Nightingale moves away from her insistence on the strict observation of phenomena in the interests of encouraging nationalist fervor for her own agenda.

Nightingale's enthusiasm for encouraging women in the arts of observation and even surveillance, which she sees as requirements for the competent nurse, ultimately requires that her rhetoric move into the metaphysical and fictional realms. Ultimately Nightingale encourages the same kind of reliance on the sensational narrative that she bemoaned earlier in *Notes on Hospitals*. Both her insistence on the need for strictly non-metaphysical approaches to disease diagnosis and prevention, and her call to eschew theoretical speculation as to the causes and means of disease transmission are undone by her own language in *Notes on Nursing*.

The easy explanation for Nightingale's motives in confusing the empiricist and metaphysical arguments she makes about bodies in *Notes on Nursing*, insisting one minute that empiricist study reveals the falsehood of contagion theory, while insisting on shocking her reader with the sensational story of moral contagion the next – perhaps she felt her language was the only way to convert people to her way of thinking?

Some may say that it is not fair to Nightingale to suggest that she was willing to sensationalize the issue of disease origins and transmission to accomplish her goal of informing the public about hygiene. But Nightingale said many things that seem uncharacteristic of her will to make a difference in the world through strict promotion of hygiene and sanitation in nursing.

Small's provocative suggestion that Nightingale may, in fact, have privately endorsed germ theory, or the theory of contagion between bodies, seems doubtful to me. However, his claim ultimately reopens the important issue of Nightingale's and others' complicated political investments in the contagion-anticontagion debate. By tracing Nightingale's rhetorical strategies in writings addressed to major political figures as well as those written for middle-class women, we can see the far-reaching effects the disease theories of the Victorians had on medicine, politics, and domestic life. Further we can recognize just how important the intersection between the languages of literature and medicine are to the political and personal worlds of Victorian men and women.

Notes

[1] See Hugh Small *Florence Nightingale: Avenging Angel.* New York: St. Martin's, 1998, 141-144. Small cites two letters previously overlooked by historians that indicate Nightingale's struggle with the knowledge that the mortality rate in her hospital was the highest of any of the Crimean hospitals by a large margin largely because they had not yet recognized that inadequate sanitation and not inadequate provisions and the weakened state of soldiers transferred to Scutari was the major cause of the high mortality rate. Additionally, he claims that the McNeil-Tulloch report, which should have exposed this fact, was doctored in the interest of preserving the honor (and the recruitment abilities) of the British War Office (Small 1-4). See James McNeil, and Alexander Tulloch. "Report of the Royal Commission into the Supplies of the British Army in the Crimea." Vol. XX, (1856). Small believes that Nightingale's distress about the high mortality rate and the government cover up explains her retreat from public life, in any fashion other than commanding major figures in public health to and from her bedside.

[2] Small, 4.

[3] Qtd. in Small, 143.

[4] *Notes on Hospitals,* 10.

[5] See Florence Nightingale, *Notes on Nursing: What it is and What it is Not.* [1860]. New York: Dover, 1969; and *Notes on Hospitals*, 3rd ed. London: Longmans, 1853.

[6] *Notes on Hospitals*, 9.

7 David Hume, *An Inquiry Concerning Human Understanding*, ed. Eric Steinberg (Indianapolis: Hackett Publishing Co., 1977).

[8] *Notes on Nursing* , 25.

[9] Nightingale wrote another version for members of the working classes entitled, "Notes on Nursing for the Labouring Classes," Pamphlet, 1861.

[10] *Notes on Nursing*, 16.

[11] Ibid., 15.

[12] Ibid., 27.

[13] Ibid., 26.

[14] Ibid., 32.

[15] Ibid., 14.

[16] William Wilkie Collins, *The Woman in White*, (New York: Oxford University Press, 1987).

[17] *Notes on Nursing*, 38.

[18] Ibid., 59.

[19] Ibid., 3.

[20] Ibid., 119-20, 120n.

[21] For more on the sensation fiction novelists and pre-Raphaelite poets' interest in following Ruskin's "truth to nature" creed, see Elaine Showalter. A great example of the obsession with "truth to nature" is the

famous anecdote about William Holman Hunt's "Light of the World" painting, in which he forced the unlucky model to stand in a chilly graveyard for hours, just so Hunt could have that particular look of a freezing man portrayed accurately.

[22] *Notes on Nursing*, 140.

[23] Kay, as he was then called, claimed in his pamphlet of 1832, *The Moral and Physical Condition of the Working Classes Employed in the Cotton Manufacture in Manchester*, that poor environmental conditions simply resulted in a *predisposition* toward the reception of epidemic diseases whose causes could be linked back to his theory of moral contagion. See *The Moral and Physical Conditions of the Working Classes Employed in the Cotton Manufacture in Manchester*, 2nd ed. (London: James Ridgeway, 1832). Strangely enough, given that statistics appear to have been the chief method of anticontagionist theory and social reform efforts of the 1830s to early 1860s, it was Kay's staunchly contagionist tract that appears to have culminated in both the founding of the Manchester Statistical Society in 1833 and, more generally, in the enormous growth of medical statistics in England. See Gary Messinger. *Manchester in the Victorian Age: The Half-Known City*, (Manchester: Manchester University Press, 1985), 45.

[24] Thomas Southwood Smith. "Plague – Typhus Fever – Quarantine," in the January-April 1825 issue of the *Westminster Review*, 499-529. See also John M. Eyler's discussion of Smith's strategy in *Victorian Social Medicine*.

[25] Nightingale's emphasis *Note on Hospitals*, 10.

[26] Nightingale goes on to claim, "With proper sanitary precautions, diseases reputed to be the most 'infectious' may be treated in wards among other sick without any danger," *Notes on Hospitals*, 10; Small, 143.

[27] Charles Dickens, *Dombey and Son*, (New York: Dell, 1963).

[28] Dickens, 669-670.

[29] Kay, 19.

[30] Ibid., 81.

[31] Ibid., 11.

[32] *Notes on Nursing*, 134.

[33] Ibid.

[34] Ibid.

[35] Ibid., 113.

Bibliography

Collins, Wilkie. *The Woman in White*. New York: Oxford University Press, 1987.

Dickens, Charles. *Dombey and Son*. New York: Dell, 1963.

Dossey, Barbara. *Florence Nightingale: Mystic, Visionary, Healer*. Springhouse PA: Springhouse Publications, 2000.

Eyler, John M. *Victorian Social Medicine: The Ideas and Methods of William Farr*. Baltimore: Johns Hopkins University Press, 1979.

Hume, David. *An Inquiry Concerning Human Understanding*. Ed. Eric Steinberg. Indianapolis: Hackett Publishing Co., 1977

Kay, James Phillip. *The Moral and Physical Conditions of the Working Classes Employed in the Cotton Manufacture in Manchester*. 2nd ed. London: James Ridgeway, 1832.

McNeil, James, and Alexander Tulloch. "Report of the Royal Commission into the Supplies of the British Army in the Crimea." Vol. XX, (1856).

Messinger, Gary. *Manchester in the Victorian Age: The Half-Known City*. Manchester: Manchester University Press, 1985.

Nightingale, Florence. *Notes on Hospitals*, 3rd ed. London: Longmans, 1853.

------------. *Notes on Nursing: What it is and What it is Not*. [1860]. New York: Dover, 1969.

-----------. "Notes on Nursing for the Labouring Classes." Pamphlet. 1861.

Showalter, Elaine. "Subverting the Feminine Novel: Sensationalism and Feminine Protest," from *A Literature of Their Own*. London: Virago, 1977.

Small, Hugh. *Florence Nightingale: Avenging Angel*. New York: St. Martin's, 1998.

Smith, Thomas Southwood. "Plague – Typhus Fever – Quarantine." *Westminster Review*. 3 (January-April 1825): 499-529.

Woodham-Smith, Cecil. *Florence Nightingale*. Edinburgh: Constable, 1950.

Note on Contributor

Louise Penner is an Assistant Professor of English at the University of Massachusetts in Boston, MA USA. Her primary research and teaching interests include intersections between the medical and literary cultures of nineteenth-century Britain and contemporary issues in medical humanities.

Part 2

Narratives and Metaphors

Making Sense of Healing: Meaning and Spirituality in Stories of Chronic Illness

Catherine Garrett

1. Healing, Spirituality and the Problem of Language

In this essay on healing, I consider some questions and ideas that contribute to a deeper understanding of what the term can mean. Without claiming definitive answers, I offer one framework within which healing might be discussed.

The word "healing" is a metaphor and, like all metaphors, it is open to multiple meanings. There are many kinds of healing: of bodies, emotions and relationships; from grief, disruption and every form of brokenness. "Healing" is to animate life as "mending" and "making" are to inanimate objects: the restoration, discovery or creation of wholeness. "Healing" in any one context always contains potential reference to the others. Becoming aware of these connections deepens our understanding of something that remains, nevertheless, a mystery. All art forms struggle to express the experience of healing, just as they struggle to represent pain itself.[1]

When poets speak of suffering, they show us that healing or salvation is mysterious, only possible through love, and always emerging from pain, grief and sorrow as something new. When anthropologists explore the rituals and beliefs through which people across cultures try to find "healing," they define it as "the redress of sickness": through cure, rehabilitation and palliation. *Cure* is the restoration of a prior healthy state, *rehabilitation* is a compensation for loss of health and *palliation* is the mitigation of suffering in the sick.[2]

Of course ideas of healing (like ideas of self and person) vary greatly in different cultural and historical circumstances. In many cultures, healing means restoring the social order when it has been broken by human disagreements or restoring the order of nature through paying homage to the gods or spirits that make life possible: sun, water, fire and so on. The self-transformation this paper explores comes closest to "palliation" but I will not use this term because today it most often refers to the care of the terminally ill, whose questions are of a related but different kind from those that arise in chronic non-fatal illness.

Faced with a chronic illness, from which cure is impossible or unlikely, people almost always ask, "What does this mean?" This question, even when it is not explicit, haunts all our attempts to talk about pain, suffering and healing. It can be approached on different levels. On the *medical* level, we ask, "What is the physical cause of this condition and can the cause be removed?" On the *existential* level, we ask "What does this condition mean, if anything, about the way I have been living my life and about how I will live it from now on?" Our answers to these existential questions can be practical ("What changes will I need to make to my diet, work or environment?"), psychological ("How can I find ways to think about what's happening that will help me endure it?"), political ("What can I do to assist greater social understanding and relief for others who suffer the same condition?") and philosophical ("What is the nature of suffering?" "How does it arise?" "Is it an inevitable part of being human?").

Spiritual questions extend the existential approach to a different level. Those who ask spiritual questions assume that there is a core aspect of each human being that can be described as his or her "spirit." They make this assumption from experience or trust in the stories of others. Some think that this spirit continues to exist after the death of the body. Some say it pre-existed this body. Spiritual questions may seek "spirit" not only within self and others but also beyond the human.

Religious questions are those which interrogate bodies of systematic spiritual thought and its expression in the artistic forms of literary, visual, tactile and performing arts. Which kinds of questions a person asks will depend partly on social background and experience and partly on differences in personality. Although not all people with chronic illness ask existential, spiritual or religious questions, the practical solutions they find to the problem of living with illness are often underpinned by unspoken answers to these philosophical issues. "Virtue" is practiced by people everywhere, in a variety of ways, with or without a theory about virtue.[3]

In contemporary society, secular or not, it is hard to talk about "spirituality" without alienating at least those listeners who call themselves atheists, agnostics or rationalists. On the other hand, people with serious and chronic illnesses do have experiences that separate them forever from the "pain-free world."[4] These experiences change the way they perceive themselves, their relations with others and the meaning of their existence. The knowledge that arises from these experiences is often referred to as "spiritual" and many clinicians and professional carers recognize its importance in the various forms of healing – nursing and occupational therapy, for instance, whose practitioners and theorists are trying to find a language of spirituality that is acceptable to their profession and those it serves.[5] Some of the more successful writings of this kind come from people involved in palliative care.[6]

Attempts to construct a "language of spirituality" that would allow dialogue across a wide range of attitudes to spirituality can only succeed by going further than the clichés people use when they first try to describe the meaning of transforming experiences of suffering. The halting, vague and stereotyped words of this struggle do deserve attention and respect, because they belong to what Arthur Frank has called the "chaos narrative" in which "meaning" is unresolved.[7] It is from such chaotic experiences and their accompanying stories that meaning is eventually created as a way out of confusion. But when people begin to construct the stories and find the symbols that will give meaning to their suffering, they invariably do so by drawing on the great myths humans have made throughout history and expressed in art and literature. Without these shared images and meta-narratives, our own narratives would be unintelligible. Since healing involves the discovery of wholeness and connection, even in the midst of suffering, it makes sense to seek it in works of art that express these connections and have the wholeness that comes from deep reflection on experience. From the language of chaos and confusion, creativity calls forth new words and symbols, which are themselves part of healing.

One artwork that reveals some of the meanings of suffering and healing is Epstein's statue of his namesake, Jacob, wrestling with the Angel. Its power comes not simply from Epstein's own life experience but also through its association with the Biblical story of Jacob's encounter with the Divine. The Angel bends his legs to support and raise Jacob, holding him beneath the shoulder blades and lifting him so that only his toes touch the ground. Jacob, slumped with exhaustion, has given in to his opponent. They are so close that a single crack of light separates them. The statue represents the moment before Jacob begs the Angel for a blessing. It is a kind of ecstasy: clasped bodies, skin on skin. It is also familiar and comforting because the bodies are pockmarked and vulnerable. The panel beside this statue in the Tate Gallery reads: "The Angel blessed Jacob because he had not abandoned the struggle. Jacob gave thanks, saying: 'I have seen God face to face and my life is preserved'." To make a sculpture is to make "an image, a fetish, something which alters human behaviour."[8]

Epstein's man and angel recreate the biblical story in stone, as if he had carved it from, as well as with, his own body and re-placed it in the world: the solid expression of what he has felt in his guts and sinews and found echoed in the Hebrew myth. It is the reflection of his whole being upon the mystery of pain and the peace that comes when we finally experience and accept a reality we have long resisted. As myth made tangible, Epstein's art alters our own understanding of the story. This image holds the potential to change forever a viewer's perceptions of suffering and healing. In music, Beethoven's late string quartets express a similar crisis, resignation and inner illumination; especially in the serenity of the Cavatina in Opus 130 and in the movement from Opus 132 that bears the superscription "Solemn song of thanksgiving of a convalescent to the Deity."

Literature exemplifies in language the changes that come about through pain and its transformation, which is why it is important to reflect carefully on the models presented by published illness narratives in fiction and non-fiction. My discussion here will be confined to the latter.

2. A New Typology for Healing Narratives

The Wounded Storyteller, Arthur Frank's influential book on illness, narrative and ethics, constructs a typology of illness narratives: chaos, restitution and quest. It is Frank's quest narrative that I will be developing below. As he explains, his three narrative "types" are not fixed, but useful devices for hearing the similarities and differences in illness stories. They often overlap in the life story of the same narrator. Each kind of narrative has its own power and each deserves recognition. The plot of the chaos narrative is an apparently shapeless "and then, and then, and then ..."[9] The restitution narrative is the one that biomedicine prefers. Its plot sounds like this: "I got sick, I had treatment (or followed regimens), I got well again."

Frank's "quest" narrative is the narrative that accompanies and creates healing. In this narrative, illness is re-framed as self-challenge. The illness is eventually understood as an opening to the other. Quest stories lead the storyteller to become a more "ethical" person: a person who lives for others. The quest story accepts contingency, acknowledging that it is impossible to control the body, life, or other people. It accepts the presence of illness but transforms its meaning. Illness becomes an opportunity for connection with others, even when they are not present. In the quest narrative, this connection is the "boon" for suffering.

Frank discusses three categories of quest narrative. The *memoir* is the gentlest of these. It combines the illness story with other events in the writer's life and illness is presented as an interruption to that life.[10] The *manifesto* is prophetic in tone. In manifestos the life story is told in order to make demands for various forms of social action on behalf of other people with similar illnesses.[11] The *automythology* is told as the mythic quest of the hero-writer.[12] It involves the reinvention of self from the fires of suffering. The hero's story becomes a paradigm of universal conflicts and concerns.[13]

I now want to extend Frank's "quest" narrative in a variety of ways. First, by emphasizing that in this narrative type, the dominant emotion is hope.[14] Hope is "desire combined with expectation."[15] Its meaning is very close to "confidence" and "trust." Confidence is an embodied experience of safety in the world. This feeling of security in the present allows us to project ourselves into the unknown future: confidence is an essential motivation for personal and social action.[16] The hope that people experience in chronic illness might include the hope of cure, but most often it is a day-by-day hope for respite from suffering. This respite and the confidence that it will recur, however unpredictably or fleetingly, is part of what I mean by healing.

Next, I want to stress that narratives of suffering and healing draw on the great myths that underpin all our stories: the lasting stories all peoples have created to try to explain the presence of suffering in the world. Ongoing discussion of theodicy and morality in religious doctrine has attempted to provide sufferers with answers across cultures throughout history. Traces of Judaic, Christian, Buddhist and Hindu theodicies can be found in most illness stories, not simply because the stories are influenced by their culture but also because the traces of these meta-narratives represent the shared human experiences of suffering and healing.[17]

Finally, I want to suggest some additional varieties of the quest narrative. Like all Frank's narrative types, these varieties may overlap and co-exist in the life of a single person. They are available to us as templates, which underpin stories of illness and healing we read and hear about in the media and from people we know. In creating this typology, my aim is not the psychological one of transforming individual stories by "telling the ill what to do." Instead, it is sociological because it is about making a variety of possibilities for healing more widely known through disseminating them as healing discourses in contemporary culture.

For each of these healing narrative "types" I name, I will give examples, explaining the aim of the narrative and the particular means through which some kind of transformation takes place within such narratives (see Appendix: Table I). The examples I have chosen include not only individual life stories but also theoretical narratives from sociology, philosophy and religion. They are "stories" too, about whole groups of people and how they suffer and are changed by their suffering. These abstract, theoretical narratives arise out of human experience but also help shape that experience by constructing some of the meta-narratives (of psychology, sociology, philosophy, spirituality and religion) upon which people may draw in creating their personal stories of healing.

A. Interpersonal Narratives: "Love Heals"

Interpersonal narratives have *love* as their main objective. They speak about healing in terms of the benefits that come to ill people from relationships with others. Their focus (the way they describe the means towards transformation) is primarily *psychological*. For example, an article by Green and Shellenberger argues that love heals, but that it does so in several different ways.[18] These authors consider a range of research studies on health and healing, all of which recognize that "health" is not simply "absence of illness" but involves a person's total "well-being." For people with chronic conditions, therefore, healing means achieving this well-being in the midst of illness.

Epidemiological studies, for instance, have found that social isolation is a "risk factor" for death and that even when people are ill, strong family ties decrease absenteeism from work. Immediate outcome studies report that supportive relations for the ill can enhance physical immunity by reducing killer cell activity. Even showing people a film about Mother Theresa's care for the poor stimulated their caring feelings and increased the levels of immunoglobulins in the bloodstream.[19] Studies of healing groups like Alcoholics Anonymous and other support groups describe the healing power of altruistic love in a forgiving community, and studies of spiritual healers show that their practices can indeed accelerate healing.[20]

In these accounts, the healing energy of love comes from partners, carers, communities and a society as a whole ("caring" societies with strong welfare policies would seem to be more "healing" than others). While these are stories about the healing associated with the love of others *for* the ill person, in *The Wounded Storyteller* Frank is most concerned with the love that comes *from* the chronically ill and is often most fully discovered through illness. In chronic illness, when there is little prospect of cure, healing is something that happens over and over, rather than once and for all. At the instant when the sick person is aware of loving or being loved, through actions, as well as gestures and words, suffering is temporarily transcended, if only for an instant. This kind of healing is not dramatic or newsworthy but love expressed daily to and by the person who suffers transforms the experience of suffering, moment by moment. It also provides a memory of transcendence to which the sufferer can turn even in total solitude.

In the film *Mask* (based on the true story of an adolescent boy with a degenerative disease that distorts his facial features and gives him severe headaches), the boy's mother teaches him to use good memories to overcome pain. Her touch, her look and the stories she tells him help him to live through the worst episodes of his illness. When he falls in love with a blind girl, he offers her the same wisdom, knowing that the memory of their embrace will alleviate their future suffering, whatever its form. Despite the film's sentimentality, this insight is genuine.

Illness narratives in the popular press usually draw on this psychological version of the quest narrative, emphasizing the reciprocal love of the sick, their family and friends as essential to the healing process. Such stories are the most common variety of the quest narrative. Stories about the other types of love (for community, for strangers, for humanity) are less prevalent and often shade into the next type of quest narrative.

B. Political Narratives: Anger and Justice

Political narratives correspond to Frank's "manifesto." Their main object is to bring about transformation in the lives of ill people through *justice*. For example, researchers at the Australian Centre for the Study of Quality of Life at Deakin University and from the (Australian) Chronic Illness Alliance, emphasize the social dimensions of chronic illness. They help articulate the desire of many chronically ill people to bring about changes in the way their illness is publicly perceived, how it is defined and treated by the medical profession, and how it is assisted, or not, by the state. They remind us that the dominant emotion in many such narratives is anger and that anger is often the impetus for improvements in society.[21] They point to the strong relationship between morbidity and socio-economic status and the need to investigate it further.[22] They draw on stories that describe the limitations and stigma of illnesses like epilepsy, diabetes, HIV, infant paralysis and Chronic Fatigue Syndrome. For example, they quote the words of a woman with epilepsy:

> I want to help other people, and it's why I speak for the Epilepsy Foundation because I want to educate people. ... It's just so misunderstood. ... And there's a lot of prejudice towards it. ... It's particularly so with employment.[23]

These authors comment that interventions designed by epidemiologists and policy-makers to improve the health status and health outcomes of people with chronic illness lose their impact or are misdirected for lack of public knowledge about the effects of a chronic condition on a person's life.[24] The personal narratives they draw upon and the public discourse they construct both advocate *political* means to bring about social justice for people with chronic illnesses. But even political narratives about illness and healing must often come from a kind of love, for without a love of others; there would be no incentive to struggle for improvements in their lives.

The life story of Father Damien de Veuster, who spent his last years in the leprosy colony of Molokai, Hawaii, is a political narrative of healing which draws on my other three narrative types as well.[25] Father Damien struggled with civil and ecclesiastical authorities on behalf of the lepers among whom he lived, demanding justice for these people who had been ostracized because of their illness. Like many of his fellow missionary priests in the Pacific, his peasant background in Europe gave him a deep understanding of poverty and injustice and their effects on the ill.[26] One historian, drawing on contemporary accounts, gives this description of the man who chose to become infected with leprosy himself, as a means of total identification with the suffering people he served:

> Damien of Molokai, who in unromantic reality was a stubborn and often angry saint, was poor among the poor; ... he exuded qualities many of his confrères demonstrated on a smaller scale; they exasperated Hawaiians by their gruff authority – and yet were much loved.[27]

His kind of self-sacrifice is not possible without an accompanying growth in self-understanding. This growth is another aspect of healing. It has its own narrative form.

C. "Inward" Narratives: Transformation through Self-Knowledge

This third kind of quest narrative refers to an "inner self" as the main source of self-transformation in the face of serious illness. I take the term "inwardness" from a paper by Heather McKenzie, in which she considers the subjective experience of cancer in Western societies.[28] She shows how the isolation that often follows a diagnosis of cancer and the "liminal status" of people with cancer "force them to rely on their own resources as they struggle to understand their situation and cope with deep-seated fears of disease recurrence." For some, this involves an inward search for self-explanations – for self-knowledge.[29] For instance: "My true self wanted to express itself in a certain way and I haven't allowed it to." McKenzie also includes people's religious searching in this "inwardness." One woman says: "You can only do it through a whole lot of self-examining. ... I really believe you get sick for a reason. It's like God telling you to wake up and look at yourself."[30] The language of inwardness, as expressed by participants in this study, included terms like "undernourished spirit" and "inner power." This "inner self" is often, unfortunately, considered personally responsible for warding off any future episodes of the disease.

Some of McKenzie's respondents identify a person's "inner self" with "spirit"; some speak of inwardness as an emotional depth and others as a place of rational deliberation.[31] These narratives, then, are sometimes "spiritual" only in the broadest sense of the word: as that which "gives life meaning" and which these people "consider to be of ultimate importance."[32] McKenzie insists that the inward orientation of her respondents is not solipsistic because they are often reflections on the connection between the self and the outer "ordinary life" of social relationships.

McKenzie argues that inwardness – the notion of attending to oneself as "inner" – is "a historically limited mode of self-interpretation, rooted in the Augustinian theoretical formulation of personhood in terms of inner and outer." She thinks that it is from within this frame of reference that modern persons attempt to find their bearings. She concludes that the psychic depths often encountered in illness are "sacred in the sense of being absolute for a given individual as well as distant and different from the 'ordinary' experience of the profane everyday life." Today, there is widespread perception that this is where we find our emotions – located at the "innermost and individuated, and hence sacred, part of the person."[33]

I also recognize in this familiar language the influence of what might loosely be called New Age discourse. This way of talking about spirituality by emphasizing the "inner search" bears the marks of oversimplified Hinduism. The concept of Self as Atman/Brahman – the aspect of self that is connected with the one true reality – has been mistranslated in consumer capitalism (through the spread of practices like yoga and transcendental meditation) in such a way that it is often equated with the ego and its desires. In spite of this, practising the ritual techniques of Hinduism (modified for Westerners) can often take practitioners beyond egocentrism to experiences of connection with others and to a sense of belonging to a sacred reality to be found both within and beyond the self.[34]

This transformation, which is also a discovery, may begin with the horrors of illness.[35] People often report finding something "sublime" in their suffering. As Alan Radley explains, this does not mean that they achieve some other-wordly, ethereal way of being. On the contrary, "the sublime is grasped in the sensual," in the body's experience of the everyday world. It is expressed in creative – aesthetic – works, of which narrative is the paradigm. The very act of creation distances the terror of death and nothingness and produces a kind of "delight" which returns the sufferer to the "zone between life and death," to a renewed appreciation of "the really real." The experience of the sublime is, therefore, at once transcendent and immanent. The Australian novelist Gillian Mears, who suffers from a mysterious paralysis of her lower limbs, has scrawled on her kitchen wall this quote: "The unendurable is the beginning of the curve of joy."[36]

These ways of talking about experiences of illness refer to a "sacred" or "spiritual" dimension. They may or may not include the terminology of religion. When illness stories emphasize a transformation that has taken place through any kind of "inner" awareness, I am calling them "spiritual narratives." The narrator's objective, consciously or not, is transformation through self-awareness and the means towards this end could be called a *spiritual search*. This variety of quest narrative shares with the next variety (the contemplative narrative) the experience of simultaneous "transcendence and immanence" that has been the foundation of all religions.

D. Contemplative Narratives: Towards Ultimate Good

Religious thought, art and music across millennia have provided ways of expressing the experience spiritual narratives are trying to describe. Religious rituals are sets of practices designed to bring us closer to that experience. At the root of religion is a concern for the well being of others, an awareness of our inter-relatedness and of our connection with the physical world (of nature and its forces). Our recognition of these connections calls forth in us a sense of responsibility that goes beyond our own personal existence. For people with chronic illnesses, the ethical question of "how not to project your own suffering onto others" is a spiritual question. It cannot be resolved through self-discipline alone: in the crisis of severe pain or uncontrollable mental and emotional changes, suffering makes this impossible. For most of us, it is a question without a final answer and in this sense forms part of a spiritual quest.

Contemplative narratives, however, offer something more than the question. They "show forth" answers in the "exemplary" lives of their authors.[37] These accounts are not examples of perfection but of beliefs and practices that assist their authors towards greater goodness. They suggest that evil can be, and often is, overcome by ultimate good.[38] In the contemplative approach to illness, this knowledge comes through personal experience and through recognition of the same experience in the great religious myths about healing.

An example of the contemplative approach is found, for instance, in the autobiography of St Teresa of Avila, who suffered almost constant illness and pain but also found comfort, and frequently rapture, in her devotional life. When she is in pain, she has a sense of her utter unworthiness, as if she and her life were trivial and meaningless. She says it is as if "the devil suddenly lays hold on my understanding, sometimes by making use of things so trifling that at any other time I should laugh at them." At such times, says Teresa, faith is quite numbed and asleep: it is useless to pray, to try to read, to engage in conversation or to seek help from a counsellor, because "the devil then makes me so peevish and ill-tempered that I seem to want to snap everyone up."[39] She links this aspect of suffering closely to her conception of "original sin" – the kind of evil that pre-exists our consciousness, and over which we have no rational control.

Teresa's physical suffering fragments her sense of self by forcing her to be aware of one of its aspects alone – her body. In this way, pain frustrates her desire for greater goodness, a higher morality, a selfless responsibility for the other: for the simultaneous knowledge of the good and the practical goodness I am calling "union with ultimate good." Her story shows how contemplation (which is quite different from rational deliberation) can help to integrate the self. During periods of contemplation she prays: "Permit my soul no longer, Lord, to be dispersed into fragments, with each fragment seeming to go its own way."[40]

Twentieth century theories about pain and suffering recognise the fragmentation of self involved, but few of them offer an account of how this fragmentation is transformed into wholeness in the process of healing which, like suffering, is a spiritual matter, concerned with what Aristotle calls "eternal truths." St Teresa was not claiming (and nor do today's "contemplative" accounts claim) total freedom from this fragmentation and the evils to which it leads. The contemplative quest narrative simply acknowledges the ideal and strives towards it.

In *The Tibetan Book of Living and Dying* (a presentation of Tibetan Buddhism to Westerners), Sogyal Rinpoche also refers to the fragmentation of self that brings about human suffering and to the way meditation reunites these fragments. He explains that the "heart" of Buddhist meditation is the Good. "In the teaching of the Buddha," he says, "there are three things that make all the difference between your meditation being merely a way of bringing temporary relaxation, peace, and bliss, or of becoming a powerful cause for your enlightenment and the enlightenment of others." They are: "Good in the Beginning, Good in the Middle, and Good at the End."[41] To realize that we have Good as our inmost essence is to be free of ignorance and hence of suffering. To be detached from the illusions in which we habitually live brings us closer to "the nature of mind" which is a truer apprehension of what is. To dedicate meditation to the liberation of all beings is to "seal the power of the meditation" to heal the whole of creation. Although this account of meditation is not given as a specific response to the sufferings of illness, it shares with other religious teachings the idea of an ultimate good and the possibility that prayer and meditation form part of the healing of a cosmos fragmented by evil.

Traces of these beliefs and their efficacy are present in many illness stories, even when they are not self-consciously religious.[42] For example, Tony Moore, the Australian surgeon who wrote, of his years of recovery from a devastating road accident, "I began to believe that (immortality) had only one dimension: the echoes of the energy I radiated to the world around me. It was my simple responsibility to try to make most of my energy contribute to a positive harmonic."[43] Moore explains that this ethical growth is closely connected with an ongoing revelation of reality: "I realised that in my general life all expectations tended to obscure what really existed."[44]

The idea of "the Good" is not necessarily associated with religion or even with techniques of meditation, as Iris Murdoch points out in her essays on *The Sovereignty of Good*. These essays are philosophical discourses of a "contemplative" kind. Her quest for a philosophical alternative to the "God" of religion begins with the problem of human suffering and evil. She comments: "That moral improvement involves suffering is usually true; but the suffering is the by-product of a new orientation and not in any sense an end in itself."[45] She makes links between what I have called the "interpersonal," the "inward" and the "contemplative" quests, by demonstrating their common search for "the real" and their common commitment to love. She is ambivalent about the value of the "political" quest because, although it is committed to justice, in the absence of any belief in a transcendent principle (one which always retains some mystery) it can too easily become merely utilitarian or romantic.

Political quests for knowledge and justice may have a "contemplative" element if they are motivated by faith in the reality of the Good and a belief that it can sometimes be connected with practical experience.[46] Murdoch's idea of goodness is derived from Plato's "form of the Good" so that although we can never know ultimate Good (her "transcendent principle"), we can see it represented in great art. By "great art" she means art that reveals reality (alterity), as opposed to the fantasies produced by a restricted focus on the individual self (a distorted inwardness). The experience Tony Moore describes experientially, Murdoch clarifies philosophically: "The attempt (usually only partially successful) to attend to goods purely, without self, brings with it an increasing awareness of the unity and interdependence of the moral world."[47]

3. Conclusions

In this essay, I have tried to show how love, justice, knowledge and good are intimately connected with the transformation of suffering into the various forms of healing. In doing this, I have used the method Iris Murdoch puts forward as the only one possible when arguing for such metaphysical matters. "All one can do," she believes, "is to appeal to certain areas of experience pointing out certain features, and using suitable metaphors and inventing suitable concepts where necessary to make these features visible."[48] I have illustrated four linked arguments. First, that the meaning of healing is most deeply understood through the creative work of writers and other artists. Second, that any "language of spirituality" will therefore be an aesthetic language in that it will reveal, not simply reproduce, understandings about healing. Third, that healing necessarily includes a mysterious element of experience that might be thought of as "faith," "hope," "spirituality" or "mysticism." Finally, that there is always more than one path towards healing.

Perhaps I should have begun by explaining what led me to write the essay, since these reasons determined its structure and some of its arguments. I wrote it in response to an experience I often have when I present my ideas to other academics at conferences and to health workers in hospitals and community centres. The audience for my presentations usually divides into groups, which become obvious from the kinds of questions people ask me and the comments they make. First, there are listeners who agree with what I have said (on love, hope and other positive emotions, on the importance of rituals, on healing without cure). This group is comfortable with my interest in what I have called here "the contemplative narrative" because it fits their own pursuit of understanding through study and practice of one or more forms of religion. Second, the importance of human relationships in living with illness is so widely accepted and so often the model for stories about chronic conditions that my category of "psychological narrative," which captures this vital aspect of healing, is uncontroversial.

Still, there are always also those who tell me that their particular experience and the experiences of those whose lives they study and wish to help do not fit the patterns of healing I have tried to identify. This group hears the stories I tell (often in the words of sick people themselves) as exhortations to behave in hopeful, joyful ways and to ignore their sufferings in favour of some kind of mystical transcendence. Although this is not the message I intend, these listeners have made me aware of another approach to suffering: a kind of stoicism which, like the existentialism of Samuel Beckett's plays, faces with courage the absurdity and pain of living. People who take this approach do not deny that others might have the kinds of spiritual experiences I have mentioned, but they reject my analysis because they do not accept that which cannot ultimately be explained in rational terms. I am moved by their response, though they do not like me saying so. It reminds me of Simone Weil, the French intellectual and contemplative who, despite her experiential faith in the God of Christianity and in the symbols of the Catholic Church, could not bring herself to be baptized into that church. Her intellectual honesty compelled her to retain the philosopher's cognitive scepticism alongside her affective spiritual life.[49] This group finds the model I call the "inward narrative" a more accurate description of the effects of illness, but does not speak in terms of "healing."

A final group of critics tell me that I seem to want chronically ill people to repress the most common emotions of illness: anger, shame, guilt and fear. They suggest that in focusing on the possibility of healing, I am helping reproduce the dominant "restitution story" of medical science with its demand that even people with chronic illnesses be "good patients" and strive towards cure. They believe that the most important response to chronic illness is to struggle with the political forces that make life even harder for sufferers. Through my category of "political narrative" I have tried to capture some of their insights.

Three important questions remain. Are these categories themselves ways of creating order out of the chaos of suffering? If so, do they themselves provide some form of healing? And, if they are only useful constructs for this purpose, do they have any other validity?[50] My answer to all three questions starts from the premise that healing is real: human beings do find respite – fleeting or extended – from their suffering, even when they are not cured from their pain, illness or disability. Healing can come from the simple presence of other people: far more than a distraction, their being near us can lift us away from pain. Children may heal us in this way and so may the company of other sufferers. Touch can heal. The presence of any living thing can be healing: lizards seen through the doorway on the path, birdsong in the early morning. Awareness of rain, sunshine, a storm, the sight of a mountain or the smell of the earth bring about sudden joy or peace, which are the opposite of suffering and cannot co-exist with it.

Creativity is not the same as healing, but it supports and maintains healing, for others perhaps even more than for ourselves. We do not need stories to find healing itself, since it can come to us without words or images. We do need them, as we need art, as mnemonics: to remind us that healing is possible. We need them, too, to express this remembering to others, as well as ourselves. Healing is a single phenomenon but the ways in which we describe it and seek to give it meaning are innumerable.

The stories through which we speak and write of illness and healing and the other works of art through which we describe these experiences do not themselves create healing out of the chaos of suffering. But they are important because they are our means of conveying something of that experience to others. Without others, we would have no existence, which is why our communication is of fundamental value. We think with stories and all our thought is social because all our stories depend on our knowing the stories of others – and how to tell stories. Telling our own stories gives others hope because it shows them they are not alone. The narrative types I have described are only useful if they serve to make our experiences more intelligible to each other. They recognize difference, which is also part of our humanity.

This essay began with the problem of language: the problem of communicating experience. It concludes with the idea that the experience of healing is beyond language yet must still somehow be shared through language. In presenting a variety of narrative types, I have tried to take a few further steps towards communication. I have tried to understand and to convey some of the differences that affect how we think and speak about illness and healing. To the extent that human connection is part of healing, these steps are part of my own healing and, I hope, might contribute to our understanding of the conditions that make healing possible.

Appendix

Table I
Varieties of the 'quest narrative' in stories of chronic illness

Type	Main aim/objective:	Means	Examples
Interpersonal	Transformation through *love*	Psychological	Shellenberger & Green. *The Mask*
Political	Transformation through *justice*	Socio-political	Millen, Peterson & Walker, Fr Damien
Inward	Transformation through *awareness of self & reality*	Spiritual search	MacKenzie, Radley, Mears
Contemplative	Transformation through *union with ultimate good*	Religious or philosophical belief and practice	Teresa of Avila, Sogyal Rinpoche, Tony Moore

Notes

[1] Elaine Scarry, *The Body in Pain: The Making and Unmaking of the World* (Oxford and New York: Oxford University Press, 1985).
[2] Robert Hahn, *Sickness and Healing: An Anthropological Perspective* (New Haven and London: Yale University Press, 1995), 7.
[3] Gareth Williams, "Chronic Illness and the Pursuit of Virtue in Everyday Life," in *Worlds of Illness: Biographical and Cultural Perspectives on Health and Disease*, ed. Alan Radley (London and New York: Routledge, 1993), 92-108.
[4] Jean Jackson, "Chronic Pain and the Tension between the Body as Subject and Object" in *Embodiment and Experience: The Existential Ground of Culture and Self*, ed. Thomas J. Csordas (Cambridge: Cambridge University Press, 1994), 201-228.
[5] Carrie Sanders, "Challenges for Spiritual Care-Giving in the Millennium," *Contemporary Nurse* 12, 2 (2002): 107-111. Loretta Do Rozario, "Spirituality in the Lives of People with Disability and Chronic Illness: A Creative Paradigm of Wholeness and Reconstitution," *Disability and Rehabilitation* 19, 10 (1997): 427-434.

[6] For example essays in Bruce Rumbold, ed., *Spirituality and Palliative Care: Social and Pastoral Perspectives* (Oxford: Oxford University Press, 2002).
[7] Arthur Frank, *The Wounded Storyteller: Body, Illness and Ethics* (Chicago: Chicago University Press, 1995).
[8] Quote from sculptor Barbara Hepworth on a Tate Gallery panel beside her work.
[9] The shapelessness of the chaos narrative is only "apparent" because this is what has been called a "hard-working narrative" in Christopher Jordens et al., "Life Disruption and Generic Complexity: A Social Linguistic Analysis of Narratives of Cancer Illness," in *Social Science and Medicine* 53, 9 (2001): 1227-1236. Their careful linguistic analysis shows that such narratives, told early in illness, are "trying out" a variety of possible ways of telling the story of this new and unfamiliar experience.
[10] Frank, 119.
[11] Ibid., 120.
[12] Ibid., 122.
[13] Ibid., 126.
[14] See also Catherine Garrett, "Sources of Hope in Chronic Illness," *Health Sociology Review* 10, 2 (2002): 99-109.
[15] *The Shorter Oxford English Dictionary* (Oxford: Oxford University Press, 1934), s.v. "hope."
[16] Jack Barbalet, *Emotion, Social Theory and Social Structure* (Cambridge: Cambridge University Press, 1998).
[17] Catherine Garrett, "Theodicies of Suffering in Narratives of Chronic Illness," paper presented at the World Congress of Sociology, Queensland University of Technology, Australia, July 6-13. See also Catherine Garrett, *Gut Feelings* (Rodopi: Amsterdam and New York), forthcoming.
[18] Judith Green and Robert Shellenberger, "The Healing Energy of Love," *Alternative Therapies* 2, 3 (1996): 46-56.
[19] Ibid., 49.
[20] Ibid., 50.
[21] Barbalet.
[22] Christine Walker et al., "Investigating Socio-Economic Status and Chronic Illness: Directions and Dilemmas," in *The Australian Sociological Association 2001 Conference Refereed Papers*, ed. Craig Browne et al., The University of Sydney (2001), CD-ROM.
[23] Ibid., 5.
[24] Ibid., 6.
[25] Gavan Daws, *Holy Man: Father Damien of Molokai* (New York: Harper and Row, 1973).
[26] John Garrett, *Footsteps in the Sea: Christianity in Oceania to World War II* (Suva, Fiji: Institute of Pacific Studies, 1992), 418.

[27] Ibid., 234.
[28] Heather McKenzie, "Inwardness: An Enduring 'Self' Concept", in C. Browne et al. (eds.), *The Australian Sociological Association 2001 Conference Refereed Papers*, The University of Sydney (2001), CD-ROM.
[29] Ibid., 3.
[30] Ibid., 5.
[31] Heather McKenzie, personal communication, June 2002.
[32] Gary Bouma, "Religion and Spirituality," in *Sociology: Australian Connections (2nd Edition)*, ed. Ray Jureidini and Marilyn Poole (Sydney: Allen and Unwin, 2000), 388.
[33] McKenzie, 6.
[34] Catherine Garrett, "Transcendental Meditation, Reiki and Yoga: Suffering, Ritual and Self-transformation," *Journal of Contemporary Religion* 16, 3 (2001): 329-342.
[35] Alan Radley, "The Aesthetics of Illness: Narrative, Horror and the Sublime", *Sociology of Health and Illness* 21, 6 (1999): 778-796.
[36] Janet Hawley, "Runaway Success – Gillian Mears," *The Sydney Morning Herald Good Weekend Magazine*, May 4, 2002: 30-33.
[37] Radley, 779.
[38] Marilyn McCord Adams, *Horrendous Evils and the Goodness of God* (Melbourne: Melbourne University Press, 1999).
[39] Teresa of Avila, *The Life of Teresa of Jesus: The Autobiography of Teresa of Avila* (New York: Image Books Doubleday, 1991), 282.
[40] Ibid., 284-285.
[41] Sogyal Rinpoche, *The Tibetan Book of Living and Dying* (Sydney: Random House, 1992), 59.
[42] Rory Williams, "Religion and Illness," in *Worlds of Illness: Biographical and Cultural Perspectives on Health and Disease* , ed. Alan Radley, (London and New York: Routledge, 1993), 71-91.
[43] Tony Moore, *Cry of the Damaged Man* (Sydney: Pan Macmillan, 1991), 94.
[44] Ibid., 131.
[45] Iris Murdoch, *The Sovereignty of Good* (London: Routledge Classics, 2001), 67.
[46] Ibid., 72.
[47] Ibid., 68.
[48] Ibid., 73.
[49] Simone Pétrement, *Simone Weil: A Life*, transl. Raymond Rosenthal (New York: Pantheon Books, 1976).
[50] I thank Harold Schweizer for raising these questions (personal communication, November 2002).

Bibliography

Barbalet, Jack. *Emotion, Social Theory and Social Structure*. Cambridge: Cambridge University Press, 1998.

Bouma, Gary. "Religion and Spirituality." In *Sociology: Australian connections (2nd Edition)*, edited by Ray Jureidini and Marilyn Poole, 386-402. Sydney: Allen and Unwin, 2000.

Do Rozario, Loretta. "Spirituality in the Lives of People with Disability and Chronic Illness: A Creative Paradigm of Wholeness and Reconstitution." *Disability and Rehabilitation* 19, 10 (1997): 427-434.

Frank, Arthur. *The Wounded Storyteller: Body, Illness and Ethics*. Chicago: University of Chicago Press, 1995.

Garrett, Catherine. *Gut Feelings: Chronic Illness and the Search for Healing*. Amsterdam, New York: Rodopi, Forthcoming.

Garrett, Catherine. "Transcendental Meditation, Reiki and Yoga: Suffering, Ritual and Self-Transformation." *Journal of Contemporary Religion* 16, 3 (2001): 329-342.

Garrett, Catherine. "Sources of Hope in Chronic Illness." *Health Sociology Review* 10, 2 (2002a), in press.

Garrett, Catherine. "Theodicies of Suffering in Narratives of Chronic Illness." *World Congress of Sociology*. Queensland University of Technology, July 6-13 (2002b).

Green, Judith and Shellenberger, Robert. "The Healing Energy of Love." *Alternative Therapies* 2, 3 (1996): 46-56.

Hahn, Richard. *Sickness and Healing: An Anthropological Perspective*. New Haven and London: Yale University Press, 1995.

Hawley, Janet. "Runaway Success – Gillian Mears." *The Sydney Morning Herald Good Weekend Magazine,* May 4 (2002): 30-33.

Jackson, Jean. "Chronic Pain and the Tension Between the Body as Subject and Object." In *Embodiment and Experience: The Existential Ground of Culture and Self*, edited by Thomas J. Csordas, 201-228. Cambridge: Cambridge University Press, 1994.

Jordens, Christopher, Miles Little, Kim Paul, and Emma Sayers. "Life Disruption and Generic Complexity: A Social Linguistic Analysis of Narratives of Cancer Illness." *Social Science & Medicine* 53, 9 (2001): 1227-1236.

McClelland, D.C. and Kirshnit, D. "Effects of Motivational Arousal on Immune Functions." In Discussion: McClelland, D.C. *Human Motivation.* Glenview Illinois: Scott Foresman & Co, 1985.

McCord Adams, Marilyn. *Horrendous Evils and the Goodness of God.* Melbourne: Melbourne University Press, 1999.

McKenzie, Heather. "Inwardness: An Enduring 'Self' Concept." In *The Australian Sociological Association 2001 Conference refereed papers*, edited by C. Browne, K. Edwards & V. Watson (eds.). The University of Sydney, CD-ROM, 2001.

Moore, Tony. *Cry of the Damaged Man*. Sydney: Pan Macmillan, 1991.

Murdoch, Iris. *The Sovereignty of Good.* London: Routledge Classics, 2001.

Radley, Alan. "The Aesthetics of Illness: Narrative, Horror and the Sublime." *Sociology of Health & Illness* 21, 6 (1999): 778-796.

Sanders, Carrie. "Challenges for Spiritual Care-Giving in the Millennium." *Contemporary Nurse* 12, 2 (2002): in press.

Scarry, Elaine. *The Body in Pain: The Making and Unmaking of the World*. Oxford and New York: Oxford University Press, 1985.

Sewell, Marilyn (ed.). *Cries of the Spirit*. Boston: Beacon Press, 1991.

Sogyal Rinpoche. *The Tibetan Book of Living and Dying.* Sydney: Random House, 1992.

Teresa of Avila. *The Life of Teresa of Jesus: The Autobiography of Teresa of Avila*. New York: Image Books (Doubleday), 1991.

Walker, Christine, C. Peterson, and N. Millen. "Investigating Socio-Economic Status and Chronic Illness: Directions and Dilemmas." In *The Australian Sociological Association 2001 Conference Refereed Papers*, edited by C. Browne, K. Edwards and V. Watson. The University of Sydney, CD-ROM, 2001.

Williams, Gareth. "Chronic Illness and the Pursuit of Virtue in Everyday Life." In *Worlds of Illness: Biographical and Cultural Perspectives on Health and Disease*, edited by Alan Radley, 92-108. London and New York: Routledge, 1993.

Williams, Rory. "Religion and Illness." In *Worlds of Illness: Biographical and Cultural Perspectives on Health and Disease*, edited by Alan Radley, 71-91. London and New York: Routledge, 1993.

Note on Contributor

Dr. Catherine Garrett is a Senior Lecturer in Sociology in the School of Applied Social Sciences, University of Western Sydney, Australia. She has written two books, Beyond Anorexia (1998) and Gut Feelings (forthcoming in 2003), and a variety of articles on illness, the body, spirituality and healing.

Entertaining Illness

Emma Govan

1. The Drama of Sickness

"Shakespeare Made Sick" was the headline for Peter Conrad's *Observer* feature on *Giulio Cesare* by Societas Raffaello Sanzio. Conrad's account of the show opened as follows:

> Antony has throat cancer, Cicero is a sumo wrestler, Brutus and Cassius are anorexic women. Will this version of Julius Ceasar be the most shocking show ever staged in Britain?[1]

It is difficult to gauge whether the show was the most shocking ever to be staged in the UK, but it certainly prompted great debate as to the ethics of productions which employ people for their particular physical conditions.

The director of Societas Raffaello Sanzio, Romeo Castellucci, formed his theatre company in 1981 and named it with ironic reference to the painter Raphael, who is celebrated for his depictions of idealised, sacred bodies. In his creative work, Castellucci can be seen to distress the bodies of his actors and push them to the limits of endurance. Rather than trained performers, Castellucci prefers to work with individuals with what he calls "physical presence" as a means to evoke "an element of truth in a system of fiction."[2] In the 1999 production of *Giulio Cesare* the cast included Dalmazio Masini as Antony/Antonius. Masini suffers from throat cancer and has had a laryngotomy which means he must speak with the aid of a voice box. A key scene within the production was where Masini delivered an edited version of Mark Antony's celebrated speech to the people following Ceasar's death. Masini spoke directly to the audience without the aid of amplification – the result being that it was very difficult to make out the words that he was saying. As Masini stood in the spotlight, the focus was on his quiet and evidently effortful speech; yet he was not performing difficulty in talking, the hole in his throat made both breathing and speaking hard to do. *Giulio Cesare* presented real sickness in order to be, what Castellucci describes as "faithful to the spirit of the drama" and Masini's speech impediment was employed to highlight the meditation on the nature of rhetoric which was at the heart of the production.[3]

While Castellucci works with ill bodies to deliver an element of truth in a system of fiction, in this essay I intend to examine texts that work with elements of fiction with a system of truth, that is texts which use a fictional representation of illness, in order to reflect on real anxieties surrounding sickness in the wider culture. While Societas Raffaello Sanzio employ an actor who really has throat cancer, I shall consider two examples of performers who seek to represent cancer. The furore surrounding *Giulio Cesare* was connected to the presence of real, suffering bodies and the presentation of illness as spectacle. In the case studies I shall discuss, however, the fictional framework is an important aspect of the efficacy of the performance event. Within the realm of live performance, professionals are often paid to play out illness, suffering and death for the entertainment of the public. Through reference to recent productions, this essay will attempt to tease out the particular pleasures that such representations may hold for an audience.

In "Thoughts for the Time on War and Death," Freud posits attraction to the representation of death (and for death we might read morbidity) in theatre as the inevitable result of a repressive culture that perceives dying as a catastrophe rather than an inevitability. Freud sees fiction as an important forum for the exploration of issues of mortality because it is the space within culture where "people still know how to die" and, as such, provides models of behaviour and an opportunity to come to an understanding of the fragility of life.[4] Reading these words within the twenty-first century and the context of a plethora of representations of ill bodies within contemporary theatre, film and TV, it is possible to understand the rise in popularity of the 'sick drama' as a response to a culture where the vulnerability of the body is repressed and sickness is removed to the enclosed space of the hospital. It may, therefore, be appropriate to understand theatre as a place where people still know how to be ill.

Freud's observations on the pleasure principle led him to conclude that all human behaviour was focused on the release of tension and he noted that tensions were kept under control through revisiting trauma in dreams. Freud connected this phenomena to the observation of his grandson whose game with a cotton reel appeared to repeatedly re-enact the disappearance (*fort*) and return (*da*) of the child's mother.[5] Through repetition, Freud argued, the child kept separation anxiety at bay. Freud developed a theory of defensive psychological response to trauma which he described as repetition compulsion and he argued that, through repetition, a person comes to terms with events which have previously shocked them. Using these theoretical insights, it is possible to understand the pleasure of viewing a 'sick drama' as either a rehearsal of trauma and an opportunity to distance that experience, or as preparation for potential events and an opportunity to develop a response. If this is true then why was *Giulio Cesare* so controversial? I would suggest that it is the reality of the suffering within that event which disturbed the audience. In "Psychopathic Characters on the Stage", Freud highlighted the importance of the fictional framework of the theatrical event. Freud's theory is that an audience member is able to enjoy the experience knowing that somebody else is suffering in their place and, on another level, that the suffering itself is an illusion. The awareness of the frame is what, Freud argues, allows for an imaginative relationship with the drama which may lead to a cathartic response. In *Catharsis in Healing, Ritual and Drama,* Scheff notes that, what he terms "aesthetic distance" is necessary within a dramatic event in order to allow for audience engagement.[6] It is arguable that the audience for *Giulio Cesare* could not imaginatively engage with the work or observe 'how to be ill' because they were too close-up to the actual illness. An event such as *Giulio Cesare* may therefore be seen to offer the shiver of excitement that a freak show might produce, rather than the shudder of catharsis that results from a tragic drama.

The case studies under discussion in this essay all relate to the presentation of cancer on stage. As Susan Sontag states in *Illness as Metaphor*, cancer has a particular currency in contemporary, Western culture. She notes that cancer is seen as threatening in that it is a non-curable, mysterious disease that remains a mortal danger in an environment that represses mortality and believes that every illness can be cured. Cancer is also seen to individuate people. Frankenburg states that cancer "se[ts] a person in relief against the environment" as people are marked out by their illness.[7] The person with cancer can be seen to assume a special status in society, which carries the stigma of falling foul of normal social codes. Sontag notes that cancer is popularly believed to be caused by the repression of emotion. She also comments that "cancer is notorious for attacking parts of the body (colon, bladder, rectum, breast, cervix, prostate, testicles) that are embarrassing to acknowledge."[8] People with cancer, Sontag argues, are viewed as obscene in that their terminal illness sets them apart and makes them taboo objects of both fear and fascination. A sick body may be understood as a body in crisis – in that it may return to health or it may expire. In contemporary, Western culture, an ill person is removed from everyday activity and allowed to inhabit a special role exempt from normal responsibilities and, often, also placed in a special space reserved for the unwell. In this way a sick person may be understood to be entering into a liminal state – or time out of time. Limen, the root of the word liminality, translates from the Latin as threshold and, when sick, a person may move out from their normal social function into the liminal state where social norms are suspended. The sickness, although it intersects with other social indicators such as status and gender, becomes the defining feature of the ill person and, as Talcott Parsons states in *Social Structure and Personality*, they are accorded a 'sick role', with the ascribed goal of getting well and returning to a functional office in public life. In this essay I shall examine different negotiations of the sick role both from the perspective of the performer and the audience.

2. Terminal Illness and Tragic Heroism: *W;t.*

W;t by Margaret Edson was first performed in 1995 at the South Coast Repertory Theater in California. The production transferred to the MCC Theater in New York in September 1998 and then went to Union Square Theater. In March 2000 the production was mounted at the Vaudeville Theatre, London and, in 2001, a film version was made. The play focuses on the fictional story of Vivian Bearing PhD, an eminent scholar of the Holy Sonnets of John Donne who is diagnosed with metastatic ovarian cancer. The piece follows the course of Vivian's treatment, including her enrolment on an experimental medical research project, and delivers a patient's perspective on the progress of cancer which culminates in Vivian's death. In the work, Edson draws on her experience on an AIDS oncology ward to develop a scenario which reflects the realities of everyday life but within a fictional framework.

The play opens as follows:

> VIVIAN BEARING *walks on [sic] the empty stage pushing her IV pole. She is fifty, tall and very thin, barefoot, and completely bald. She wears two hospital gowns – one tied in the front and one tied in the back – a baseball cap, and a hospital ID bracelet. The house lights are at half strength.* VIVIAN *looks out at the audience, sizing them up.*
>
> VIVIAN *(in false familiarity, waving and nodding to the audience)*. Hi. How are you feeling today? Great. That's just great.[9]

In the London production the lights were up in the house as well as on the stage for this section, which enabled the performer to make eye contact with the audience. This direct address from the stage is not only startling in its acknowledgement of the audience as witnesses to the event, but it also resists the convention of the passive patient as much of the information about Vivian is gathered from the character herself. In placing Vivian as narrator of her own story, Edson structures her work in a different way from the conventional TV medical dramas, where bodies of patients come and go and are seen from the medical perspective.[10] Also, unlike TV drama where the cliff-hanger is often whether a life can be saved, in *W;t* the audience are told what the outcome will be from the beginning. Vivian says in her opening speech: "It is not my intention to give away the plot; but I think I die at the end."[11] This acknowledgement of an inevitable fate is concurrent with a classical, tragic schema which charts a hero/ine's inevitable downfall and serves to prompt the audience to pay attention to the process of illness rather than its outcome.

The hospital setting is of particular significance within this piece for several reasons. Firstly it throws the action into stark relief as the audience witness human suffering set against an officious, clinical backdrop. As Elaine Scarry notes in *The Body in Pain,* it is difficult to represent pain in a concrete manner and it would seem that the image of a once great person stripped down to near nakedness in a bleak environment serves to highlight, but also to a certain extent give visual expression to, the psychic process that the character of Vivian is meant to be undergoing. It can, however, also be seen to create a neutral space that the audience can imagine themselves inhabiting. The generic hospital ward is often the scene for sickness and this play uses this setting to provide authenticity but also to allow for a fairly blank canvas that allows for imaginative access to the piece. In this text then, the visual aesthetic of the piece appears to be about creating intimacy with a particular character, rather than serving as spectacle.

Illness is not only physically situated within this piece, but it is also given a temporal context. Unlike *Giulio Cesare* where Masini is observed as a 'physical presence' with particular characteristics, in *W;t* illness is regarded as a process through one state and into another; albeit a process foreshortened within the structure of the play. As Aristotle noted, the craft of theatre-making relates to the selection and employment of materials, ordered in terms of aesthetic time and, within *W;t,* the time-out-of-time nature of illness is structured through the narrative of the drama. This point is brought to the fore at the beginning of the text when Vivian states: "They've given me less than two hours" and the scope of the play is seen to be within the time that it takes the character to die.[12] The temporal dimensions of the piece allow for sensitivity to the deprivations in the shift from health to illness that the character is undergoing, yet it also serves to remind the audience of the theatrical nature of the event and, in so doing, engender distance. Vivian comments:

> In this dramatic structure you will see the most interesting aspects of my tenure as an in-patient receiving experimental chemotherapy for advanced metastatic ovarian cancer. But as I am a *scholar* before…an impresario, I feel obliged to document what it is like here most of the time, between dramatic climaxes. Between the spectacles. In truth it is like this: *She ceremoniously lies back and stares at the ceiling.*…If I were writing this scene, it would last a full fifteen minutes. I would lie here and you would sit there. *She looks at the audience, daring them.*[13]

This speech, spoken directly to the audience, serves to remind the spectator that they are witness to a theatrical presentation which is being staged for their benefit and that the process of terminal illness has been edited and made easily accessible, even entertaining, through enacting aesthetic distancing. Yet the audience are also encouraged to reflect upon the reality of illness and the fact that sickness is not in itself inherently enjoyable.

Like *Giulio Cesare*, *W;t* uses the shocking, what we might call abject, aspects of illness to engage the audience. Spectators are witness to the ravages of the cancer on Vivian's body demonstrated through shaking, vomiting and baldness. Yet, although emotional involvement was courted within the production, the overall frame of the play promoted distance. A key example of how this functions is a section where Vivian is discussing with the character of Susie, her primary nurse, whether she should be DNR (do not resuscitate). In production it was very intimate moment, played with soft voices and small gestures passing between the two women. As Susie leaves, the stage directions indicate that:

> VIVIAN *sits upright, full of energy and rage.*
> VIVIAN. That certainly was a *maudlin* display ... I can't believe my life has become so ... *corny.*[14]

This moment provides a reflection on the liminal state of the process of sickness from the perspective of the patient, yet the passion with which Kathleen Chalfant delivered her lines brought pity into check, through rupturing emotional engagement and reminding the audience that this was only a performance. Within text, as well as the production, the representation of Vivian played across absence and presence. For example, in one sequence Vivian is examined by the clinical fellow while at the same time critically discussing that procedure with the audience. This splitting of subjectivity can be read as a demonstration that the character is both present within the action and distant from it. The fact that Vivian can step out of her pain to comment on the progression of her illness can be seen to encourage the audience to recognise the fictional nature of the events and so promote critical engagement with the piece. It also reminds the audience that Kathleen Chalfant is a performer who has developed a technical delivery that signals illness but also has an awareness of the dramatic impact she wishes to create. Unlike Masini, Chalfant can leave the illness behind at the end of the performance. This is most striking at the curtain call. Although, within the text, the character dies, the curtain call allows for a resurrection into the reality of the performer. Freud's notion of the importance of fiction for the audience's enjoyment of the representation of death can also be seen to be linked to such a *fort/da* (disappearance/appearance) situation. Within the moment of the curtain call, the ill body is present in that it was presented by Chalfant's body but it is also absent as it has been killed off. The audience can have a sense of having faced their fear of sickness and learnt from the experience of being with suffering within a safe, and distanced, environment.

The piece appears to work in the same way as a tragic drama with the character of Vivian as a tragic heroine. Vivian certainly is the fullest drawn character within the piece. The programme notes for the London production even offered commentary on her research work as if she were a real person. Her status as an academic is important beyond the need to tie in literary conceits. In a television interview Edson stated: "I wanted her to be someone very powerful and I thought she could be a senator or a judge, or a doctor even."[15] I suggest that the character had to be of a certain status in order to be able to fulfil the role of tragic hero. Vivian can also be seen to display tragic hubris and brings about her fate in the play, through the repression of emotion that Susan Sontag documents in *Illness as a Metaphor* as being commonly believed to cause cancer.[16] In this way the tragic heroine of *W;t* can be seen to speak to conservative social values and acts as a cautionary figure as to the results of a particular course of action and, in so doing, encourages the audience to engage in emotional responses that will affirm their 'health'. The focus on Vivian's fortitude of character in the face of death also can be seen to link with contemporary western beliefs about cancer. Sontag notes that people are often measured by their behaviour when confronted with terminal illness. It could be seen that the contemporary tragedies of illness are the episodes that offer the tests of great character and that *W;t* (re)presents an example against which to measure behaviour. Vivian says of herself "In everything I have done, I have been steadfast, resolute – some would say in the extreme. Now, as you can see, I am distinguishing myself in illness."[17]

Sheridan Morley's review states that "there is something maddeningly tutorial and distanced about the whole venture," yet others found the play too emotionally manipulative.[18] Gore-Langton's review in *The Express* is indicative. It states that "if you like bathing in the sorrows of prolonged illness, then you'll love this."[19] For all his cynicism, Gore-Langton's comments raise an interesting point. The self-selection of an audience to attend a show about terminal cancer in the West End, and making that choice over more obvious 'good nights out' such as a musical, must mean that people are attending the show for a particular reason and to make particular use of the product.

Kathleen Chalfant suggests that those with personal experience of cancer – patients and carers – have been drawn to the show. She talks of the collective experience of the theatre as being a place where concerns and emotions could be aired. She says "Playing her for four years, I have looked out into the audience to see other bald people sitting with their loved ones amid lots of weeping and laughing."[20] Chalfant also talks of the many carers who have come to speak to her after the show to discuss their experiences, often for the first time. The cathartic power of the public forum appears to be sought out by those who have experienced private grief, often crying for the first time during the performance. They may seek to use the foreign body (or transitional object) of the character of Vivian through which to play out their tension and reconcile themselves to the notion of death. The reviews, however, generally displayed an aversion to the subject matter and anecdotal evidence shared by Kathleen Chalfant and my own observations suggest whilst many people spend their evenings watching people dying on TV or films, there is something about the fictional representation of death within theatre that is unsettling. I suggest that it is about the live representation of this story and the proxemics – or 'in-the-same-room-ness' – of theatre that may make people feel so uncomfortable with the piece as they are, literally, brought face-to-face with simulated suffering. In *W;t* the audience are not presented with a body to be gazed at as in *Giulio Cesare*, but a character to be interacted with.

3. Distancing Emotion: *A Lump in My Throat.*

Having considered a conventional dramatic representation of illness, I will now consider a more experimental manner of representing cancer within the framework of the theatre. *A Lump in My Throat: John Diamond and Me*, was first performed on the 1st February 2000 at the Grace Theatre in Battersea. It was then revived for a season at the New End Theatre in Hampstead, before going up to the Edinburgh Fringe Festival 2000. It was adapted for television in 2002. Robert Katz was the instigator of the project. Katz was an avid reader of weekly columns by John Diamond which documented Diamond's encounter with cancer. Katz conceived of a theatre adaptation of Diamond's writings due to a belief that they would translate into effective monologic material. In developing the piece, Katz collaborated with Victoria Coren a friend of Diamond's. Coren states her emphatic support for the project in her programme notes. She states: "Of course John Diamond's work should be staged."[21] It appears that Coren views the public sharing of a personal illness narrative as being an undeniably good thing, although the reason for this is less clear. The justification for the work appears to come from the closeness to the source material – that is its relationship to John Diamond and his authentic illness experience. Coren was a person who was personally touched by John Diamond's illness and thus it has a particular significance for her. Katz's relationship with Diamond is further removed but he states in the programme that, although he has only met John Diamond once, "I feel as if I know him."[22] This relationship appears to have been developed through his reading of the column and the identification he formed with Diamond's writing. The sub-title *John Diamond and Me*, highlights the identification that underpins the production. The publicity for the show gave visual emphasis to this element in that the marketing depicted photographs of Katz alongside John Diamond.

In performing this piece, Katz was in a very different situation to Kathleen Chalfant in *W;t*. Rather than bringing a fictional character to life, Katz was working to transfer John Diamond's writing from the written word to a spoken dialogue. In representing a real person, Katz chose not to impersonate the author but instead to draw parallels between himself and John Diamond. Within *A Lump In My Throat,* the framing of the piece highlighted the reality of Katz's narrative and of his real-time relationship with the audience. The identification between the narrator and the subject of the story was a key force of the story-telling and infused the piece with a sense of authenticity. Another important impulse in the performance event would seem to be the personal relationship that audience members had with the figure of John Diamond. In his column of 19th February 2000, John Diamond describes how many of his friends had attended the show and these people obviously, like Coren, had a personal relationship with the subject matter. Others, like Katz, had a relationship with John Diamond through his writing and, like Katz, they may feel that they know John Diamond. Certainly on the evening that I attended the production in Hampstead, the audience seemed to view their theatre-going as an extension of their emotional engagement with John's story with pre-show conversations discussing the situation. Within *A Lump in My Throat,* Katz appeared to invite the audience to engage with his mimetic negotiation of John Diamond's narrative.

The work was simple in format – a one man show where Robert Katz delivered pieces of text taken from John Diamond's writing. The structuring of *A Lump in My Throat* can be seen to embody the relationship that readers enacted every week in making connections between their own experience and that of the writer from a critical distance. At the beginning of the piece, following an opening sequence where a light went up on a picture of John Diamond on the wall and highlighted Diamond's absence, Robert Katz entered the playing space and delivered a monologue which detailed his similarities to Diamond. He commented to the audience that he and Diamond are both from North London, they are both agnostic Jews, they both work in the media, they both have small children and they both "play Russian roulette with their immune systems."[23] What is interesting is that many of the audience in Hampstead were also from North London and, on the evening I attended the performance, many were also Jewish. The make up of the audience made the Jewish jokes within the piece an important point of connection. This is thrown into relief by the television adaptation of the production which places the Jewish material in the middle of the text, rather than the theatrical usage which sought to make a connection at the beginning of the piece in a manner that acknowledged and encouraged identification both with Katz and John Diamond.

I would suggest that, through Katz, the audience could see a reflection of their own negotiation of the subject matter. This situation was heightened by the mirror which hung above the set and reflected the audience back to themselves. Katz own mirroring, however, was within the playing space. At the end of his opening monologue Robert Katz stated with reference to Diamond: "We could be the same person,"[24] yet they obviously are not, and what really differentiates them within the social context, is the fact that one has throat cancer and the other is healthy.[25] What the piece highlights, however, is the fine line of differentiation between Diamond and Katz, health and illness. Indeed, one reviewer mistook an extract from Diamond's column as Katz's own words because of the possibility of shared experience. It seemed that this tension was the fulcrum on which the piece pivoted, with the setting for the show appearing to indicate the separate, yet parallel spaces of what Sontag terms, the kingdoms of the well and the sick.[26] One half of the stage space was painted red and furnished with coke cans, butt ends, magazines, etc. while the other half was painted blue and furnished with pill boxes and medical dictionaries. Katz, it could be said, enacted Sontag's claim of dual citizenship as he moved between the two, negotiating his current state as a smoker and the potential that, like Diamond, he could find himself with throat cancer. His first move into the blue section was as he said in the words of John Diamond, "I had cancer all along."[27] This seemed to highlight Katz's claim that he inhabits a psychic terrain where Diamond once resided while Diamond has moved to the liminal space of illness where Katz (and indeed the audience) might yet go in the future.

Hemming's review stated: "There is something unsettling about the whole experience."[28] I would suggest that the unsettling element stems from the sense of hysterical identification between Katz and his subject matter. In "Mourning and Melancholia," Freud describes how the loss of a love object may lead to a keen awareness of one's own mortality. While a healthy mourning process leads to the re-establishment of the ego and the recognition of the death of the separate object, hysterical identification remains with the sense of 'that could happen to me' and a meditation on the mechanics of loss. *A Lump in My Throat: John Diamond and Me* appears hysterical in its recapitulation of the process of dying and suggests a mourning process that enters into identification and demonstrates the influence of the lost object through emphasizing commonality. For the audience, however, I suggest that the differences between the two men remain significant as the sense of distance is what allows for a meditation on the story of John Diamond. In practical terms the fact that Katz could speak while John Diamond has had surgery which has left him without a tongue, worked against suspension of disbelief in the audience, maintaining a continual Brechtian awareness that, although in the first person, this was reported speech. Yet, more than that, the engaged tone of Katz's presentation allowed the audience to identify with his identification.

In John Diamond's writings there is a wealth of medical information. Indeed, one of the chapters in his book *C: Because Cowards Get Cancer Too,* contains a detailed list of drugs, equipment and symptoms that he is in possession of. In compiling *A Lump in My Throat*, Victoria Coren edited out much of that material, focusing instead on the personal and emotional journey of cancer, within the domestic sphere – an experience that could elicit a more generalised identification. The domestic setting could also be seen to echo the environment in which the audience may be used to relating to Diamond's work as they read his columns in the privacy of their own homes. To place the activity in the medical setting would have meant an attempt at mimesis of the reality rather than a repetition of the reports that Diamond gives of the events and, as such, would have disrupted the dynamic of the piece and potentially alienated the audience. A section that clearly indicated the distance between the reality of John Diamond's life and the theatrical representation was a piece where John Diamond's words describe him not being able to storm out of the marital bedroom after an argument because of the amount of equipment he would have to take with him. The 'argument scene' was one of the few moments within the piece when clinical references were made and Katz brought on the items that Diamond's text described – oxygen bottle, tubing and so forth. Each item was placed at the front of the stage, remaining there for the rest of the performance. In making reference to the physical difficulties that Diamond encountered, these items seemed to highlight the difference between Katz and Diamond. Katz was able to comment on the action unencumbered by medical equipment, and the audience were drawn into a relationship with Katz which may not have been possible with either the reality of, or realistic representation of, a sick person linked to tubes and unable to speak. Instead, an imaginative relationship with the narrative was possible and pity and fear were allowed their full scope in the pity for the reality of Diamond's situation and the fear that it might happen to them. This was in stark contrast to *Giulio Cesare* that presented stark reality that left no room for imaginative engagement or aesthetic distance. Indeed, some viewers found it the intensity of the piece too much to cope with and ended up having emotional "breakdowns" in the interval.[29]

A Lump in My Throat, however, also manipulated its core subject matter to foreground the meaning of the event. In developing this piece, Victoria Coren can be seen to have constructed John Diamond as a pathetic figure (in the Aristotelian sense of the word). Diamond's column was an immediate piece of journalism, reporting events of the past week with an emphasis on the drama of living and no knowledge of what is going to happen next. In an after-show discussion on 25 July 2000, Coren discussed how she was aware of constructing a narrative of Diamond's illness with the knowledge of how the arc of the story progressed. Coren worked to build the tension, to deliver punch-lines and draw the audience into the action, as well as framing it with a neat beginning, middle and end. The majority of the pieces that Coren had selected were focused on cancer, emphasising a cancer-defined personality although, within his column, Diamond wrote about a wide range of issues. Coren also chose many positive sections which could give an unbalanced account of work that seeks to document the highs and lows of a personal narrative. Prior knowledge of the narrative by the audience could allow for a reading where, knowing how the story will develop, hope is seen as optimism in the face of despair, whereas, within a continuous commentary hope may be a rational response. This particular framing of the story creates a tragic figure who courageously faces death and it could be argued that hysterical identification by Coren served to re-shape Diamond's experiences in its own image.

4. Conclusion: Identification and Aesthetic Distance

It is difficult to explain why people may be drawn to enter into a relationship with a stranger who is terminally ill, or even with a representation of a stranger who is terminally ill, but perhaps there is a masochistic element to this exposure. In "Mourning and Melancholia," Freud recognised masochism as a significant element in melancholia – the state which characterises hysterical identification. Certainly Emily Mumford's comments in a letter to *The Guardian*, suggests the desire to undergo the psychic trauma elicited by the experience of terminal illness. She states "John Diamond's decision to make his experience available to millions allowed people to feel the intense and conflicting emotions evoked by a life-threatening illness."[30]

The experience, however is always that of a witness, as Mumford et al. are able to access the experience from a distance.[31] Freud's later work *The Ego and the Id* revisits the notion of melancholia and he argues that identification may allow for psychic health as the Other is incorporated into the ego. In the light of this later work, hysterical identification may be seen as positive action with Katz (and those who identify with him) preserving personal health through integrating Diamond's illness into their own experience. *A Lump in My Throat* may then be read as a kind of theatrical 'talking cure' where Katz articulates and attempts to come to terms with moments of trauma while the audience act as witnesses and interpreters, moving towards a healthy resolution.

In her survey of contemporary American theatre, Schulman posits that "We [are] seeing more work about plagues, about other illnesses, about other people … with metaphoric diseases, mostly cancer."[32] I want to suggest that there may be a growing interest in the public representation of cancer because the representation of terminal illness within performance offers the opportunity to explore private emotions and psychic landscapes which a person might otherwise leave uncharted.

Illness is seen as abject in contemporary Western culture and cancer holds particular fears. While productions such as *Giulio Cesare* appear to use the unwell body as means to shock, other dramatic presentations appear to be interested in exploring, and to some extent resolving, the process of illness. Each text discussed in this paper offers a different type of experience to the audience, but all work through bringing people together around the common trauma of sickness in a culture which seeks to repress mortality. Unlike television, the theatre event offers the possibility of a live, collective experience. The theatre pieces I have discussed all seek to engender a communal response which is, nevertheless, individualised as audience members respond in the light of their own experience and fears.

The events considered in this essay would appear to support Freud's assertion that theatre can be an effective forum for the examination of distressing material. "I am learning how to suffer" states Vivian in *W;t* and I would suggest that this is also the process that the audience are engaged in as they explore the process of dying within the safe forum of the play.[33] Although they share similar psychical function I suggest that the different dramas offer different lessons. Lyn Gardner describes the emotional landscape of *Giulio Cesare* as follows: "The suffering goes on and on, stretching into the future with no relief."[34] Mimetic representations of suffering in dramas such as *W;t* and *A Lump in My Throat,* however, appear to allow safe space for reflection and the release of emotion that may actually help audience members to feel better.

Notes

[1] Peter Conrad, "Shakespeare Made Sick," *Observer*, 6th June 1999, (3 June 2002).
http://www.guardian.co.uk/Archive/Article/0,4273,3872256,00.html.

[2] Quoted in Dominic Cavendish, "Giulio Cesare," in LIFT'99 Programme. London: LIFT, 1999, 15.

[3] Cavendish, 15.

[4] Sigmund Freud, "Thoughts for the Times on War and Death." In *Civilization, War and Death,* ed. John Rickman, 1-25. (London: Hogarth Press, 1939), 17.

[5] The words in brackets are those used by Freud's grandson and translated as the German for 'gone' and 'there'.

[6] Thomas Scheff, *Catharsis in Healing, Ritual and Drama*, (Berkley: University of California, 1979), 40.

[7] Ronald Frankenberg, "Sickness as Cultural Performance: Drama Trajectory, and Pilgrimage Root Metaphors and the Making of Disease," *International Journal of Health Services*. 16, 4, (1986), 609.

[8] Susan Sontag, *Illness as Metaphor: AIDS and its Metaphors,* (Harmondsworth: Penguin, 1991), 18.
[9] Margaret Edson, *W;t*, (London: Nick Hern Books, 2000), 1.
[10] TV medical dramas generally focus on the individual acting upon rather than the recipient thus, the cameras follow the movements of the medical staff. This is partly to do with their role as active agents within the drama and also connected to the fact that they are the points of continuity, the characters that are seen every week and that keep the attention of the audience.
[11] Edson, 2.
[12] Edson, 2.
[13] Edson, 21/22.
[14] Edson, 45.
[15] Jim Lehrer, Interview with Margaret Edson, 14 April 1999, (8 September 2000). http://www.pbs.org/newshour/bb/entertainment/jan-june99/edson_4-14.html.
[16] Sontag, 25.
[17] Edson, 34.
[18] Sheridan Morley, "Fine Fiennes," *Spectator,* 22 April 2000, 40.
[19] Robert Gore-Langton,, "Theatre," *Express,* 7 April 2000, 49.
[20] Kathleen Chalfant, Personal Interview with author, 11 May, 2000.
[21] Victoria Coren, "From Victoria Coren," Programme notes, Pluto Productions, 2000 b.
[22] Robert Katz, "From Robert Katz." Programme notes, Pluto Productions, 2000.
[23] Victoria Coren, *A Lump in My Throat: John Diamond and Me*, Unpublished Script, London, 2000 c.
[24] Coren, 2000 c.
[25] At the time of the performance Diamond was still alive. He died on 2 March 2001.
[26] Sontag, 3.
[27] Coren, 2000 c.
[28] Sarah Hemming, "Painfully Articulate Voice of an Unquenchable Spirit," *Financial Times*, 8 February 2000, accessed via CD Rom.
[29] Conrad, 3.
[30] Emily Mumford, "Letter to the Editor," *Guardian*, 6 March 2001, 21.
[31] Ibid.
[32] Sarah Schulman, *Stagestruck: Theater, AIDS and the Marketing of Gay America*, (Durham: Duke University Press, 1998), 51.
[33] Edson, p.19.
[34] Lyn Gardner, "Imperial Horror Show," *Guardian*, 17 June 1999, 20.

Bibliography

Aristotle. *The Poetics*. Trans. Theodore Buckley. New York: Prometheus Books, 1992.

Billington, Michael. "Death is Not Academic." *Guardian,* 4th April 2000, 20.

Cavendish, Dominic. "Giulio Cesare." In LIFT'99 Programme. London: LIFT, 1999, 15.

Chalfant, Kathleen. Personal Interview with author. 11 May, 2000.

Conrad, Peter. "Shakespeare Made Sick." *Observer*, 6 June 1999. http://www.guardian.co.uk/Archive/Article/0,4273,3872256,00.html (3 June 2002).

Coren, Victoria. After-show discussion. New End Theatre, London, 25th July 2000 a.

---. "From Victoria Coren." Programme Notes. Pluto Productions, 2000 b.

---. *A Lump in My Throat: John Diamond and Me*. Unpublished Script. London, 2000 c.

Diamond, John. *C: Because Cowards Get Cancer Too*. London: Vermillion, 1998.

Edson, Margaret. *W;t*. London: Nick Hern Books, 2000.

Frankenberg, Ronald. "Sickness as Cultural Performance: Drama Trajectory, and Pilgrimage Root Metaphors and the Making of Disease." *International Journal of Health Services*. 16, 4, (1986): 603-626.

Freud, Sigmund. "Mourning and Melancholia." In *On Metapsychology: The Theory of Psychoanalysis*. Trans. James Strachey, 251-268. Harmondsworth: Penguin, 1955; 1991.

---. "Psychopathic Characters on the Stage." In *Art and Literature*. Trans. James Strachey, 121-127. Harmondsworth: Penguin, 1985; 1990.

---. "The Ego and the Id." In *On Metapsychology: The Theory of Psychoanalysis*. Trans. James Strachey, 339-408. Harmondsworth: Penguin, 1955; 1991.

---. "Thoughts for the Times on War and Death." In *Civilization, War and Death.* Ed. John Rickman, 1-25. London: Hogarth Press, 1939.

Hemming, Sarah. "Painfully Articulate Voice of an Unquenchable Spirit." *Financial Times*, 8 February 2000, accessed via CD Rom.

Gardner, Lyn. "Imperial Horror Show." *Guardian*, 17 June 1999, 20.
Gore-Langton, Robert. "Theatre," *Express,* 7 April 2000, 49.

Katz, Robert. "From Robert Katz." Programme Notes, Pluto Productions, 2000.

Lehrer, Jim. Interview with Margaret Edson, 14 April 1999. http://www.pbs.org/newshour/bb/entertainment/jaan-june99/edson_4-14.html (8 September 2000).

Lichtenstein, Olivia (dir). *A Lump in My Throat.* BBC2, 15 July 2001.

Morley, Sheridan. "Fine Fiennes." *Spectator,* 22 April 2000, p. 40.

Mumford, Emily. "Letter to the Editor." *Guardian*, 6 March 2001, 21.

Parsons, Talcott. *Social Structure and Personality*. London: The Free Press, 1964.

Scarry, Elaine. *The Body in Pain*. Oxford: Oxford University Press, 1985.

Scheff, Thomas *Catharsis in Healing, Ritual and Drama*. Berkley: University of California, 1979.

Schulman, Sarah. *Stagestruck: Theater, AIDS and the Marketing of Gay America.* Durham: Duke University Press, 1998.

Sontag, Susan. *Illness as Metaphor: AIDS and its Metaphors.* Harmondsworth: Penguin, 1991.

Myths and Metaphors of Illness Reconsidered: Nancy versus Sontag

Sofie Vandamme and Arko Oderwald

About 25 years ago, Susan Sontag published *Illness as Metaphor*,[1] a book considered to be a standard work on illness narratives. In this essay, Sontag strips away the mythologies that surround experiences of illness as they are expressed in metaphors. According to Sontag, metaphors of illness are imposed from what she calls "the country of the healthy people." "The healthiest way of being ill," she argues, "is one purified of metaphorical thinking."

According to Sontag, metaphorical thinking should be avoided when talking and writing on personal experiences of illness because metaphorical language colours the 'real' experience of illness. An authentically 'healthy' way of writing on personal experiences of illness is for her one freed from metaphorical language. Using a metaphor-free language in illness accounts is for Sontag the only way to do justice to the personal experience of being ill. Sontag knows very well what she is talking about, because she experienced personally what it means to be ill. She had cancer.

The same goes for the French philosopher Jean Luc Nancy. In 2000 Jean-Luc Nancy wrote *L'intrus,* an autobiographical illness account of his heart transplantation followed by a cancer provoked by the use of immuno-suppressors. In contrast to Sontags' thesis, Nancy elaborates in his account the metaphor of the 'intruder' as the only possibility to reconstruct what happened to him.

In confronting both views on using metaphors in illness narratives, we want to question the nature of metaphors in illness accounts: are they, as Sontag claims, literary vehicles, literary techniques fit to transport the cultural myths of illness? Or is illness, as Nancy explains in his personal narrative, a thoroughly metaphorical experience?

1. Myths of Heart Transplantation Reconsidered

In contrast to Sontag who wants to exclude all mythical connotations of illness, Nancy's illness account shows how his personal coping with his illness is ingrained in the social image and mythology surrounding disease, such as in his personal case heart failure and heart transplantation.

In the past, popular media played an important role in the creation of the image of heart transplantation. We are all familiar with the images of the hospital television series such as *E.R.* or *Chicago Hope* where doctors, carrying the famous cool box, sprint into the operating room in order to replace the heart of the patient as it simply were the motor of a car.

The daily medical practice of heart transplantation is maybe less glamorous then the television serials, but nevertheless still spectacular. According to Lex Maat,[2] a Dutch heart surgeon, a heart transplantation is in the first place a spectacular operation because it is a high-tech medical performance.

> A heart is a pump. The most spectacular moment of heart transplantation is the moment where the heart is lifted out of the body and the surgeon has it in his hands. That is the moment of the most oh's and ah's. Because at that very moment the whole team –the surgeon, the assistants, the nurses, the anaesthetist, the perfussionist and the cardiologist – they are all looking into a yawning gap." It's spectacular how huge such a cavity can look like.

Every medal has its reverse. So does the medical-technical success story of heart transplantation. Although heart transplantation takes away the acute threat of dying, the battle against rejection turns the immediate danger of heart failure into a chronic disease.

From the patients' point of view, having a heart transplantation is not merely a question of living with somebody else's heart. What really matters is how to live with the continuous fear that the new heart might be rejected. In other words, the so-called spectacular fact of receiving somebody else's heart on the surgery table does not equate with living with a transplanted heart. The post operational period is not as spectacular as the social or the technical side of this event.

Living with a transplanted heart leads to a less spectacular life, but not to lesser fundamental questions: How can one accept the strangeness of a donor heart, an organ that touches one's very personality? How can a person be seen as a store of replaceable components, as a collection of 'things', as mere donation material? How can one recompose his identity after having had heart transplantation? How can one live with this strange element in his body while knowing that this 'stranger' is a contentious threat?

Trying to live with these existential questions is inextricably connected to the symbolic meaning of the heart in Western culture and therefore cannot be viewed purely on the individual level. On the one hand the heart is indeed the motor of the body. But on the other hand, a heart cannot be considered as being purely a physiological organ. It is not only a matter of pumping blood though the body's veins. The heart is just as well the epicentre of love, passion, tenderness, happiness, grief, pain and anger. It is the very spot where all human feeling is nested. Over and above this, the heart is the seat of the soul; it is what goes beyond human corporeality in the metaphysical sense. By having a heart transplantation one's personal identity is totally confused because the illusion of interchangeability of souls is never far away. Having had a heart transplantation is far more than a physical experience and for that reason it can also be described in terms of a metaphysical adventure. It is a heartbreaking experience because it shows how close body and soul are connected. Having had a heart transplantation means that one loses the symbolic centre of feeling and of the soul in exchange for an alien body part. One has to believe that the previous heartbeats of the donor heart linger on in the body of its former and now deceased owner of the heart. He has to believe that his heart, his new heart is only an empty cartridge that accommodates his own unchanged feelings and as well as his very own soul.

The former implies that talking and writing about experiences of illness can never be isolated from any existing cultural ideas. That is the essence of Nancy's argument. To a certain extent Susan Sontag shares this idea. According to her, experiencing illness is culturally determined in so far as certain ideas on being ill are socially imposed. In her essay she stresses the negative connotations that are connected to illnesses such as tuberculosis and cancer. Sontag does not mention heart disease, despite its prominent place among causes of death when *Illness as Metaphor* was published. Heart disease, cancer and tuberculosis have strong symbolic connotations. One may view this shortcoming as an indication of Sontag's aim to prove that myths surrounding illness imply accusation of the ill. She therefore restricts herself to those diseases with a purely negative image. Heart disease does not fit into her framework that illness myths are socially imposed and stigmatise the ill. Sontag focuses instead on why people use illness metaphors rather than on describing the personal use of metaphors. Thus she is rejecting the idea that myths surrounding certain illnesses fundamentally shape the personal perception and experiences of illness. Consequently, Sontag would reject Nancy's viewpoint that personal experience and the very expression of this experience are fundamentally determined by social myths and by metaphors of illness. According to Nancy, personal meaning of illness is not a self-reliant entity. It is for him, on the contrary, a complex of medical, personal and symbolical indications of illness. In his personal experience, the various meanings of his own heart disease and heart transplantation are entangled in the metaphor of the intruder.

2. The Metaphor of the Intruder Reconsidered

In *Illness as Metaphor* Sontag quotes Thomas Paynell who describes cancer in 1528 using the metaphor of the intruder: "A cancer is a melancolye impostume, eatynge partes of the body."[3] Nancy deploys the metaphor of the intruder to understand heart transplantation. Similarities between Nancy and Sontag stop here because the authors have diametrically opposed views of metaphorical thinking. In *Illness as Metaphor*, Sontag argues that metaphors are to be isolated from 'other' speech behaviour, assuming that there should be such a thing as a 'neutral' and 'objective' language. This implies that being ill is considered to be a pre-linguistic actual fact. According to Sontag, metaphoric language is a linguistic problem, a style concept often used in illness narratives unrelated to the reality of being ill. Precisely that is the point in the recent critique of Sontag's work.[4]

We in turn, want to show through analysing Nancy's illness account *The intruder,* how performing metaphors as a literary technique stirs the imagination. Of course, a skilled writer like Nancy is a natural in using sharp metaphors. But the main goal in our analysis of *The intruder* is to show how the author tries to get a grip on his life by using metaphors. For Nancy, metaphorical language is not merely a way to understand what has happened to him. He describes how it is through the very image created by the metaphor that the relationship and consistency between the events is re-constructed. The metaphor of illness as being used by Nancy does not have a one-dimensional meaning but rather shifts throughout the process of illness. Nancy's illness account is the story of the never-ending process of alienation that is pointing in no direction whatsoever. For Nancy, this feeling corresponds with the process of intruding: penetrating, pushing forward and permeating.

A. The Penetration of the Intruder Affects One's Singularity

According to Nancy, illnesses have strange characteristics insofar as they are imperceptible or first appear through harmless symptoms. Subsequently, they loom up in one part of the body obtrusively calling for attention. "All of the sudden," Nancy describes his first awareness of his heart disease, "my heart presented itself as a red lump of meat surrounded by a number pipelines of which I had no awareness."

Typically, we are not conscious of our own body's functions, such as our heartbeat. Yet, a malfunctioning organ is no longer an element in the bodily machinery that can be ignored. Nancy describes how that particular organ is suddenly the focus of all attention; the engine is now sputtering. Something is terribly wrong. According to Nancy, the heart no longer is an anonymous element functioning in the totality of the human body but it has become an autonomous and therefore 'strange' bodily part that has become different from other organs. The sick organ has become unreliable and unpredictable and because of that, the whole body is not functioning as a whole any longer.

For Nancy, the way the illness is manifesting is comparable to an intruder who enters the house as a thief in the night. One has to resolve this malfunctioning in order to continue daily life. The intruder has to be driven out.

B. The Intruder is Pushing Itself into the Very Core of the Self

In the next stage of the illness process, Nancy describes how the intruder imposes itself. From the deficient organic heart the intruder points at the symbolic connotations of the heart, hitting the sick into the very core of his existence. According to Nancy, this particular meaning of the intrusion already exists when one becomes conscious that the little defect is not an innocent occurrence. Life will not resume its normal course any longer. From that moment on it no longer is the normality but the abnormality of corporal functioning that dominates daily life.

For Nancy this physical experience is a pure personal experience: *my* body loses its familiarity; *my* body behaves in a strange way. But it is not only a matter of physical changes. Because my own body – the body I *have* – is changing, my whole identity is changing. The sick heart, the heart that has to be removed, distorts and ruptures 'the person I am' from 'the body I have.' Because the body is the vital condition of the self, it forces itself upon the self. More precisely, the poor physical condition intrudes as if it were a new identity. It is an identity that imposes itself on Nancy. Obviously, he had no choice. Nancy describes how his body determines his self-image because his whole existence is focussed on his dysfunctional corporal existence. At that moment, the sick body has become the representation of the self.

According to Nancy, the strange conjunction of physical oddity and particularity exceeds this alienation of one's physical condition. At first, it is the physical dependence that is alienating the *usual* identity. But subsequently this alienation resulting from physical deficiency is assimilated and becomes the basis for a new peculiar identity. Nancy points out a paradoxical inversion: the involvement in oneself, the intensity of one's own identity is proportional to the alienation towards one's own body. The more I am confronted with the person I no longer am, the more I become conscious of my own identity. Step by step it is put on par with the physical condition. 'I' and 'sick' become 'I am sick' and finally 'Being ill, is what I am.'

For Nancy, this paradoxical situation of alienation contributing to identification with the physical condition, results in an ambiguous attitude towards the heart. The heart, the symbolic shelter of personal identity, has been diminished to an ordinary corporal organ. And at the same time, this organ is because of its vital function, cherished and nourished as never before.

Life is for Nancy, like for all of us, more than the heartbeats of the well functioning heart. But in a critical situation like he has experienced, one cannot escape from identification with that failing heart.

Nancy describes how he is ceaselessly aware of this ill-fated dependence. Slowly the self loses touch with the older, familiar self-image. In addition 'my' heart as symbolical epicentre is exchanged for a mechanised physiological stranger: the heart as a pump. The self is confronted with a heart that has lost all its symbolic connotations. The dysfunctional heart can no longer be the place of love, of passion, happiness or grief. The heart can no longer have metaphysical connotations because it is precisely that heart which is going to be cut out.

Although the intimate and personal place of the heart is perceived in Western culture as the shelter of our identity, in the case of transplantation it is reduced to only a vital physiological organ. At this stage the heart is only a pump, a motor of our body and of our alleged identity that has to be replaced. As Nancy's story shows, to depict something like this is impossible because the physiological and the symbolical meaning of the heart are inextricable connected in the awareness of identification of the self:

> Quel vide ouvert soudain dans la poitrine ou dans l'âme – c'est la même chose- lorsqu'on me dit: "il faudra une transplantation"... Ici, l'esprit se heurte à un object nul: rien à savoir, rien à comprendre, rien à sentir. L'intrusion d'un corps étranger à la pensée.[5]

It is precisely because we have no idea about what is going to happen, that makes heart transplantation such a difficult decision. Nevertheless, according to Nancy, it is precisely this 'unthinkable reality' that everything is about. There simply is no choice because at this stage the intruder has penetrated the very core of existence, threatening the foundations of one's particular being: life. The intruder is death itself. Death is dominating individual life through persecuting one's existence with the ultimate question: How much time to go?

In this threat of death, personal existence is reduced to a beating piece of meat necessary to stay alive. In this struggle for life every symbolic or existential meaning is subject to survival. All typical characteristics of the symbolic heart have to be exchanged for the strangeness of the demystified donor heart. Only then, the decision to undergo this type of operation is feasible.

C. The Intruder is Permeating All Individuality

Nancy's story demonstrates that successful heart transplantation is not sufficient to continue daily life. Despite the fact that receiving a donor heart was in his case a life saving operation, the intrusion has not stopped altogether. As Nancy describes, the donor heart will permeate life like the perfume of a rose that saturates the air or like a stench that affects its surroundings. In numerous side effects that go along with a heart transplant, the intruder has a solid base to dominate the total existence of the patient.

> Il semblerait plutôt que s'expose une loi générale de l'intrusion: il n'y a jamais eu une seule intrusion: dès qu'il s'en produit une, elle se multiplie, elle s'identifie dans ses differences internes renouvelées. [6]

For Nancy, mentally, his heart transplantation is an ambiguous success. Immediately after operation an equivocal relationship develops towards the donor heart. Every beat of the donor heart is an extension of life, which creates an intimate feeling of solidarity towards it. The new heart gives birth to life and triumphs over death. While the original heart cannot be considered purely a physiological organ before the heart transplantation, the donor heart cannot be seen as merely a mechanical pump giving life neither.

Nancy mentions that most of the patients are haunted by thoughts of mixing up the organic and symbolic hearts during the transplantation process. Some people are obsessed by the idea that not only the heart but also the soul of the dead person has been removed. This idea of metamorphosis renders the new organ into a phantom gnawing at every feeling of authenticity and individuality. The intrusion of transplantation is not just a physical transfiguration but also a mental transgression. The terrifying thought Nancy was afraid of before the operation has come true: the strange donation gets through heart and soul.

That is not the only way in which the strangeness of the donor heart is manifesting itself. Living with a donor heart is, for Nancy, entering into a never-ending struggle against rejection, the natural reaction of the immune system to defend the body against intruders. Paradoxically, the rejection of the donor heart, of this strange corporal element, is to retain one's own immunity. This lifelong treatment is focused on the neutralization of one's own immune system to accept the strange element of the donor heart. Once again there is a new process of alienation going on, leading to a blurring of the borders between singularity and strangeness, between intruder and individuality, between visitor and host. This alienation caused by another intruder identifies itself as a different being: the medical existence.

The medical dependence to maintain the donor heart, to control the rejection and the infinite complications of decreased immunity, becomes a constant factor in daily life. Continuing medical interventions are permeating life and the whole existence with the consequences of living with a donor heart. As the effects of rejection are not immediately perceptible, the corporal is subdued to a never ending measuring and testing in order to evaluate the situation. Nancy describes how life depends on what he calls 'a continuous exteriorization,' because of its being dependent of external follow up. The new individual living through the donor heart becomes totally dependent on the medical alienation.

> Quel étrange moi!
> Ce n'est pas qu'on m'ait ouvert, béant, pour changer le coeur. C'est que cette béance ne peut pas être refermée. Je suis ouvert fermé. Il y a là une ouverture par où passe un flux incessant d'étrangeté: les médicaments immuno-dépresseurs, les autres médicaments chargés de combattre certains effects dits secondaires … les contrôles renouvelés, toute l'existence mise sur un nouveau registre, balayée de part en part ...[7]

Eventually an all-devastating accomplice of the initial intruder will turn up, as Nancy describes his cancer, provoked by the ciclosporine. His completed being, already permeated by medical intervention, is now being absorbed by ongoing medical treatment. Nancy describes throughout the exhausting cancer treatment and how he did not merely become a physical patchwork being both scared and dependent on tubes, but how his total existence turned into a mute sensation of suffering. His individuality has been torn to pieces, leaving behind a mechanized body under medication.

Despite living with a transplant for more than ten years, Nancy's *L'intrus* does not have a happy ending. In Nancy's illness account, which is predicated on the patient experience, the heart transplantation is not just simply a medical-technical miracle. Nevertheless, Nancy invokes the same image as the surgeon to represent his personal experience of transplantation, the image of the gaping hole in the cavity that appears at the moment of the extraction of the heart. Whereas for the surgeon that particular dark cave is the most fascinating aspect of the craft of heart transplantation, for Nancy it is the frightening image smoothing the path for the intruder. It is that particular image of a hole, which at first glance he would not have been able to grasp, but that afterwards cannot be filled. It is the place of laceration and estrangement provoked by the intruder.

> Simplement, le sensation physique d'un vide déjà ouvert dans la poitrine, avec une sorte d'apnée ou rien, strictement rien, aujourd'hui encore, ne pourrait démêler pour moi l'organique, le symbolique, l'imaginaire, ni démêler le continu de l'interrompu: ce fut comme un même souffle, désormais poussé à travers une étrange caverne déjà imperceptiblement entrouverte, et comme une même représentation, de passer par-dessus bord en restant sur le pont. [8]

That dark cave, the focus of the medical doctor and the transplant recipient, illustrates two sides of the same experience. For the surgeon it is mainly a matter of technique. It is the image of his fascination for medical craftsmanship. On the other hand, the patient experiences it as a matter of technique and metaphysics. For Nancy the organic and the symbolic are intermingled, the former being the consequence of the latter.

In his approach, Nancy is questioning this medical fascination with technical control over the body. The technical possibilities to save lives with the help of medical achievements have for Nancy a definite reverse side. Particularly the chronic consequences of the heart transplantation diminish the illusion of control over the body. According to Nancy, the patient pays heavily for his life extension.

> Je suis la maladie et la médecine, je suis la cellule cancéreuse et l'organe greffé, je suis les agents immuno-dépresseurs et leurs palliatifs, je suis les bouts de fil de fer qui tiennent mon sternum et je suis ce site d'injection cousu en permanence sous ma clavicule. Je deviens comme un androïde de science- fiction, ou bien un mort-vivant.[9]

3. Metaphor of Illness Reconsidered

We can conclude that the metaphor of the intruder helped Nancy to make sense of the experience of having heart transplantation and especially of the aftermath of the operation. But *L'intrus* is not merely an ultimate reflection upon the history of his illness and on the medical success story in which he plays a main role. The reverse is true. Nancy's most intimate conviction in *L'intrus* comes down to the infinite yearning for control over life by medical support and the myth of immortality. We are all humans driven to reshape the natural world and bend it to our own will in order to rule the world. This is particularly the case in medicine, where the application of technology enables us to understand and to manipulate existence. Due to their medical experiences, Nancy and others, having had similar experiences, are the living examples of this successful ambition.

The way in which Nancy presents his personal experiences indicates that the medical success is only a myth, but a myth that is part of life. Notwithstanding his being particularly lucky to survive for more than ten years with a donor heart, he describes, through this metaphorical use of the intruder, how devastating this life saving operation has been and how it lingers to the present. Through the intrusion, Nancy has experienced how vulnerable 'his' body and 'his' being are. Through the intruder, he has experienced the finality of all being, in which also the ultimate sparkle of individuality is permeated by alienation.

The metaphor of the intruder is not the philosopher's Jack in the Box who, through metaphorical byways, shuffles off this mortal coil. Neither is it a 'healthy' way to describe the utter meaning of illness, to quote Susan Sontag.

For Nancy however, the ultimate confrontation with illness or whatever the significance of the intrusion might suggest is inherent to life because life, for Nancy, is impregnated by alienation, which makes it particularly felt in illness. Illness strengthens the strangeness, which always has been part of life and therefore becomes insolvable, neither through tracing the causes of illness, nor by enhancing the possibilities of medical treatment, as Sontag claims.

For Sontag, illness cannot possibly be an intruder because there remains a possibility for the medical treatment of the disease. Fear of death, according to her, is one of the main reasons in using hard metaphors to describe illness. On the other hand Nancy's story indicates that the cure itself is partly the cause of using the metaphor of the intruder. Using metaphors of illness is for Nancy the only way of living with disease.

The metaphorical language of Nancy describes life itself, which is constructed of various facts. Through all this, life may seem often glorious and successful, sometimes hard, but definitely final.

Notes

[1] Susan Sontag, *Illness as Metaphor*, (London: Penguin Books, 1977).
[2] Eveline Brandt, "Een pomp, meer niet," *De Groene Amsterdammer*, 1 November 1998.
[3] Thomas Paynell, quoted in Sontag, *Illness as Metaphor,* 15.
[4] Barbara Clow, "Who's Afraid of Susan Sontag?" *Social History of Medicine*, 14 (2001): 293-312.
[5] Jean-Luc Nancy, *L'intrus*, (Paris: Galilée, 2000), 17.
[6] Ibid., 31-32.
[7] Ibid., 35.
[8] Ibid., 15.
[9] Ibid., 43.

Bibliography

Brandt, Eveline. "Een pomp, meer niet." *De Groene Amsterdammer*, 1 November 1998.

Clow, Barbara. "Who's Afraid of Susan Sontag?" *Social History of Medicine*, 14, (2001): 293-312.

Sontag, Susan. *Illness as Metaphor.* London: Penguin Books, 1977.

Note on Contributors

Sofie Vandamme is working on a PhD-research entitled “(Re)presentation of illness in stories” at the Department Metamedica, Vrije Universiteit, Amsterdam.
Arko Oderwald is associate-professor of Medical Philosophy and Ethics at the department Metamedica, Vrije Universiteit, Amsterdam.

Acknowledgements

I would like to express my gratitude to Joël Dely for his comments on the English translation of this text.

Part 3

Healing Practices Today

"Shades of Grey": A Qualitative Inquiry of Evidence and Contemporary Family Practice

Peter L. Twohig, Wayne Putnam, Lois Jackson, Fred Burge and Jafna Cox

1. Introduction

Health care in Canada has been characterized by rapid change and innovation in recent years that have important implications for family practice. Health care services, once largely organized at the level of the single practitioner (such as a family physician), have been replaced by a complex labyrinth of health and social services comprised of different kinds of health care providers, discharge planners, social workers, and others. Primary care has been one of the most important settings for the development of multiprofessional practice in Canada, the United States and Great Britain. In Canada, areas such as diabetes, gerontology, and palliative care, to name only a few, involve myriad professionals, including family doctors, specialists, patient educators, nurses, pharmacists, and others. How health professions work together, or fail to work together, is one of the fundamental questions facing the Canadian health care system in the current period of reform. In Canada, the introduction of health care providers such as nurse practitioners, licensed practical nurses and the "re-emergence" of midwifery has prompted questions about "appropriate" tasks, levels of education and training and, of course, compensation for a wide range of health care professions.[1] Established professions are trying to re-assert their jurisdiction over elements of health care delivery from which they were alienated.[2]

Creating, defending and negotiating professional boundaries, in Canada and elsewhere, are contentious debates with deep historical roots. Such debates involve not only the organization of health services, but also the ways in which disciplines are structured internally. One of the most important developments through the 1990s has been the rise of "evidence-based medicine." This paper seeks to explore the ways in which "evidence," the dominant discourse within medicine today, has been incorporated into day-to-day family practice.[3] A view from family practice, using the vehicle of an evidence-based Canadian cardiovascular clinical guideline, provides much needed insight into the ways in which a dominant discourse is incorporated into contemporary medical practice and the ways in which family doctors transform that discourse to continue to meet their patient's interests and needs.

2. The Birth of Family Medicine

Family medicine is among the newest of medical specialties, although general practice has a long history.[4] There are rich historical studies of family practice in Canada, though these overwhelmingly focus on the nineteenth and early twentieth centuries.[5] Studies of professional medicine's internal organization in Canada include Shephard's study of the Royal College of Physicians and Surgeons and Woods' study of the College of Family Physicians of Canada (CFPC) published more than twenty years ago.[6] There are many biographical studies. The most notable for this study is W. Victor Johnson's autobiography.[7] Johnson was an early organizer of family medicine in Canada, and served as the executive director of the College of General Practice of Canada from its founding in 1954 until 1965. In more general works, family physicians usually merit only brief mention, despite their longstanding position as the entry point for much of health care.[8] The two most comprehensive studies of family physicians remain Clute's work, published four decades ago and Badgely and Wolfe's study, which is thirty years old.[9] Outside of Canada, there are more, and more sophisticated analyses of family (or general) practice during the nineteenth and twentieth centuries.[10] The best of these studies attempt to situate family practice in the broader context of inter-professional relations within medicine, to changes in the patterns of care and to the changing relationship between the state and family medicine, to name a few examples.[11]

Ian McWhinney has provided much description and analysis of family medicine's clinical methods that provide both a philosophical and scientific rationale for the discipline of family medicine.[12] Similarly, since 1985, the College of Family Physicians of Canada has promulgated the "principles of family medicine." These principles declare that family physicians are skilled clinicians, family medicine is a community-based discipline, family physicians are a resource to their practice population and the patient-physician relationship is at the centre of family physician's role. Expressed another way, family medicine is characterized by continuity and comprehensiveness. Family physicians also have an important role in providing access to care and co-ordinating aspects of patient care. Their role is both bound by context and relationships. As Irwin Bean, President of the College of General Practice in the early 1960s, noted "the family physician in Toronto is different from the one in Moose Factory."[13] In other words, family practice can vary greatly depending upon the setting and the population being served. Family medicine is, therefore, a discipline that is well suited to detailed analyses that seek to explicate the influence of particular settings on broad questions such as the role of evidence.

3. Evidence in Family Practice

One of the most significant transitions in contemporary medicine is the rise of "evidence-based medicine" (EBM) through the 1990s. Evidence is an important constituent element of family practice in countries such as Canada, the United States and Great Britain, and elsewhere.[14] While there has been pithy debate about how much of medicine is actually "evidence-based," we now live in the "age of evidence-based medicine."[15] Evidence-based medicine (EBM), defined and articulated through the 1990s, has been defined by Sackett et al., as "the conscientious, explicit, and judicious use of current best evidence in making decisions about the care of individual patients."[16] Viewed in the broadest sense, EBM seeks to integrate research findings into daily clinical practice whenever possible. EBM encourages physicians to pose answerable clinical questions and search out and critically appraise pertinent research findings in an effort to help patients make appropriate decisions.[17] There is a large body of research that describes the development and expansion of medical research during the 20th century.[18] Nevertheless, the relationship between science, medical research, and clinical practice remains poorly understood.

Concurrent with the ascendancy of EBM, a number of articles appeared documenting physicians' slow uptake of evidence.[19] Since that time, discussions of the best ways to "translate the results of medical research into clinical practice" have become ubiquitous among clinicians, educators and policy makers.[20] Much of the debate, however, continues to take place through vehicles such as editorials.[21] Specialized journals such as *Evidence Based Medicine*, initiatives such as the Cochrane Collaboration and a plethora of guidelines are all intended to facilitate the uptake of evidence, but the impact of these efforts is still a source of much debate.[22]

There have been several studies of the uptake of evidence among family physicians/general practitioners.[23] In their national survey of Australian GPs, for example, Gupta, Ward and Hayward (1997) found "positive views towards guidelines and supports [for] an evidence-based approach to health care. However, GPs are cautious about the relevance of guidelines for everyday practice, and there is patchy awareness of different guidelines and unconvincing evidence of their adoption."[24] Beyond clinical practice, evidence is also viewed as a critical component in shaping policy, through optimising care and rationalizing increasingly precious resources.[25] Finally, even in this age of evidence-based medicine, there remain important debates about the reification of "scientific" knowledge or using presumably "objective" research to advance political agendas.[26]

Within many areas of contemporary medicine, science generates and tests hypotheses; clinical research produces and validates these for clinicians, while EBM provides the tools to translate research findings for practice. Underpinning the entire enterprise is a fundamental belief that medical science provides answers that are both neutral and generally applicable. Critics of this model, particularly medical sociologists, have argued that "the values underlying medical research, practice, theories and knowledge are deeply biased by the practice situations and the social characteristics of the dominant group of medical professionals – physicians."[27] This seems to presume that all of medicine is an undifferentiated mass, without regard to sub-specialties. A more nuanced understanding is required, one that acknowledges that much of what underpins evidence-based medicine, particularly in the form of clinical practice guidelines or recommendations, is generated by people removed from day-to-day family practice. Moreover, much writing about "paradigms" is overly deterministic and, significantly for this inquiry, leaves front-line practitioners out of any consideration of how paradigms are formed and re-formed. In other words, we might re-state Lorber's assertion thusly: medical research and the production of evidence are deeply biased, because the production of evidence occurs through particular (and limited) clinical content areas and with highly selected study participants. Furthermore, evidence does reflect the "practice situations" of dominant medical professionals but this does not encompass all physicians. Rather, EBM is often promulgated and supported by the activities of élite physician groups or organizations, academic physicians, or specialists in particular clinical content areas.

4. Study Design

In 1999, funding was received by the Medical Research Council of Canada (now the Canadian Institutes of Health Research) to explore evidence-based cardiovascular recommendations drawn from the Canadian Cardiovascular Society's 1997 consensus statement with family physicians in Nova Scotia.[28] Building on the research team's prior experience conducting focus groups in the same geographic setting, we believed that focus groups presented a unique opportunity to understand the range of experiences and opinions regarding ischemic heart disease in the community setting.[29] We believe, following Morgan that focus groups "are useful when it comes to investigating *what* participants think, but they excel at uncovering *why* participants think as they do."[30] Focus groups are an effective method for ascertaining the blend of attitudes, knowledge, past experiences and the flow of information, all of which shape physician behaviour.

Nine focus groups conducted between March 1 and June 6, 2000 in communities throughout the Canadian province of Nova Scotia, including three each in rural, town and urban settings. Family physicians were eligible to participate if they had practiced in their community for more than one year and had patients with ischemic heart disease. The researchers also theoretically sampled eligible physicians to ensure an appropriate mixture of male and female physicians, and varying lengths of time since graduation from medical school. In sum, 66% of all the eligible physicians approached actually participated in the focus groups, ranging from 50% to 100%. Each focus group followed a consistent structure. An investigator who was also a physician facilitated all of the sessions, while a second team member co-facilitated. The author was present for eight of the nine sessions. Sessions were guided by a moderator's guide developed by the research team following three preliminary groups conducted as part of an earlier pilot study. While the research team was prepared to present up to seven recommendations to the group, this proved overly ambitious. Typically, sessions were able to grapple with three or four recommendations. We rotated the recommendations to ensure that each one was discussed in each of the three geographic settings. To complete the process, the researchers debriefed with one another immediately after the session. Audiotapes were transcribed within forty-eight hours and the researchers read the transcripts as soon as they were available, to clarify any muffles or add contextual information felt to be important. The transcripts were then finalized and imported into QSR N4 for later analysis. This mode of dealing with the focus group transcript enabled the researchers to read and reflect on a session before conducting another one.

Each transcript was read independently by members of the research team, who identified key passages for further consideration. Two of the team members then compared and contrasted their emerging ideas and developed larger conceptual categories. Other researchers reviewed the transcripts independently and critiqued and confirmed the preliminary categories. Disagreements were resolved through team discussion and this process was repeated until the categories were clear. These categories became the basis for a coding structure within QSR N4, software designed for textual analysis. The author coded all of the transcripts, while other team members checked the coding carefully to ensure accuracy and to ensure that the spectrum of experience was represented. The researchers also actively searched for disconfirming examples.

The analysis was guided by grounded theory methodology.[31] As an approach, grounded theory seeks to develop and understand connections. It is therefore excellent for examining complex social realities, such as family practice. Specifically, this approach helped reveal the varied and interesting ways in which family physicians in our study now think about EBM. Members of the research team created and revised numerous categories to accommodate the data adequately.

5. Findings and Interpretation

The evidence explosion is one component of a broader challenge of the expansion of research in the clinical literature. In an oft-cited BMJ editorial from 1995, for example, Davidoff et al. identified "20 clinical journals in adult internal medicine that report studies of direct importance to clinical practice and in 1992 these journals included over 6000 articles with abstracts: to keep up the dedicated doctor would need to read about 17 articles a day every day of the year."[32] Clinical practice guidelines, one of the important vehicles for transmitting evidence, have appeared for a large range of conditions. The explosion of evidence has a couple of effects on the clinical encounter. The proliferation of evidence, its rapid production and dissemination poses challenges for physicians. A participant suggested that "If I really believe that this medication is going to help, [then] I'm probably more aggressive about pushing it" (Town 2). Many factors affect belief in or "comfort" with evidence, including the longevity of the recommendation. For example, few of the participants in our study questioned the blood pressure target for patients with ischemic heart disease. One participant noted that the recommendation was "around for many years," while another said simply "HOT trial …" (City 3). Large and important trials that address an important patient outcome, such as HOT, 4S or HOPE, are remembered clearly by physicians and may even be cited to patients.[33] But even with these large and memorable studies, family physicians maintain a reflective posture. Reflecting on the effort to reduce LDL's, an urban participant said "Every once in a while you have to think …how true is this? How do we know?" (City 1).

The changing nature of evidence may also introduce uncertainty for the patient regarding a particular course of action. One participant described this:

> And the evidence is always changing, too, so a lot of patients say, well look, if I start on this medication this year, three years from now there's going to be something different out and they're going to say this medication in this many long-term studies caused this problem and I shouldn't have been on it in the first place, so maybe I'm better off not even trying medication and see what happens. (Town 2)

While there were general comments about the applicability of trials to family practice, family doctors recognized that the authority of EBM helps to frame advice and treatment options, reinforcing decisions or promoting particular paths. This is, however, done in a very particular way. Participants told us that they rarely quoted *specific studies* to patients but that they were more "evidence-minded" during the clinical encounter and did discuss evidence in a general sense with patients.[34] One participant articulated it thusly: "I think it helps to be able to quote some information you gather from studies or specialists that say this drug is going to help you live longer or be freer from disease. In this situation, I think you can state things like that and they're more likely to heed your advice and take their medication" (Town 3). Studies were described as medicine's "ace-in-the-hole" and the authority of EBM served to differentiate the physician's recommended treatment from "what you got off the net last night, or what your complementary practitioner told you, or what your neighbour told you. It's not just my opinion. … and it's not just my experience…" (Town 3). The implication here is that evidence makes decisions appear neutral and objective (i.e., not just the personal opinion of the physician). This may take on heightened significance in the context of family practice because of the emphasis on cultivating open and respectful relationships with patients that break down the physician's "expert" authority.

In other words, family physicians must deal with evidence in the context of the doctor-patient relationship, one of the defining principles of family practice (cite). Participants throughout our study acknowledged the many ways in which evidence in family practice is contextually bound. A rural participant argued that "Medicine is as much an art as it is a science. And that includes … applying evidence" (Rural 1), a comment that resonates with many analyses of EBM. In a general sense, studies were criticized for the failure to consider that family physicians must abide by patient choices and decisions, and that the result is a process of negotiation. Studies "don't take into any consideration the relationship … all the studies are with specialists and everybody's just a number" (City 1).

Ideally in family practice, evidence-based recommendations are never applied without due consideration to other patient-centred questions, including co-morbidities, patient preferences or behaviours, or other broad questions. For example, Oswald and Bateman found in their study of evidence application in atrial fibrillation that in the "great majority of cases, the reasons for not anticoagulating with warfarin were based on the conscious medical judgements of GPs or consultants to whom patients had been referred."[35] Physicians, too, make choices about when and whether to adhere to specific recommendations. In our study, a participant intimated that he had "a real problem with starting people on statins when they're still smoking. …it's like you're in a boat, right, and there's a hole here, so you're plugging up the cholesterol hole, but buddy in the meantime is drilling another hole, he's smoking a cigarette." (City 1) Later during the same session, another participant said, "You have to use your common sense. It doesn't make any sense at all to feed drugs to somebody who's porking out [i.e., eating excessively]" (City 1). It is important to note that the recommendations do not apply only to non-smokers or to those watching what they eat. While these assumptions may make perfect sense to clinicians and to the population at large, they nevertheless stand as interesting examples of the ways in which non-evidence based decision-making or judgements can shape the application of even well evidenced recommendations.

The contextual nature of evidence in family practice is perhaps most clearly illustrated regarding treatment targets or goals. Age is one of the important contextual factors. A participant suggested that "If I have an elderly person that comes into my practice and has a systolic at 220, if I get them to 180 or 170 I generally stop before I make them dizzy … the same logic applies that if I reduce the systolic by 40 mm of mercury I don't want them being dizzy all the time so I am not going to push it even though the standards are probably higher [i.e., the treatment targets are lower] than that." (Rural 2) The same participant also considered age when recommending drug therapy for high cholesterol. "If an elderly person comes into me and they are 90, as they often do they go to [the local drugstore] and have their cholesterol checked and their LDL [low-density lipoprotein] is 3.6, 3.8 or 4.2 or something like that I am less inclined to start them on a [medication]" (Rural 2). In both cases, this physician weighed particular treatment goals against the overall wellness of the patient (the "well-elderly"). The physician indicated that although he may be "less prone to be aggressive" in recommending the use of medications, decisions were made in consultation with the patient. Other participants indicated that they, too, viewed recommendation through the lens of the whole patient and in some instances that this took them "away a little bit from the evidence … and so you break the guidelines" (Town 1). A participant described a clinical scenario in which the patient's LDL was 2.7 or 2.8 and posted the question "Are you really going to increase their dose of medication to get it below the 2.5?" (Town 1). Such is the contextual nature of family practice.

Viewed superficially, evidence-based medicine seems to limit the autonomy of individual practitioners. Guidelines present clear recommendations to guide treatment, for referral to consultants, or for myriad other issues. Some commentators, physicians and others, feared that EBM was an assault on medicine's clinical tradition, and they dismissed EBM as 'cookbook medicine.' But the leading promulgators of EBM always acknowledged that the movement was "about integrating individual clinical expertise and the best external evidence." The authors added, "Clinicians who fear top down cookbook [medicine] will find the advocates of evidence based medicine joining them at the barricades."[36] Despite these assurances, David Armstrong has recently argued that EBM threatened to divide medicine's corporate body between a group of elite physicians (who designed, defined and evaluated evidence-based recommendations) and those charged with applying the evidence to real patients.[37]

It is clear that contemporary family physicians weigh evidence, whether in the form of clinical practice guidelines or other vehicles, against any number of other considerations, including such things as the cost of medications, side effects, patient desires. Rather than striving to achieve a particular (and optimal) treatment goal such as an LDL level or blood pressure target, family physicians may stop short rather than adding another medication or risking other side effects (such as dizziness or falls). Sometimes, close is good enough for the family physicians and their patients. This finding likely has applicability to a range of clinical content areas, including cholesterol levels, blood pressures, or glycaemic control, to name only a few. More importantly, however, is that such decisions indicate the on-going importance of clinical autonomy. In making decisions about the applicability of evidence, weighing treatment paths against other factors (such as cost or risks), or establishing treatment goals that deviate from recommendations but are more manageable for individual patients, family physicians are asserting their clinical autonomy. Furthermore, these choices are made in concert with patients or consultants, in the midst of patients who have not simply one disease, but many. As long as guidelines remain disease-centred, and not patient-centred, there will always be opportunities for clinical autonomy.

6. Conclusion

In 1989, Jonathon Lomas et al. concluded that clinical practice was largely untouched by guidelines.[38] More recently, Salisbury et al., wrote that in the UK, "GPs are being bombarded with advice, and their reaction is to ignore most of it."[39] A more optimistic view is that today's family physicians recognize that evidence is an important component of daily clinical practice but are confronted with the continuing need to apply evidence in their real world practice setting, a setting that must account for a person's ability to pay for a medication, patient values, comorbidities, and a wide range of other factors. Some of these competing priorities can be resolved because of the family physician's long-term relationship with patients, part of the core identity of Canadian family practice.[40] But there is a tension in the clinical encounter. On the one hand, the doctor-patient relationship permits physicians to reinforce messages across repeated visits or work toward a treatment goal over time. On the other hand, the family physician must find ways to accommodate patient preferences.

In one of their 1993 "Users' Guides to the Medical Literature," the Evidence-Based Medicine Working Group observed, "Evidence comes in shades of gray. Often results may be valid, perhaps demonstrate an important effect, and might improve patient care."[41] This paper, and the broader research effort, sought to explore family physicians' views of evidence, in contradistinction to much of the research that focuses on other questions, such as how to influence the behaviour of physicians or their knowledge. It complements other inquiries and joins with them in raising several questions: Do research evidence and guidelines frame unreasonable expectations of family physicians who must, after all, deal with evidence in context? When we are evaluating the "failure" of physicians to achieve particular treatment goals do we pay enough attention to contextual explanations? How is the rise of evidence-based medicine reshaping family medicine's professional identity, relationships between academic centres and community-based practitioners, between specialists and family physicians, or between family physicians and other health care providers? What seems to be clear is that family physicians view the application of evidence not in exclusively black and white terms but rather in the many shades of grey that constitute daily family practice.

Notes

[1] S.J. Cavanagh and M. Bamford, "Substitution in Nursing Practice: Clinical, Management and Research Implications," *Journal of Nursing Management*, 5, 6 (November 1997): 333-39; A. DiCenso, "The Neonatal Nurse Practitioner," *Current Opinion in Pediatrics*, 10, 2 (April 1998): 151-5; B. Burtch, *Trials of Labour: The Re-Emergence of Midwifery* (Kingston and Montreal: McGill-Queen's University Press, 1994).

[2] L. Gilbert, "Dispensing Doctors and Prescribing Pharmacists: A South African Perspective," *Social Science and Medicine*, 46, 1 (January 1998): 83-95; F.J. Ritchey and D.G. Sommers, "Medical Rationalization and Professional Boundary Maintenance: Physicians and Clinical Pharmacists," *Research in the Sociology of Health Care*, 10 (1993): 117-139; Sydney A. Halpern, "Medicalization as Professional Process: Postwar Trends in Pediatrics," *Journal of Health and Social Behavior*; 31, 1 (March 1990): 28-42.

[3] Family medicine is the discipline, or sub-specialty in medicine, encompassing clinical areas such as medicine, obstetrics and gynecology, psychiatry, surgery, and the social and behavioural sciences, among others. Family practice is the application of this knowledge to a particular community. See William Victor Johnson, *Before the Age of Miracles* (New York: Paul S. Eriksson, Inc., 1972), 204.

[4] Jacalyn Duffin, *History of Medicine: A Scandalously Short Introduction* (Toronto: University of Toronto Press, 2000), 337-359;

[5] Robert D. Gidney and W.J.P. Millar, *Professional Gentlemen: The Professions in Nineteenth-Century Ontario* (Toronto: University of Toronto Press, 1994); Jacalyn Duffin, *Langstaff: A Nineteenth-Century Medical Life* (Toronto: University of Toronto Press, 1993); A. Duncan, *Medicine, Madams and Mounties: Stories of a Yukon Doctor, 1933-1947* (Vancouver: Raincoast Books, 1989); J.T.H. Connor, "A Sort of Felo-De-Sec": Eclecticism, Related Medical Sects, and Their Decline in Victorian

Ontario," *Bulletin of the History of Medicine*, 65 (1991): 503-27; Robert D. Gidney and W.J.P Millar. "The Origins of Organized Medicine in Ontario, 1850-1869," in *Health, Disease and Medicine: Essays in Canadian History*, ed. Charles G. Roland (Toronto: Hannah Institute for the History of Medicine, 1982), 65-95; Charles G. Roland, "The Diary of a Canadian Country Physician: Jonathan Woolverton (1881-1883)," *Medical History* 14 (1971): 168-80; Charles G. Roland and B. Rubashewsky, "The Economic Status of the Practice of Dr. Harmaunus Smith in Wentworth County, Ontario, 1826-1867," *Canadian Bulletin of Medical History*, 5 (1988): 29-49; Terri Romano, "Professional Identity and the Nineteenth-Century Ontario Medical Profession," *Histoire Sociale/Social History* 23 (1995): 77-98; S.E.D. Shortt, "Before the Age of Miracles: The Rise, Fall, and Rebirth of General Practice in Canada, 1890-1940" in *Health, Disease and Medicine: Essays in Canadian History*, ed. Charles G. Roland (Toronto: Hannah Institute for the History of Medicine, 1982), 123-52.

[6] David A.E. Shephard, *The Royal College of Physicians and Surgeons of Canada: The Pursuit of Unity* (Ottawa: Royal College of Physicians and Surgeons of Canada, 1985) and David Woods, *Strength in Study: An Informal History of the College of Family Physicians of Canada* (Toronto: College of Family Physicians of Canada, 1979).

[7] Johnson, *Before the Age of Miracles*.

[8] Edward Shorter's *Bedside Manners: The Troubled History of Doctors and Patients* (New York: Touchstone, 1985), despite its focus on examining the roots of the doctor-patient relationship and dedicating about one-third of the text to contemporary medicine, only briefly mentions family physicians. Conversely, David Gagan and Rosemary Gagan's recent analysis of Canadian hospitals, nicely integrates the concerns of family doctors. See Gagan and Gagan, *For Patients of Moderate Means: A Social History of the Voluntary Public General Hospital in Canada, 1890-1950* (Montreal & Kingston: McGill-Queen's University Press, 2002), 99, 107-8, 127.

[9] Kenneth F. Clute, *The General Practitioner; A Study of Medical Education and Practice in Ontario and Nova Scotia* (Toronto: University of Toronto Press, 1963) and Samuel Wolfe and Robin F. Badgley, *The Family Doctor: Has he Disappeared? Can we Get him Back?* (Toronto: Macmillan, 1973).

[10] D.P. Adams, "Community and Professionalization: General Practitioners and Ear, Nose and Throat Specialists in Cincinnati, 1945-1947," *Bulletin of the History of Medicine*, 68 (1994): 664-84; Anne Digby, *The Evolution of British General Practice, 1850-1948* (Oxford: Oxford University Press, 1999); W.J. Doherty, C.E. Christianson, M.B. Sussman, eds. *Family Medicine: The Maturing of a Discipline* (New York: Haworth Press, 1987); John P. Geyman, "Family Practice in

Evolution: Progress, Problems, and Projections," *New England Journal of Medicine*, 298 (1978): 593-601; D.P. Gray, "History of the Royal College of General Practitioners: The First Forty Years," *British Journal of General Practice*, 42 (1992): 29-35; Irvine Loudon, "The Concept of the Family Doctor," *Bulletin of the History of Medicine*, 58 (1984): 347-362; Irvine Loudon, *Medical Care and the General Practitioner* (Oxford: Oxford University Press, 1986).

[11] Toby Gelfand, "The Decline of the Ordinary Practitioner and the Rise of the Modern Medical Profession," in *Doctors, Patients, and Society: Power and Authority in Medical Care*, eds. M. Staum and D.E. Larsen (Waterloo: Wilfrid University Press, 1981); Wendy Mitchinson, *Giving Birth in Canada, 1900-1950* (Toronto: University of Toronto Press, 2002); P. Day, "The State, the NHS and General Practice," *Journal of Public Health Policy* 13 (1992): 165-79.

[12] McWhinney, *A Textbook of Family Medicine* (New York: Oxford University Press, 1997; McWhinney, "General Practice as an Academic Discipline," *Lancet* 1 (February 19, 1966): 419-23; McWhinney, "General Practice in Canada," *International Journal of Health Services*, 2, 2 (1972): 229-237;
McWhinney, "The Importance of Being Different: The Marginal Status of Family Medicine," *Canadian Family Physician*, 43 (1997): 193-95, 203-05.

[13] Quoted in David Woods, *Strength in Study: An Informal History of the College of Family Physicians of Canada* (Toronto: College of Family Physicians of Canada, 1979), 81.

[14] C. Salisbury et al., "The Implementation of Evidence-Based Medicine in General Practice Prescribing," *British Journal of General Practice,* 48, (1998): 1849-1851.

[15] P. Gill et al., "Evidence Based General Practice: A Retrospective Study of Interventions in one Training Practice," *British Medical Journal*, 312 (1996): 819-821.

[16] David L. Sackett et al., "Evidence Based Medicine: What it is and What it isn't. It's about Integrating Individual Clinical Expertise and the Best External Evidence," *British Medical Journal*, 312 (1996): 71-72.

[17] A.C. Freeman and K. Sweeney, "Why General Practitioners do not Implement Evidence: Qualitative Study," *British Medical Journal,* 323 (2001): 1-5; S.E. Strauss and D.L. Sackett, "Using Research Findings in Clinical Practice," *British Medical Journal*, 317 (1998), 339-42.

[18] Richard Shyrock, *American Medical Research: Past and Present* (London: Oxford University Press, 1947); A. McGehee Harvey, *Science at the Bedside: Clinical Research in American Medicine, 1905-1945* (Baltimore: Johns Hopkins University Press, 1981); V.H. Harden, *Inventing the NIH: Federal Biomedical Research Policy, 1887-1937* (Baltimore: Johns Hopkins University Press, 1986); D. Stetten and W.T.

Carrigan, eds., *NIH: An Account of Research in Its Laboratories and Clinics* (New York: Academic Press, 1984); William G. Rothstein, *American Medical Schools and the Practice of Medicine: A History* (New York: Oxford University Press, 1987); C.C. Booth, "Clinical Research," in *Companion Encyclopedia of the History of Medicine, Vol. 1*, eds. W.F. Bynum and Roy Porter (London: Routledge, 1993), 205-229;
J.V. Pickstone, R.J. Cooter and C.C.S. Murphy, "Exploring 'Clinical Research': Academic Medicine and the Clinicians in Early Twentieth-century Britain," *Society for the Social History of Medicine Bulletin*, 37 (1985): 79-81; C. Lawrence, "Clinical Research," in *Science in the Twentieth Century*, eds., J. Krige and D. Pestre (Amsterdam: Harwood Academic, 1997), 439-59.

[19] H. Fineberg, "Clinical Evaluation: How does it Influence Medical Practice?" *Bulletin on Cancer*, 74 (1987), 333-46.
E.M. Antman et al., "A Comparison of Results of Meta-Analyses of Randomized Control Trials and Recommendations of Clinical Experts," *Journal of the American Medical Association*, 268 (1992): 240-48; J. Lau et al., "Cumulative Meta-Analysis of Therapeutic Trials for Myocardial Infarction," *New England Journal of Medicine*, 327 (1992): 248-54.

[20] A.D. Oxman et al., "Users' Guides to the Medical Literature," *Journal of the American Medical Association*, 270 (1993): 2093-2095.

[21] Chris van Weel, C.V. and J. André Knottnerus, "Evidence-Based Interventions and Comprehensive Treatment," *Lancet*, 353 (1999): 916-918; W.W. Rosser, "Application of Evidence from Randomised Controlled Trials to General Practice," *Lancet*, 353 (1999): 661-664; Larry Culpepper and Thomas T. Gilbert, "Evidence and Primary Care: Evidence and Ethics," *Lancet*, 353 (1999): 829-831; David Mant, "Evidence and Primary Care: Can Randomised Trials Inform Clinical Decisions about Individual Patients?" *Lancet,* 353 (1999): 743-746.

[22] J.M. Young and J.E. Ward, "General Practitioners' Use of Evidence Databases," *Medical Journal of Australia*, 170 (1999): 56-58.

[23] K. Fairhurst and G. Huby, "From Trial Data to Practical Knowledge: Qualitative Study of how General Practitioners have Accessed and Used Evidence about Statin Drugs in their Management of Hypercholesterolemia," *British Medical Journal*, 317 (1998): 1130-1134; A. McColl et al., "General Practitioners' Perceptions of the Route to Evidence Based Medicine: A Questionnaire Survey," *British Medical Journal*, 316, (1998): 361-365; J. Mayer and L. Piterman, "The Attitudes of Australian GPs to Evidence-Based Medicine: A focus Group Study," *Family Practice*, 16 (1999): 627-632.

[24] L. Gupta, J.E. Ward and R.S.W. Hayward, "Clinical Practice Guidelines in General Practice: a National Survey of Recall, Attitudes and Impact," *Medical Journal of Australia*, 166, (1997): 69-72.

[25] P. Davies and R. Boruch, "The Campbell Collaboration," *British Medical Journal*, 323 (2001), 294-295; L.W. Niessen, E.W.M. Grijseels, and F.F.H. Rutten, "The Evidence-Based Approach in Health Policy and Health Care Delivery," *Social Science and Medicine*, 51 (2000): 859-869.
[26] M. Mentzel and M. Rutgers, eds., *Science and Public Policy* [Special Issue], 26 (1999); E.J. Power and J.M. Eisenberg, "Are we Ready to Use Cost-Effectiveness Analysis in Health Care Decision-Making? A Health Services Research Challenge for Clinicians, Patients, Health Care Systems, and Public Policy," *Medical Care*, 36 (1998): S10-S14; R. Raine, "Evidence-Based Policy: Rhetoric and Reality," *Journal of Health Services Research and Policy*, 3 (1998): 251-253.
[27] Judith Lorber, *Gender and the Social Construction of Illness* (Thousand Oaks: Sage, 1997), 2.
[28] Canadian Cardiovascular Society, "1997 Consensus Conference on the Evaluation and Management of Chronic Ischemic Heart Disease," *Canadian Journal of Cardiology*, 14, Supplement C (1998): 2C-23C.
[29] Wayne Putnam et al., "Asthma in Primary Care: Making Guidelines Work," *Canadian Respiratory Journal*, 8, Supplement A (2001): 29A-34A; Frederick Burge et al., "Palliative Care by Family Physicians in the 1990s: Resiliency Amid Reform," *Canadian Family Physician*, 47 (2001): 1989-1995.
[30] David L. Morgan, *Focus Groups As Qualitative Research* (Newbury Park: Sage, 1988), 25.
[31] Barney G. Glaser and Anselm L. Strauss, *The Discovery of Grounded Theory* (Chicago: Aldine, 1967); Barney G. Glaser, *Theoretical Sensitivity: Advances in the Methodology of Grounded Theory* (Mill Valley, CA: Sociology Press, 1978); Anselm L. Strauss and Juliet Corbin, *Basics of Qualitative Research: Grounded Theory Procedures and Techniques* (Newbury Park: Sage, 1990); Anselm L. Strauss and Juliet Corbin, eds., *Grounded Theory in Practice* (Thousand Oaks: Sage Publications, 1997).
[32] D. Davidoff et al., "Evidence Based Medicine," *British Medical Journal*, 310 (1995): 1085-1086.
[33] Wayne Putnam et al., "Evidence in Primary Care: What the Practitioners are Saying," *Canadian Medical Association Journal*, 166, 12 (2002): 1525-30.
[34] Ibid.
[35] N. Oswald and H. Bateman, "Applying Research Evidence to Individuals in Primary Care: A Study Using Non-Rheumatic Atrial Fibrillation," *Family Practice*, 16 (1999): 414-419.
[36] David L. Sackett et al., "Evidence-Based Medicine: What it is and What it isn't," *British Medical Journal*, 312 (1996): 71-72.

[37] David Armstrong, "Clinical Autonomy, Individual and Collective: The Problem of Changing Doctors' Behaviour," *Social Science and Medicine*, 55 (2002): 1171-77.
[38] J. Lomas, G.M. Anderson, and K. Domnick-Pierre, "Do Practice Guidelines Guide Practice? The Effect of a Consensus Statement on the Practice of Physicians," *New England Journal of Medicine*, 321 (1989): 1306-1311.
[39] Salisbury et al., 1851.
[40] McWhinney, *A Textbook of Family Medicine*, 16.
[41] Oxman, 2093.

Bibliography

Adams, D.P. "Community and Professionalization: General Practitioners and Ear, Nose and Throat Specialists in Cincinnati, 1945-1947." *Bulletin of the History of Medicine*, 68 (1994): 664-84.

Antman, E.M. et al. "A Comparison of Results of Meta-Analyses of Randomized Control Trials and Recommendations of Clinical Experts." *Journal of the American Medical Association*, 268 (1992): 240-48.

Armstrong, David. "Clinical Autonomy, Individual and Collective: The Problem of Changing Doctors' Behaviour." *Social Science and Medicine*, 55 (2002): 1171-77.

Booth, C.C. "Clinical Research." In *Companion Encyclopedia of the History of Medicine, Vol. 1*, eds. W.F. Bynum and Roy Porter, 205-229. London: Routledge, 1993.

Burge, Frederick, et al. "Palliative Care by Family Physicians in the 1990s: Resiliency Amid Reform." *Canadian Family Physician*, 47 (2001): 1989-1995.

Burtch, Brian. *Trials of Labour: The Re-Emergence of Midwifery*. Kingston and Montreal: McGill-Queen's University Press, 1994.

Canadian Cardiovascular Society. "1997 Consensus Conference on the Evaluation and Management of Chronic Ischemic Heart Disease." *Canadian Journal of Cardiology*, 14, Supplement C (1998): 2C-23C.

Cavanagh, S.J. and M. Bamford. "Substitution in Nursing Practice: Clinical, Management and Research Implications." *Journal of Nursing Management*, 5, 6 (November 1997): 333-39.
Clute, Kenneth F. *The General Practitioner; A Study of Medical Education and Practice in Ontario and Nova Scotia*. Toronto: University of Toronto Press, 1963.

Connor, J.T.H. "A Sort of Felo-De-Sec": Eclecticism, Related Medical Sects, and Their Decline in Victorian Ontario." *Bulletin of the History of Medicine*, 65 (1991): 503-27.
Culpepper, Larry and Thomas T. Gilbert. "Evidence and Primary Care: Evidence and Ethics." *Lancet*, 353 (1999): 829-831.

Davidoff, D. et al. "Evidence Based Medicine." *British Medical Journal*, 310 (1995): 1085-1086.

Davies, P. and R. Boruch. "The Campbell Collaboration." *British Medical Journal*, 323 (2001), 294-295.

Day, P. "The State, the NHS and General Practice." *Journal of Public Health Policy* 13 (1992): 165-79.

DiCenso, A. "The Neonatal Nurse Practitioner." *Current Opinion in Pediatrics*, 10, 2 (April 1998): 151-5.

Digby, Anne. *The Evolution of British General Practice, 1850-1948*. Oxford: Oxford University Press, 1999.

Doherty, W.J., C.E. Christianson, M.B. Sussman, eds. *Family Medicine: The Maturing of a Discipline*. New York: Haworth Press, 1987.

Duffin, Jacalyn. *History of Medicine: A Scandalously Short Introduction*. Toronto: University of Toronto Press, 2000.

Duffin, Jacalyn. *Langstaff: A Nineteenth-Century Medical Life*. Toronto: University of Toronto Press, 1993.

Duncan, A. *Medicine, Madams and Mounties: Stories of a Yukon Doctor, 1933-1947*. Vancouver: Raincoast Books, 1989.

Fairhurst, K. and G. Huby. "From Trial Data to Practical Knowledge: Qualitative Study of how General Practitioners have Accessed and Used Evidence about Statin Drugs in their Management of Hypercholesterolemia." *British Medical Journal*, 317 (1998): 1130-1134.

Fineberg, H. "Clinical Evaluation: How does it Influence Medical Practice?" *Bulletin on Cancer*, 74 (1987), 333-46.

Freeman, A.C. and K. Sweeney. "Why General Practitioners do not Implement Evidence: Qualitative Study." *British Medical Journal,* 323 (2001): 1-5.

Gagan, David and Rosemary Gagan. *For Patients of Moderate Means: A Social History of the Voluntary Public General Hospital in Canada, 1890-1950*. Montreal & Kingston: McGill-Queen's University Press, 2002.

Gelfand, Toby. "The Decline of the Ordinary Practitioner and the Rise of the Modern Medical Profession." In *Doctors, Patients, and Society: Power and Authority in Medical Care*, eds. M. Staum and D.E. Larsen. Waterloo: Wilfrid University Press, 1981.

Geyman, John P. "Family Practice in Evolution: Progress, Problems, and Projections." *New England Journal of Medicine*, 298 (1978): 593-601.

Gidney Robert D. and W.J.P. Millar. *Professional Gentlemen: The Professions in Nineteenth-Century Ontario*. Toronto: University of Toronto Press, 1994.

Gidney, Robert D. and W.J.P Millar. "The Origins of Organized Medicine in Ontario, 1850-1869." In *Health, Disease and Medicine: Essays in Canadian History*, ed. Charles G. Roland, 65-95. Toronto: Hannah Institute for the History of Medicine, 1982.

Gilbert, Leah. "Dispensing Doctors and Prescribing Pharmacists: A South African Perspective." *Social Science and Medicine*, 46, 1 (January 1998): 83-95.

Gill P., et al. "Evidence Based General Practice: A Retrospective Study of Interventions in one Training Practice." *British Medical Journal*, 312 (1996): 819-821.

Glaser, Barney G. and Anselm L. Strauss. *The Discovery of Grounded Theory*. Chicago: Aldine, 1967.

Glaser, Barney G. *Theoretical Sensitivity: Advances in the Methodology of Grounded Theory*. Mill Valley, CA: Sociology Press, 1978.

Gray, D.P. "History of the Royal College of General Practitioners: The First Forty Years." *British Journal of General Practice*, 42 (1992): 29-35.

Gupta, L., J.E. Ward and R.S.W. Hayward. "Clinical Practice Guidelines in General Practice: a National Survey of Recall, Attitudes and Impact." *Medical Journal of Australia*, 166, (1997): 69-72.

Halpern, Sydney A. "Medicalization as Professional Process: Postwar Trends in Pediatrics." *Journal of Health and Social Behavior*; 31, 1 (March 1990): 28-42.

Harden, V.H. *Inventing the NIH: Federal Biomedical Research Policy, 1887-1937*. Baltimore: Johns Hopkins University Press, 1986.

Harvey, A. McGehee. *Science at the Bedside: Clinical Research in American Medicine, 1905-1945*. Baltimore: Johns Hopkins University Press, 1981.

Johnson, William Victor. *Before the Age of Miracles*. New York: Paul S. Eriksson, Inc., 1972.

Lau, J. et al. "Cumulative Meta-Analysis of Therapeutic Trials for Myocardial Infarction." *New England Journal of Medicine*, 327 (1992): 248-54.

Lawrence, C. "Clinical Research." In *Science in the Twentieth Century*, eds., J. Krige and D. Pestre, 439-59. Amsterdam: Harwood Academic, 1997.

Lomas, J., G.M. Anderson, and K. Domnick-Pierre. "Do Practice Guidelines Guide Practice? The Effect of a Consensus Statement on the Practice of Physicians." *New England Journal of Medicine*, 321 (1989): 1306-1311.

Lorber, Judith. *Gender and the Social Construction of Illness*. Thousand Oaks: Sage, 1997.

Loudon, Irvine. "The Concept of the Family Doctor." *Bulletin of the History of Medicine*, 58 (1984): 347-362.

Loudon, Irvine. *Medical Care and the General Practitioner*. Oxford: Oxford University Press, 1986.

Mant, David. "Evidence and Primary Care: Can Randomised Trials Inform Clinical Decisions about Individual Patients?" *Lancet,* 353 (1999): 743-746.

Mayer, J. and L. Piterman. "The Attitudes of Australian GPs to Evidence-Based Medicine: A Focus Group Study." *Family Practice*, 16 (1999): 627-632.

McColl, A. et al. "General Practitioners' Perceptions of the Route to Evidence Based Medicine: A Questionnaire Survey." *British Medical Journal*, 316, (1998): 361-365.

McWhinney, Ian. "General Practice in Canada." *International Journal of Health Services*, 2, 2 (1972): 229-237.

McWhinney, Ian. *A Textbook of Family Medicine*. New York: Oxford University Press, 1997.

McWhinney, Ian. "General Practice as an Academic Discipline." *Lancet* 1 (February 19), 1966: 419-23.

McWhinney, Ian. "The Importance of Being Different: The Marginal Status of Family Medicine." *Canadian Family Physician*, 43 (1997): 193-95, 203-05.

Mentzel, M. and M. Rutgers, eds., *Science and Public Policy* [Special Issue], 26 (1999).

Mitchinson, Wendy. *Giving Birth in Canada, 1900-1950*. Toronto: University of Toronto Press, 2002.

Morgan, David L. *Focus Groups As Qualitative Research*. Newbury Park: Sage, 1988.

Niessen, L.W. E.W.M. Grijseels, and F.F.H. Rutten. "The Evidence-Based Approach in Health Policy and Health Care Delivery." *Social Science and Medicine*, 51 (2000): 859-869.

Oswald, N. and H. Bateman. "Applying Research Evidence to Individuals in Primary Care: A Study Using Non-Rheumatic Atrial Fibrillation." *Family Practice*, 16 (1999): 414-419.

Oxman, A.D. et al. "Users' Guides to the Medical Literature." *Journal of the American Medical Association*, 270 (1993): 2093-2095.

Pickstone, J.V., R.J. Cooter and C.C.S. Murphy. "Exploring 'Clinical Research': Academic Medicine and the Clinicians in Early Twentieth-Century Britain." *Society for the Social History of Medicine Bulletin*, 37 (1985): 79-81.

Power, E.J. and J.M. Eisenberg. "Are we Ready to Use Cost-Effectiveness Analysis in Health Care Decision-Making? A Health Services Research Challenge for Clinicians, Patients, Health Care Systems, and Public Policy." *Medical Care*, 36 (1998): S10-S14.

Putnam, Wayne et al. "Asthma in Primary Care: Making Guidelines Work." *Canadian Respiratory Journal*, 8, Supplement A (2001): 29A-34A.

Putnam, Wayne et al. "Evidence in Primary Care: What the Practitioners are Saying." *Canadian Medical Association Journal*, 166, 12 (2002): 1525-30.

Raine, R. "Evidence-Based Policy: Rhetoric and Reality." *Journal of Health Services Research and Policy*, 3 (1998): 251-253.

Ritchey, F.J. and D.G. Sommers. "Medical Rationalization and Professional Boundary Maintenance: Physicians and Clinical Pharmacists." *Research in the Sociology of Health Care*, 10 (1993): 117-139.

Roland, Charles G. "The Diary of a Canadian Country Physician: Jonathan Woolverton (1881-1883)." *Medical History* 14 (1971): 168-80.

Roland, Charles G. and B. Rubashewsky. "The Economic Status of the Practice of Dr. Harmaunus Smith in Wentworth County, Ontario, 1826-1867." *Canadian Bulletin of Medical History*, 5 (1988): 29-49.

Romano, Terri. "Professional Identity and the Nineteenth-Century Ontario Medical Profession." *Histoire Sociale/Social History* 23 (1995): 77-98.

Rosser, W.W. "Application of Evidence from Randomised Controlled Trials to General Practice." *Lancet*, 353 (1999): 661-664.

Rothstein, William G. *American Medical Schools and the Practice of Medicine: A History*. New York: Oxford University Press, 1987.

Sackett, David L. et al. "Evidence Based Medicine: What it is and What it isn't. It's about Integrating Individual Clinical Expertise and the Best External Evidence." *British Medical Journal*, 312 (1996): 71-72.

Sackett, David L., et al. "Evidence-Based Medicine: What it is and What it isn't." *British Medical Journal*, 312 (1996): 71-72.

Salisbury, C. et al. "The Implementation of Evidence-Based Medicine in General Practice Prescribing." *British Journal of General Practice*, 48, (1998): 1849-1851.

Shephard, David A.E. *The Royal College of Physicians and Surgeons of Canada: The Pursuit of Unity*. Ottawa: Royal College of Physicians and Surgeons of Canada, 1985.

Shorter, Edward. *Bedside Manners: The Troubled History of Doctors and Patients*. New York: Touchstone, 1985.

Shortt, S.E.D. "Before the Age of Miracles: The Rise, Fall, and Rebirth of General Practice in Canada, 1890-1940." In *Health, Disease and Medicine: Essays in Canadian History*, ed. Charles G. Roland, 123-52. Toronto: Hannah Institute for the History of Medicine, 1982.

Shyrock, Richard. *American Medical Research: Past and Present*. London: Oxford University Press, 1947.

Stetten D. and W.T. Carrigan, eds., *NIH: An Account of Research in Its Laboratories and Clinics*. New York: Academic Press, 1984.

Strauss, Anselm L. and Juliet Corbin, eds. *Grounded Theory in Practice*. Thousand Oaks: Sage Publications, 1997.

Strauss, Anselm L. and Juliet Corbin. *Basics of Qualitative Research: Grounded Theory Procedures and Techniques*. Newbury Park: Sage, 1990.

Strauss, S.E. and D.L. Sackett. "Using Research Findings in Clinical Practice." *British Medical Journal*, 317 (1998), 339-42.

van Weel, Chris, C.V. and J. André Knottnerus. "Evidence-Based Interventions and Comprehensive Treatment." *Lancet*, 353 (1999): 916-918.

Wolfe, Samuel and Robin F. Badgley. *The Family Doctor: Has he Disappeared? Can we Get him Back?* Toronto: Macmillan, 1973.

Woods, David. *Strength in Study: An Informal History of the College of Family Physicians of Canada*. Toronto: College of Family Physicians of Canada, 1979.

Young, J.M. and J.E. Ward. "General Practitioners' Use of Evidence Databases." *Medical Journal of Australia*, 170 (1999): 56-58.

Note on Contributors

Peter L. Twohig is Canada Research Chair in Atlantic Canada Studies at Saint Mary's University. At the time of this study he was, together with Wayne Putnam and Fred Burge, a member of the Department of Family Medicine, Dalhousie University, Halifax, Nova Scotia, Canada; Lois Jackson is a faculty member in the School of Health of Human Performance, Dalhousie; and Jafna Cox is a member of the Division of Cardiology, Dalhousie.

Acknowledgments

This project was funded by the Medical Research Council of Canada (now the Canadian Institutes of Health Research).

Narratives of Domestic Violence Cases: GPs Defining Their Professional Role

Jarmila Mildorf

General practitioners today face a wide array of psychosocial problems in their practice work, of which domestic violence constitutes a significant part. If one considers that one in four women experience physical abuse by a partner,[1] it becomes clear that this is a universal problem which is likely to be presented to doctors at some point. In Scotland alone, where the present study was conducted, it is estimated that between 87,000 and 136,000 general practice consultations are related to domestic violence per annum.[2] However, studies on the disclosure of domestic abuse in general practice have shown that GPs frequently do not discover domestic abuse in patients,[3] while victims have expressed their dissatisfaction with the help offered by medical professionals.[4] This clearly indicates a lack of communication between doctors and patients, the root problems of which need to be identified so that changes can be initiated.

Over the past four decades, linguistic research has contributed immensely to the identification as well as the solution of social problems, e.g., in the areas of forensic linguistics,[5] emergency calls[6] and doctor-patient communication.[7] Given the vast background of sociolinguistic research, the current article attempts to make a further contribution by focusing on a hitherto under-researched problem area, namely general practitioners' conceptualisation and subsequent discursive presentation of domestic violence and their possible implications for actual medical practice. Although more recent research on domestic violence has also taken into account the work and viewpoints of health care professionals,[8] a linguistic approach has not featured strongly in the literature yet. This article takes a step in that direction by focusing on the discursive practices by which GPs draw upon but also reinforce culturally codified concepts.

One of the problems surrounding the perception and treatment of domestic violence cases in primary care, I would argue, is the way GPs define domestic abuse and, ultimately, their own role as health care professionals who have to deal with this issue. One elementary way of ordering one's life and of defining one's identity is by following the "narrative principle," i.e., the "readiness of human beings both to organize their experience and to interpret their social lives according to narrative plots."[9] Sarbin contends that:

> The plans we make, our rememberings, even our loving and hating, are all guided by narrative plots. Survival in

> a world of meanings would be problematic in the absence of skill to make up and to interpret stories about interweaving lives.[10]

In a similar vein, Herman defines narrative not only as a discourse genre but also as a "cognitive style," and he contends that "stories both have a logic and are a logic in their own right,"[11] i.e., narratives are not only structured in specific ways in order to be understood but they also constitute a "logic by virtue of which people (including writers) know when, how, and why to use stories to enable themselves and others to find their way in the world."[12] It is therefore not surprising that in recent years narrative has received a lot of interest from researchers in a number of disciplines.[13] As Dittmar and Bredel's analysis of East and West Berliners' narratives about the fall of the Berlin wall reveals, narrative not only reflects people's perceptions of and attitudes towards events or other people but it also supports these cognitive processes and thus ultimately shapes people's view of the world.[14] In this sense, the GPs' narratives can be viewed as a means of "making sense" of domestic violence cases since they also set up explanatory frameworks. Moreover, since the GPs' narratives constitute what Linde calls an "institutional memory,"[15] i.e., the sum of narratives that are related to (re)produce the identity and culture of institutions in bureaucratic settings – in this case, the primary care sector – they indirectly also inform further policy and practice. Thus, the GPs' narratives have wider social and political implications and therefore deserve, if not demand, closer investigation.

Taking the narrative paradigm as a theoretical backdrop, this study investigates GPs' narratives about their experiences with abuse victims with a view to identifying the discursive strategies by which the doctors set up defining parameters and explanatory frameworks. As Schiffrin points out, "the agentive and epistemic selves that we display linguistically, through reported actions and beliefs in a story world, provide a sensitive index to our ongoing relationships with others in that story world."[16] In other words, the GPs' narrative reconstruction of their relationships with domestic abuse victims reveals the role format they conceptualise for themselves and their patients in a consultation. The paper highlights three constitutive elements of this role format, namely: 1. the "spacetime regions"[17] in which doctors and patients are located; 2. the confining boundaries of the biomedical model;[18] and 3. the discourse of the social which allocates certain rights and responsibilities to social actors.[19] The narratives which form the foundation for this study were elicited in twenty in-depth interviews with eleven male and nine female GPs conducted in the city of Aberdeen between March and July 2000. Three narratives and other material from the sample were selected for this article to exemplify the interplay among the above-mentioned concepts.

1. Spatio-Temporal Mapping and the Consultation

When people experience the world, they are inevitably confronted with the dimensions of time and space. Downs and Stea refer to people's organised representations of some part of the spatial environment as "cognitive maps," i.e., mental images of the environment which have been transformed into, for example, sketch maps showing the route to one's house, travel brochures, etc. "Cognitive mapping," by contrast, is the dynamic thought process by which such mental images and models are conjured up.[20] However, cognitive mapping encompasses more than simply a means of orientation. Notions of time and space are also necessary in our lives because they help us structure mentally not only the environment in which we live, but also our everyday experiences of events, encounters with other people, etc.[21] Through communication, spatio-temporal mapping becomes translated into language and is encoded in linguistic signs expressing space-time relationships. As Lakoff and Johnson demonstrate, spatial and temporal expressions can be metaphorically extended to other areas concerning human experience and have thus become an essential means of constituting as well as conveying general concepts of life, society and culture.[22] If space and time pervade people's lives to such an extent, one can assume that space-time parameters are also essential in personal narratives. Herman argues that "such cognitive mapping is fundamental and obligatory for narrative understanding, not a derivative or optional aspect of telling and comprehending stories."[23] One therefore has to address the question which "space-time regions"[24] the GPs conceptualise in their narratives.

The normal workplace for GPs, except when they conduct house calls, is the practice and, within the practice, the consultation room. Patients usually go to the practice to present their problems, and both the examination of the patient and the GP's diagnosis, as well as the initiation of treatment, takes place within this confined space. Thus, the location of medical interviews is relatively fixed, and the doctor as one actor in this setting is also a more or less fixed "object." The patient, on the other hand, appears as a variable and mobile actor. "Come" is by far the most commonly used motion verb in the GPs' discourse, and it is normally combined with the spatial adverbs "in" or "along" to delineate the patients' movements: "Occasionally people *come in* and present their bruises"; "on occasions people will *come along* with stories of physical violence." In addition, locatives such as "through the door" ("unless they see it as a medical problem they're not probably gonna *walk through the door* with that"; "I certainly do have a lot of depressed patients *coming through my doors*") create a mental image of the practice as an enclosed place, as they evoke the "container metaphor."[25] The practice is envisaged as a kind of "container" with an opening, the door, through which patients move in and out. The point of view taken up is the one of the GP, who is located at the centre of the practice environment and experiences the patients' movements as constant "passing by." The consultation, in turn, is often realised by means of the "path schema," which is "one of the most common structures that emerges from our constant bodily functioning"[26] and thus serves as a basis for a number of metaphors. Paths are important since they connect the spatial world around us.

The GPs in my sample regularly used spatial language in order to depict the way they would try to find out more about underlying issues or, once domestic abuse had been established, what their next steps would be:

1. a) you're obliged to ask how things are at home and to *follow that avenue* in addition to what's happening at work.
b) we probably don't *go out [of our way]* because we know, we know it's a *difficult area*, we don't feel we can do much.
c) it causes offence to ask these questions whereas it doesn't cause offence to, to *go down the physical route*.
d) I sympathised with her, I *sent her on her way*.
e) even if it's just a few girls that we *could set off in the right direction*, give them a fresh start it'd be worth it.
f) you have to hope that if they're coming then they actually are looking to *find a way through* to talk about it.
g) I think, if, er, if they've got information about *places that they could go* so then, even if they *go home* to the same situation and do nothing, if they've got those numbers, should it recur or should there be a crisis then at least they feel they've got a safety net or they've got an *escape route*.

What strikes one immediately in these responses is the fact that the GPs conceptualise different paths for patients and for themselves in their cognitive mappings. The answers in (1a) to (1c) represent paths taken by GPs in their practice work, while the answers in (1d) to (1g) illustrate the paths GPs envisage for their patients. Thus, doctors can "go down the physical route" in a consultation, i.e., examine a patient merely with regard to physical problems, or they can follow the "avenue" of more private questions in order to discover more hidden issues. However, there is sometimes also a reluctance to ask questions concerning violence. As the GP in (1b) admits, "we probably don't go out of our way" because domestic violence is a "difficult area" and thus potentially dangerous.

A notion of danger as well as of adventure and risk-taking is not only evoked through the verb phrase "go out of our way," but also through the mentioning of the "escape route" that women can access once they have obtained sufficient information on "places that they could go" (1g). One way of avoiding "dangerous ground" is to disentangle mentally the spatial networks of doctors and patients and to pass the responsibility of finding appropriate paths onto the woman. Thus, GPs can set patients "off in the right direction" (1e) but, ultimately, the victim is "on *her* way" (1d) and she has to "go forward and get help," as another GP put it. Victims of domestic violence have to "find a way through" (1f) to their GP, which again implies a distance between doctors and patients, as the "way" or "path" described is not one that the GP equally enters and follows. By linguistically creating different "route" maps for their patients and for themselves, GPs reinforce the spatial distance that is already in place through the layout of the consultation room, which is secluded from the life world of the patient. Although the practice environment is permeable to the extent that patients can come in and present their problems, this "intrusion" is only temporary and is usually remedied by the installation of a ritual "ceremonial order," i.e., a bureaucratic role format with rules for talk and interaction in medical interviews, according to which the encounter between doctor and patient can take place smoothly and without major disturbances.[27] Domestic violence poses a threat in that it cannot usually be dealt with in the same ritual manner as a "normal" case of illness. In order to decrease the disrupting effect of disclosure, GPs can either pass over the issue altogether, whether deliberately or unintentionally, or they can attempt to formalise the situation and make it more "orderly," as it were, by following the "paths" currently available in general practice, which mainly involve treatment of physical injuries and onward referral to other agencies. This also means, however, that GPs' paths are clearly demarcated and indeed separated from the paths of their patients. Historically, this separation of doctors' and patients' spheres was put in place and has been reinforced through the so-called "biomedical model," upon which most of today's mainstream medical practice is based.

2. The Biomedical Model and GPs' Restricted Role

The history of medicine and of conceptual models used in medical practice was highly influenced by two major developments: firstly, the rise of the hospital as a medical institution, initially in France in the early 19th century;[28] and secondly, the emergence of "laboratory medicine" in the mid-nineteenth century, i.e., medicine which was informed by increasing scientific knowledge of physio-chemical processes.[29] While, up until the 18th century, medical practitioners worked within a "person-oriented cosmology,"[30] the patient gradually became part of the mass of hospital patients waiting for treatment and was almost reduced to a material entity to be analysed. As Annandale puts it, in "the eighteenth century the sick person was conceived as a 'whole person'; today the body is typically viewed as a complex machine apart from the mind."[31] Moreover, the control over medical knowledge was entirely passed from the patient to the doctor and interpretations of illness were no longer mutually negotiated.

The biomedical model is rooted in three assumptions: reductivism, the doctrine of specific aetiology, and scientific neutrality. In line with the reductivist approach, "biomedicine assumes that health and disease are natural phenomena which exist in the individual body, rather than in the interaction of the individual and the social world."[32] The doctrine of specific aetiology holds that disease is produced by the intrusion of a single specific factor, e.g., a virulent micro-organism, into a healthy body. Finally, a claim to scientific neutrality is made, which means that "medicine can be rational, objective and value-free, treating each individual according to their need and irrespective of any sense of moral worth."[33] When it comes to identifying and treating problems which do not match the biomedical model alone but which have psychosocial origins, however, the above assumptions obviously pose difficulties. In the case of domestic violence, the reductivist approach, for example, implies that abuse cannot, strictly speaking, be viewed as an illness and thus does not fall within the duties and responsibilities of medicine. Furthermore, since the causes of abuse are not definable within a biophysical framework, i.e., there is no "specific aetiology," GPs may find it puzzling to identify their own role as suitable to deal with this problem. As one young female GP in my sample put it, "from the medical point of view it [i.e., domestic violence] doesn't fit the medical wardrobe. … So, as you can't treat it, uhm, you know, we don't have a very big role to play in that." The main reason for GPs' lack of agentive power is the mismatch between the biomedical model and the psychosocial model. In other words: if there is nothing physically wrong with a patient, the GP cannot do much. Consider the following responses where GPs define their role:

2. a) I think giving them sympathy but *that's about it.*

b) it's difficult 'cause it's not, *there's not like a cure for it.*

c) I kind of think: 'Oh, heaven's sakes, *what am I going to do here?*' because it's not really something you can, you can help people with in a kind of 'sorting it' way, you know, you can help and support them but *you can't really fix it for them.*

d) you feel a bit *powerless* actually. There's *not an awful lot you can do* for them.
e) *I don't feel there's an awful lot practical we can do* to support them. It's usually referring on to other agencies.
f) *Social services may be better placed* to deal with this type of thing.
g) Something I'm *ill-equipped to deal with.*

In (2b), (2c) and (2e), the presuppositions of the medical framework shine through, which assign doctors the power to deal with a physical problem "practically" by means of "fixing it" with "cures." These responses reveal GPs' implicit expectations of their job, which involves adhering to the biomedical model and treating the symptoms the patient presents with and thus avoiding further involvement. It is not surprising that the vocabulary most of the GPs used when they spoke about their role also conveyed a sense of the "clinical" approach to domestic violence:

3. a) Well, if she's got *signs* of physical abuse I would *examine her* and find out if she's got any injuries, the *nature of the injuries*, the *extent of the injuries.*
b) So, often at a first disclosure, it's only appropriate to *note it*, to ask a little bit more about the circumstances, what's happening *in terms of physical stuff.*
c) Yes, my role is mainly, I suppose, *medical or supportive.*
d) And in that situation obviously, uhm, we listen, we *record* what happened, we *record any injuries.*
e) I think as GPs, our job is to try and *identify it.*
f) I think for the GP the main job is to *detect the problem.*
g) Most of the women have come to *have injuries catalogued.*
h) What can you do? What are the *immediate needs*? You know, is there *anything broken*, is there anything that needs some sort of *treatment*?
i) We're not mind readers and if we're having a busy surgery and, all we see is the *pink page in front of us.* We're not looking through notes all the time and analyse everybody's consultation. So *if they come in with a sore throat we deal with their sore throat* and then they go.
j) And then you know, depending on what they want to do, we would see them as regularly after that even if it's just as *support capacity* or *treating a depression.*

> k) I have *documented the intrusion* and I have said to her I'd be willing to support her.

The responses illustrate to what extent the GPs' narratives are informed by scientific and bureaucratic discourses surrounding medical practice. Thus, domestic violence has to be "identified" (3e) and "detected" (3f) through physical "signs" (3a) just like other diseases caused by natural aggressors such as bacteria or viruses, and a normal institutional procedure is to "examine" (3a) the patient and to "document" (3k), "record" (3d) or "catalogue" (3g) any physical injuries. The patient is thus implicitly reduced to the "pink page" (3i) in front of the doctor, i.e., the "medical gaze"[34] is more or less restricted to the signs and symptoms that have entered the medical record and thus, medical discourse, on the patient's case history. In the case of psychosocial symptoms, however, GPs are "ill-equipped" and feel "powerless," as the doctors in (2g) and (2d) admitted. By drawing upon a medical discourse, GPs not only prove to be immersed in concepts of the biomedical model but they also reinforce professional boundaries which delimit their scope of intervention. A number of GPs explicitly defined themselves as "generalists" or even "general practice specialists" who were "just expected to do too many things" and therefore did not regard it as their task to prioritise domestic violence. As one male GP put it: "I don't want to be a specialist in domestic violence." The GPs thus reinforced a clear divide between "medical" and "social" problems and they indirectly delegated agency to other service providers or to the victims. Another element which is thus at stake in the construction of the GPs' professional role in domestic violence cases is the discourse of the social.

3. Social Frameworks and the Role of the Patient

Goffman distinguishes between "natural" and "social" frameworks in which actors participate, and the main difference between these two is the way individuals are conceptualised with regard to agency:

> In the case of natural perspectives, individuals have no special status, being subject to the same deterministic, will-less, nonmoral way of being as any other part of the scene. In the case of social frameworks, individuals figure differently. They are defined as self-determined agencies, legally competent to act and morally responsible for doing so properly.[35]

An important factor in the consultation frame, I contend, is the way illness is perceived by both doctor and patient. Illness and disease can undoubtedly be located in a "natural framework" since they are usually caused by bacteria or viruses, which have a harmful impact on the physical condition of a person. In that sense, people are seen as being involuntarily exposed to disease and they are not normally attributed an active role in the process of falling ill. The role of the doctor, as a health care professional, is to help the individual patient who does not have the expertise to overcome the problem alone. In the case of domestic violence, the natural framework is no longer applicable, since one cannot, strictly speaking, diagnose a biological cause for the injuries sustained, for example. Moreover, women are often regarded as adults who ought to be sensible enough to leave a violent relationship in order to protect themselves. Victims are thus implicitly interpreted within a social framework where they are given a role that entails free will and decision-making as well as a legal and moral obligation to take responsibility. This way of conceptualising women who suffer domestic violence places them outside the sphere of intervention by the doctor:

4. a) a lot of that is *within the woman's own hand.* I just try and give her the confidence and try to empower her but *she should take some sort of action.*

b) I can't get too involved in that. There are too many things going on. Er, but people, I guess, have some *responsibility to themselves* and their own actions.

c) You can't make somebody leave somebody, it's *not your responsibility*. People *have to make their own decisions.*

d) *patients have choices* themselves or, you know, they can get in touch with the police or social work

e) And you can say to them and say to them and say to them and they won't want to change it. You just say: "*Well, that's their lot.*"

f) I think it's very much *up to the patient* or, what they want to do about it.

g) But I think, I think *they've got to decide* what to, what to do about it themselves.

A common denominator of all these responses is the theme of choice and the women's responsibility to take decisions themselves. The modal auxiliary "should" in (4a) and the quasi-modal "have got to" in (4c) and

(4g) are significant in this respect since they imply not only the women's choices in making decisions but in fact their obligation to do so. This attitude makes it easier for GPs to distance themselves from their patient's problem and to avoid a feeling of frustration if the patient does not accept their advice, as one can see in (4e): it is "their lot," not the doctor's. Occasionally, GPs expressed the concern that some patients might regard open questions about domestic abuse posed by their GP as intrusive or that it was impossible to impose one's own opinions on other people. Interestingly enough, these points were mostly elaborated through notions of distance and separation, as I demonstrated above. In order to analyse how the three constitutive elements of the domestic violence role format, spatio-temporal mapping, the biomedical model and the social framework, combine and support each other in the GPs' narratives, let us consider three exemplary narratives from the sample.

4. Narratives of Domestic Violence Cases

The interview narratives were told either in response to a question posed by the interviewer (e.g., "Can you tell me about your experiences?" or "Is there any case that's particularly vivid in your memory?") or, in most cases, spontaneously in contexts where the interviewer had not specifically asked for a story. The narratives were analysed following Labov's "narrative grammar"[36] and Labov and Waletzky's diamond model with "orientation," where general information on the participants, the setting and initial actions is provided; "complicating action," which contains clauses that answer the question "What happened then?"; "resolution," which, as the name suggests, resolves the story; and "coda," a final section which returns the narrative to the actual time of speaking.[37]

The following story was related by an older female doctor in the context of a discussion of the status of domestic violence in the health care setting. The narrative refers to an incident which occurred while the GP was on duty with the regional emergency doctors (G-Docs = Grampian Doctors).

Narrative A

1. I was in G-Docs, er, just a few weeks ago,
2. and, er, I was called out to something with, you know, that was a domestic violence situation.
3. Uhm, it was kind of given a lower status than or a low-, lower priority than say, maybe an elderly person with a stroke or a heart attack or something like that.
4. So, you know, it was kind of a nuisance that we had to go out and see it

5. and, er, then they got the social workers involved
6. and I say I think they kind of think, "Well, it's the social workers' problem, it's not ours", you know,
7. and the police were involved as well, so,
8. they left it with the social workers, so.
9. Poor social workers, that's not fair [laughs].

The narrative consists of a very brief orientation section (line 1), a complicating action sequence (lines 2 to 4), a lengthy resolution (lines 5 to 8), and a little coda in line 9, which provides an evaluative commentary on the entire episode. In this narrative, the GP openly, albeit tentatively, addresses the fact that domestic violence is often given low priority by doctors. The hedge "kind of" in lines 3, 4 and 6 ("kind of given lower status," "kind of a nuisance," "they kind of think…") indicates that the GP implicitly wishes to downplay the fact that domestic violence was not taken too seriously by the doctors, and thus to maintain her "face wants,"[38] namely not to be viewed critically herself by the interviewer. Higher up on GPs' agenda and thus presumably also at the forefront of their attention, as the GP hypothesizes by using the modal adverbial "maybe" in line 3 ("maybe an elderly person with a stroke"), one can find diseases which are easily identifiable as prototypical "medical" problems, e.g., a "stroke" or a "heart attack" (line 3). Interestingly enough, the GP compartmentalises such diseases by placing them in the same category, as can be seen in the extended noun phrase "something like that" (line 3). Although the category remains unspecified, the GP nonetheless indirectly draws a distinctive line between "medical" and "other" problems.

In the case of domestic violence, the emergency doctors find it "a nuisance" to "go out and see it" (line 4). The postposition "out" in "called out" (line 2) and "go out" (line 4) evokes both the container metaphor and the path schema whereby the doctors are forced to leave their secluded medical sphere ("*in* G-Docs"), especially as the roles are reversed in this particular setting and doctors now assume the part of the "moving actor" who approaches the patient. This spatio-temporal condition combined with the above-mentioned separation of "medical" and "other" problems discursively creates a seemingly valid reason for doctors' discontent. In other words: Since domestic violence is not a medical problem, it does not justify that they are called out. Consequently, the GP expresses her own feeling of irritation in that situation, and she establishes a division of duties for doctors and social workers in the direct quotation of her colleagues' alleged thoughts: "Well, it's the social workers' problem, it's not ours" (line 6). The quote has as its central theme the delegation of further responsibility to other agencies, and the fact that the GP uses the alleged thoughts of others to express this view reveals again the mechanisms of "face work": In order to avoid potential criticism on the part of the interviewer and to save her own face, the GP "hides" her own opinion behind the one of her colleagues. The shift from the deictic centre "I" (line 2) to "we" (line 4) to "they" (lines 5, 6 and 8) and the use of passive constructions, which usually blur agency,[39] in lines 3 and 7 ("it was kind of given a lower status," "the police were involved") contribute to a certain discursive "self-defence."

At the same time, however, the narrative itself reinforces on a micro-linguistic level exactly those concepts which the GP seems to acknowledge as being problematic or at least open to criticism. Thus, for example, the delegation of responsibility to other "social actors" is captured by the contrast between the frequently and fully spelt out noun phrase "social workers" in lines 5, 6, 8 and 9, and the replacement of the noun phrase "G-Docs" by its reduced form, the personal pronoun "they" in lines 5, 6 and 8. In a sense, the social workers are thus granted fuller cognitive presence in the narrative and hence, more importance, while the GPs appear only as marginal actors in this situation. Likewise, the domestic violence case as such is marginalized in the narrative by means of underspecification through the vague pronoun "something" and the indefinite determiner "a" in line 2 ("a domestic violence situation") as well as its further linguistic reduction through the pronoun "it" (lines 3, 4, 6 and 8). These rather tentative descriptors indicate the GP's reluctance to label the incidence in terms of domestic violence and perhaps also her embarrassment to speak about the issue. Despite the GP's awareness that doctors' refusal to prioritise domestic violence can be problematic, which becomes obvious in the fact that she actually highlights the issue by verbalising it as the "reportable event," i.e., the most noteworthy or outstanding event of the story,[40] the narrative undermines this message by linguistically replicating the same refusal. It also demonstrates how deeply the GP's discourse is immersed in and informed by the models I explained above, which combine very subtly to justify the low priority of domestic violence on GPs' agenda, namely because it leads doctors away from the clearly demarcated "pathway" prescribed by the biomedical model and thrusts on them a responsibility which they do not perceive as part of their social role as medical professionals.

Other narratives in my sample did not necessarily address the question of priority explicitly but they also demonstrated medicine's difficulty in "grasping" domestic violence. The following story about a young girl who finally disappeared illustrates the limitations of the "medical gaze."[41]

Narrative B

1. we had a little girl who was a drug addict
2. and her boy-friend was a drug addict
3. and that was really sad

4. and she was coming in with black eyes and, you know, bruises and all sorts of things
5. and she was different in that she just couldn't do anything about it.
6. You know, no matter what we suggested she...wasn't able to, to break away from this guy.
7. Unless while he was in prison, which was alright, she was much better then
8. and she just, she didn't finish her degree
9. and she just looked iller and iller and more and more tired
10. and eventually she just disappeared
11. and we don't know what's happened to her.
12. She left Aberdeen
13. and goodness knows where she is now.

In the orientation section, the GP already draws upon a social discourse of domestic violence by emphasising through parallel sentence structure and repetition the drug addiction of the two partners involved: "we had a little girl who was a drug addict and her boy-friend was a drug addict" (lines 1 and 2). Most of the narratives in my sample are similar in that they often presuppose a causal connection between social factors and domestic violence. Although a causal link between drug addiction and domestic violence is not established explicitly, it is implied by the way these two items are interlinked linguistically right from the beginning of the narrative. As in the previous narrative, biomedicine is also evoked by the noun phrases "black eyes" and "bruises" (line 4). Interestingly enough, the GP points in the noun phrase "all sorts of things" towards other problems the patient presented with, but these problems remain unspecified while, again, physical and thus, typically "medical," issues are foregrounded.

The narrative also draws upon the "practice as a container" metaphor and establishes the typical spatial vector underlying the patient's movement into the practice by using the verb phrase "coming in" (line 4). The continuous form signifies an unspecified period in time, during which the girl repeatedly visited the practice. What is more important, however, is the GP's own stationary position within the practice, which makes it impossible for her to know "what's happened" (line 11) to the girl after she left and hence did not visit the practice anymore. In a sense, the "medical gaze" thus proves to be too restricted. The girl's gradual movement out of the GP's sight is linguistically enacted in the description of her physical decline by means of comparatives in line 9: "iller and iller," "more and more tired," and finally by her almost literal physical vanishing in line 10: "she just disappeared."

The linguistic "layout" of the practice with the girl's movements is supplemented by the GP's expectations concerning the girl's role as patient, which again draws on the biomedical model as well as the discourse of the social. Thus, the negative modal auxiliaries in the GP's statements that the girl "just couldn't do anything about it" and "wasn't able to break away from this guy" (lines 5 and 6) imply the GP's expectation that the girl ought to have assumed responsibility and a more active role. At the same time, a sense of frustration is conveyed in view of the fact that the girl did not fulfil her role as patient and thus did not accept the GP's advice: "no matter what we suggested..." (line 6). As in narrative A, the three elements of spatio-temporal mapping, the biomedical model and the social framework thus combine to set up a narrative frame which explains the ultimate failure of this medical encounter instead of questioning the explanatory models and their impact on the consultation.

In contrast to narrative B, the following narrative relates a successful outcome of a domestic violence case. Nevertheless, the GP's part in it still remains limited and somewhat dissatisfactory.

Narrative C

1. Uhm, so, I suppose, there was one girl in particular
2. I remember her being really quite a hard thing for me.
3. She was always at the surgery, minor, usually minor, minor complaints
4. or she'd drag along her little boy
5. and it'd be something very minor with him, uhm,
6. and they were here all the time
7. and then, one day, basically she admitted that, you know,
8. I, I'd actually visited her at home as well, in the presence of this very 'loving' in inverted commas boy-friend
9. and then one day she admitted to me that he'd been abusing her for years
10. but her son was out of, as a result of a rape,
11. and it was just horrendous.
12. Now, since that has come up I have never, I see her once a year.
13. So, in the long run, I've saved a lot of time
14. and she's perhaps, she's got rid of the boy-friend which was the real cure,
15. there was nothing medical I could do for her, uhm,
16. but that really sticks in my mind, that case.

Narrative C provides a short orientation section (lines 1 and 2), followed by a fairly detailed complicating action sequence (lines 3 to 8), which culminates in the resolution (lines 9 to 11). Finally, a lengthy coda (lines 12 to 16) recapitulates the episode by presenting its consequences and by justifying its "reportability" in the final evaluative statement: "that really sticks in my mind, that case" (line 16). The spatio-temporal map used as a background to this story draws upon the same space-time parameters displayed in narrative B and supports the build-up of suspense in the complicating action sequence. The practice forms the enclosed centre indicated by the spatial deictic "here" (line 6) to which the patient even "drags along" (line 4) her son. The spatial postposition "along" once again points towards the path schema envisaged for the patient. The time grid in the narrative encompasses a lengthy period marked by the phonetically stressed prepositional phrase "for years" (line 9), and frequent repeat visits, which can be seen in the use of the durative modal auxiliary "would" in lines 4 and 5 as well as the temporal adverbials "always" (line 3) and "all the time" (line 6). The regularity of this spatio-temporal pattern is only disrupted when the GP mentions her house call(s) in line 8, where she assumes the part of the "moving actor" and visits her patient "at home," i.e., outside the actual medical sphere.

Interestingly enough, this change in spatial behaviour is used as the climax of a series of events which lead up to the "reportable event" of the narrative, namely the patient's disclosure of domestic violence. In the resolution, the GP emphasises that, despite the regular contact between doctor and patient, the GP failed to notice that domestic violence was the underlying issue in this particular case. Here, the discourse of the social becomes visible in that it is the woman who finally takes action. Only when the patient shows courage to open up does the GP realise what is going on, but even then the GP's role remains confined to the biomedical realm: "there was nothing medical I could do for her" (line 15). The noun phrase "the real cure" (line 14) also points towards a biomedical discourse and implies the limitations of medical practice in the context of psychosocial problems. It meshes with the discourse of the social since the "real cure" ironically consisted in the fact that the patient "got rid of the boy-friend" (line 14), i.e., she fulfilled her duty as social actor by assuming an active role and responsibility both for herself and her son. After the disclosure, the "medical gaze" becomes more restricted again, which is emphasised by a new continual time frame: "I see her once a year" (line 12). What the narrative demonstrates is that the "medical gaze" can be limited even if signs are presented to the doctor and if the spatio-temporal setting allows for a "wider" view of the woman's family background. This indicates that a lack of awareness in GPs may also impede the discovery or disclosure of domestic violence, and part of this lack of awareness, I would argue, stems from the restricted view GPs have of their own professional role, which manifests itself in the discursive self-definitions in their narratives.

5. Conclusion

The transactional nature of medical encounters requires that participants' expectations of the interaction are met, otherwise they can lead to misunderstandings and disappointment. If different preconceptions by doctor and patient impede a successful encounter, both may feel frustrated and powerless in that situation. As I mentioned at the outset of this article, research has already unravelled some of the reasons for the dissatisfaction both women and doctors experience during consultations in which domestic violence is an issue. This article illuminates the problem from a discourse-analytical perspective and looks more closely at GPs' professional self-definitions as one possible source for problems in doctor-patient interaction. The analysis of the GPs' narratives about their experiences with domestic violence victims demonstrates that doctors build their role on at least three conceptual "pillars": spatio-temporal mappings in which doctors and patients are located with reference to the practice environment; the biomedical model, which restricts GPs' sphere of activity; and the discourse of the social, which defines women's role with regard to their own agency and responsibility. These three elements combine to constitute the role format GPs set up for themselves and their patients, a role format they may not be conscious of but which informs their discursive and, I would argue, ultimately their professional practice. The narratives produced in the interviews function as "conceptual windows," i.e., they provide "a limited current view of the story world, like a moving window establishing a perspective from and through which events in the story world are viewed."[42] In telling their stories, the GPs enabled the interviewer and ultimately, us as recipients of these narratives, to glance at the "conceptual windows" and at the story worlds with their "story logic"[43] displayed therein. If one accepts the view that stories do not only *have* a logic but also *are* a logic in the sense that they order one's life experiences and structure one's perceptions and beliefs of the world, the GPs' narratives also represent their conceptualisations and definitions of their own professional role in domestic violence cases. Thus, for example, GPs apply a strategy of distancing themselves from the life world of their patients in their narrative creation of "spacetime regions," which indirectly reflects GPs' cognitive placement of patients on the other side of the doctor-patient, as well as the "wellness-illness divide."[44] This division can lead to conflicting narratives about disease, which ultimately impede successful doctor-patient interaction:

> One type of conflict arises from an ontological mismatch between the sufferer's actual experience of illness and the health professional's reformulation of it as disease. For example, while the patient might *feel* pain, fever and an aching throat, the clinician *sees* viral proliferation of influenza.[45]

Similarly, patients who suffer domestic violence perhaps bring to the consultation expectations, emotions and anxieties they might wish to communicate to their GP, while the doctor attempts to concentrate on fulfilling the requirements implicitly set forth by the biomedical model, namely to diagnose illness and to initiate remedial treatment. That the biomedical model indeed has a strong hold on GPs' conceptual frameworks can be seen in the way the doctors' narratives are steeped in the vocabulary of a biomedical discourse. Likewise, the discourse of the social pervades the narratives and thus points towards conceptual definitions of victims within social frameworks, which in turn widen the gap between doctors and patients.

By drawing upon these predetermined cognitive models in their narrative discourse, the GPs not only recycle but in fact reinforce them, and thus they perpetuate conceptions which impede necessary paradigm shifts and, consequently, an improvement in the medical service provision offered to battered women. As long as GPs consider themselves "ill-equipped" to deal with domestic violence because it is not a "medical" problem, and as long as they repeat this argument in their narratives, they implicitly establish it as an unchallengeable "fact." At the same time, they preclude the emergence of other narratives, where, for example, GPs step beyond the boundaries of the biomedical realm and create different notions of "social actors" which match and reflect more accurately the real-life experiences of domestic violence victims. Furthermore, rigid institutional narratives can also prove detrimental in the consultation itself, where, in the worst case, the patient's narrative is simply "rewritten" and replaced by the medical case narrative. As Trinch showed for protective order interviews with Latina survivors of abuse, communication problems and misrepresentations of cases occur when women and professionals adhere to different expectational frameworks and use divergent narrative strategies.[46] Thus, the "institutional memory as it is stored in various types of narrative genres, in this case in a domestic violence report, can only be as complete as the interaction that went into its production."[47] Conversely, if the narratives that constitute GPs' institutional memory of domestic violence are already informed by and further emphasise restrictive concepts, they are likely to influence the consultation and lead to the non-detection or even neglect of domestic violence in general practice.

It is therefore imperative to change GPs' narrative discourse on domestic violence and thus also their self-definitions. After all, "what is recorded in institutional memory can change over time and not surprisingly, the new information remembered will have an impact on the mission and identity of the institution."[48] As I argue elsewhere, one possible starting point for changes can be found in the "narrative paradigm."[49] On the one hand, it is essential that GPs learn about their own narrative strategies and to what extent these might hinder successful doctor-patient encounters. On the other hand, they ought to become familiar with the emotional and psychological processes women undergo when they experience violence. These two tasks could be accomplished by means of a narrative teaching module which incorporates both sociolinguistic narrative and discourse analysis as well as a literary teaching module as is already applied in approximately one third of American universities.[50] The ultimate aim of (re)introducing the narrative paradigm into the "scientific" realm of medicine must be to encourage a more holistic, person-led approach, which helps validate women's experiences and thus empowers them. To conclude with the words of one of the doctors in my sample, the aim must be to reintroduce life into medical training: "there are medical problems and there are other problems … but that's really fiction. Life is not like this. And the moment you step out of medical school and you're a doctor, you deal with life again."

Notes

[1] Elizabeth A. Stanko, ed., *Taking Stock. What Do We Know About Violence?* (London: ESRC Violence Research Programme, 1998).
[2] D. Young, *The Economic Implications of Domestic Violence in Greater Glasgow* (University of York: Unpublished MSc thesis, 1995).
[3] Pamela Abbott and Emma Williamson, "Women, Health and Domestic Violence," *Journal of Gender Studies* 8/1 (1999): 83-102. Borkowski, Margaret et al., *Marital Violence. The Community Response* (London: Tavistock, 1983).
[4] Danielle Mazza et al., "Physical, Sexual and Emotional Violence Against Women: A General Practice-Based Prevalence Study," *Medical Journal of Australia* 164 (1996): 14-17. Jan Pahl, "Health Professionals and Violence Against Women," in *Family Violence and the Caring Professions*, ed. Paul Kingston and Bridget Penhale (Basingstoke:

Macmillan, 1995), 127-148. Emma Williamson, *Domestic Violence and Health. The Response of the Medical Profession* (Bristol: The Policy Press, 2000).

[5] Peter Tiersma and Lawrence M. Solan, "The Linguist on the Witness Stand: Forensic Linguistics in American Courts," *Language* 78/2 (2002): 221-239.

[6] Alison Imbens-Bailey and Allyssa McCabe, "The Discourse of Distress: A Narrative Analysis of Emergency Calls to 911," *Language and Communication* 20 (2000): 275-296.

[7] Glyn Elwyn and Richard Gwyn, "Stories We Hear and Stories We Tell: Analysing Talk in Clinical Practice," in *Narrative Based Medicine: Dialogue and Discourse in Clinical Practice*, ed. Trisha Greenhalgh and Brian Hurwitz, (London: BMJ Books, 1998), 165-175. Candace West, "Medical Misfires: Mishearings, Misgivings and Misunderstandings in Physician-Patient Dialogues," *Discourse Processes* 7 (1984): 107-134.

[8] Emma Williamson, *Domestic Violence and Health* (Bristol: The Policy Press, 2000). Bradley, Fiona et al., "Reported Frequency of Domestic Violence: Cross Sectional Survey of Women Attending General Practice," *British Medical Journal* 324 (February 2002): 271-273.

[9] Theodore R. Sarbin, "Believed-In Imaginings: A Narrative Approach," in *Believed-In Imaginings. The Narrative Construction of Reality*, ed. Joseph De Rivera and Theodore R. Sarbin (Washington: American Psychological Association, 1998), 15.

[10] Ibid.

[11] David Herman, *Story Logic. Problems and Possibilities of Narrative* (Lincoln: University of Nebraska Press, 2002), 22.

[12] Ibid., 24.

[13] Michele L. Crossley, *Introducing Narrative Psychology: Self, Trauma and the Construction of Meaning* (Buckingham, UK: Open University Press, 2000). Eric Laurier, "Talking about Cigarettes: Conversational Narratives about Health and Illness," *Health* 3/2 (1999): 189-207. Jane Perkins and Nancy Blyler, eds., *Narrative and Professional Communication* (Stamford: Ablex, 1999).

[14] Norbert Dittmar and Ursula Bredel, *Die Sprachmauer. Die Verarbeitung der Wende und ihrer Folgen in Gesprächen mit Ost- und WestberlinerInnen* (Berlin: Weidler, 1999).

[15] Charlotte Linde, "The Transformation of Narrative Syntax into Institutional Memory," *Narrative Inquiry* 9/1(1999): 139-174.

[16] Deborah Schiffrin, "Narrative as Self-Portrait: Sociolinguistic Constructions of Identity," *Language in Society* 25/2 (1996): 196.

[17] David Herman, "Spatial Reference in Narrative Domains," *Text* 21/4 (2001): 515-541.
[18] Ellen Annandale, *The Sociology of Health and Medicine. A Critical Introduction* (Cambridge: Polity Press, 1998).
[19] Erving Goffman, *Frame Analysis* (Harmondsworth: Penguin, 1974).
[20] Roger M. Downs and David Stea, *Maps in Minds. Reflections on Cognitive Mapping* (New York: Harper and Row, 1977), 6.
[21] Ibid., 27.
[22] George Lakoff and Mark Johnson, *Metaphors We Live By* (Chicago: University of Chicago Press, 1980).
[23] Herman, "Spatial Reference in Narrative Domains," 518.
[24] Ibid.
[25] Lakoff and Johnson.
[26] Mark Johnson, *The Body in the Mind. The Bodily Basis of Meaning, Imagination, and Reason* (Chicago: University of Chicago Press, 1987), 116.
[27] Phil M. Strong, *The Ceremonial Order of the Clinic* (London: Routledge and Kegan Paul, 1979).
[28] Michel Foucault, *The Birth of the Clinic*, trans. A.M. Sheridan, (London: Tavistock, 1973).
[29] Annandale, chapter 1.
[30] Ibid., 5.
[31] Ibid., 6.
[32] Ibid.
[33] Ibid., 7.
[34] Foucault.
[35] Goffman, *Frame Analysis*, 188.
[36] William Labov, "Some Further Steps in Narrative Analysis," in *Oral Versions of Personal Experience: Three Decades of Narrative Analysis*, ed. Michael G. W. Bamberg (Mahwah, NJ: Lawrence Erlbaum, 1997), 396-415.
[37] William Labov and Joshua Waletzky, "Narrative Analysis: Oral Versions of Personal Experience," in *Essays on the Verbal and Visual Arts. (Proceedings of the 1966 Annual Spring Meeting of the American Ethnological Society)*, ed. June Helm (Seattle: University of Washington Press, 1967), 12-44.
[38] Erving Goffman, *Interaction Ritual. Essays on Face-To-Face Behaviour* (London: Allen Lane and Penguin, 1967).
[39] Ray Jackendoff, *Foundations of Language. Brain, Meaning, Grammar, Evolution* (Oxford: Oxford University Press, 2002).

[40] Labov, 406.
[41] Foucault, see chapter 6 ("Signs and Cases").
[42] David A. Zubin and Lynne E. Hewitt, "The Deictic Center: A Theory of Deixis in Narrative," in *Deixis in Narrative. A Cognitive Science Perspective*, ed. Judith F. Duchan et al. (Hillsdale, NJ: Lawrence Erlbaum, 1995), 129-155: 131.
[43] Herman, *Story Logic*.
[44] Anne Donald, "The Words We Live In," in *Narrative Based Medicine*, ed. Trisha Greenhalgh and Brian Hurwitz (London: BMJ Books, 1998), 17-26.
[45] Ibid., 23.
[46] Shonna Trinch, "Managing Euphemism and Transcending Taboos: Negotiating the Meaning of Sexual Assault in Latinas' Narratives of Domestic Violence," *Text* 21/4 (2001): 567-610.
[47] Ibid., 600.
[48] Ibid., 578.
[49] Jarmila Mildorf, *General Practitioners' Narrative Discourse on Domestic Violence: A Sociolinguistic Study* (University of Aberdeen: Unpublished Doctoral Thesis, 2002).
[50] Harriet A Squier, "Teaching Humanities in the Undergraduate Medical Curriculum," in *Narrative Based Medicine*, ed. Trisha Greenhalgh and Brian Hurwitz (London: BMJ Books, 1998), 128-139.

Bibliography

Abbott, Pamela and Emma Williamson. "Women, Health and Domestic Violence." *Journal of Gender Studies* 8/1 (1999): 83-102.

Annandale, Ellen. *The Sociology of Health and Medicine. A Critical Introduction*. Cambridge: Polity Press, 1998.

Borkowski, Margaret, Mervyn Murch and Val Walker. *Marital Violence. The Community Response*. London: Tavistock, 1983.

Bradley, Fiona, Mary Smith, Jean Long and Tom O'Dowd. "Reported Frequency of Domestic Violence: Cross Sectional Survey of Women

Attending General Practice." *British Medical Journal* 324 (February 2002): 271-273.

Crossley, Michele L. *Introducing Narrative Psychology: Self, Trauma and the Construction of Meaning*. Buckingham, UK: Open University Press, 2000.

Dittmar, Norbert and Ursula Bredel. *Die Sprachmauer. Die Verarbeitung der Wende und ihrer Folgen in Gesprächen mit Ost- und WestberlinerInnen*. Berlin: Weidler, 1999.

Donald, Anne. "The Words We Live In." In *Narrative Based Medicine. Dialogue and Discourse in Clinical Practice*, edited by Trisha Greenhalgh and Brian Hurwitz, 17-26. London: BMJ Books, 1998.

Downs, Roger M. and David Stea. *Maps in Minds. Reflections on Cognitive Mapping*. New York: Harper and Row, 1977.

Elwyn, Glyn and Richard Gwyn. "Stories We Hear and Stories We Tell: Analysing Talk in Clinical Practice." In *Narrative Based Medicine: Dialogue and Discourse in Clinical Practice*, edited by Trisha Greenhalgh and Brian Hurwitz, 165-175. London: BMJ Books, 1998.

Foucault, Michel. *The Birth of the Clinic*. (Translated by A.M. Sheridan). London: Tavistock, 1973.

Goffman, Erving. *Interaction Ritual. Essays on Face-To-Face Behaviour*. London: Allen Lane and Penguin, 1967.

Goffman, Erving. *Frame Analysis*. Harmondsworth: Penguin, 1974.
Herman, David. "Spatial Reference in Narrative Domains." *Text* 21/4 (2001): 515-541.

Herman, David. *Story Logic. Problems and Possibilities of Narrative*. Lincoln: University of Nebraska Press, 2002.

Imbens-Bailey, Alison and Allyssa McCabe. "The Discourse of Distress: A Narrative Analysis of Emergency Calls to 911." *Language and Communication* 20 (2000): 275-296.

Jackendoff, Ray. *Foundations of Language. Brain, Meaning, Grammar, Evolution*. Oxford: Oxford University Press, 2002.

Johnson, Mark. *The Body in the Mind. The Bodily Basis of Meaning, Imagination, and Reason*. Chicago: University of Chicago Press, 1987.

Labov, William. "Some Further Steps in Narrative Analysis." In *Oral Versions of Personal Experience: Three Decades of Narrative Analysis*, edited by Michael G. W. Bamberg, 396-415. Mahwah, NJ: Lawrence Erlbaum, 1997.

Labov, William and Joshua Waletzky. "Narrative Analysis: Oral Versions of Personal Experience." In *Essays on the Verbal and Visual Arts. (Proceedings of the 1966 Annual Spring Meeting of the American Ethnological Society)*, edited by June Helm, 12-44. Seattle: University of Washington Press, 1967.

Lakoff, George and Mark Johnson. *Metaphors We Live By*. Chicago: University of Chicago Press, 1980.

Laurier, Eric. "Talking about Cigarettes: Conversational Narratives about Health and Illness." *Health* 3/2 (1999): 189-207.

Linde, Charlotte. "The Transformation of Narrative Syntax into Institutional Memory." *Narrative Inquiry* 9/1(1999): 139-174.

Mazza, Danielle, Lorraine Dennerstein and Vicky Ryan. "Physical, Sexual and Emotional Violence Against Women: A General Practice-Based Prevalence Study." *Medical Journal of Australia* 164 (1996): 14-17.

Mildorf, Jarmila. *General Practitioners' Narrative Discourse on Domestic Violence: A Sociolinguistic Study*. University of Aberdeen: Unpublished Doctoral Thesis, 2002.

Pahl, Jan. "Health Professionals and Violence Against Women." In *Family Violence and the Caring Professions*, edited by Paul Kingston and Bridget

Penhale, 127-148. Basingstoke: Macmillan, 1995.
Perkins, Jane and Nancy Blyler, eds. *Narrative and Professional Communication*. Stamford: Ablex, 1999.

Sarbin, Theodore R. "Believed-In Imaginings: A Narrative Approach." In *Believed-In Imaginings. The Narrative Construction of Reality*, edited by Joseph De Rivera and Theodore R. Sarbin, 15-30. Washington: American Psychological Association, 1998.

Schiffrin, Deborah. "Narrative as Self-Portrait: Sociolinguistic Constructions of Identity." *Language in Society* 25/2 (1996): 167-203.

Squier, Harriet A. "Teaching Humanities in the Undergraduate Medical Curriculum." In *Narrative Based Medicine. Dialogue and Discourse in Clinical Practice*, edited by Trisha Greenhalgh and Brian Hurwitz, 128-139. London: BMJ Books, 1998.

Stanko, Elizabeth A., ed. *Taking Stock. What Do We Know About Violence?* London: ESRC Violence Research Programme, 1998.
Strong, Phil M. *The Ceremonial Order of the Clinic*. London: Routledge and Kegan Paul, 1979.

Tiersma, Peter and Lawrence M. Solan. "The Linguist on the Witness Stand: Forensic Linguistics in American Courts." *Language* 78/2 (2002): 221-239.

Trinch, Shonna. "Managing Euphemism and Transcending Taboos: Negotiating the Meaning of Sexual Assault in Latinas' Narratives of Domestic Violence." *Text* 21/4 (2001): 567-610.

West, Candace. "Medical Misfires: Mishearings, Misgivings and Misunderstandings in Physician-Patient Dialogues." *Discourse Processes* 7 (1984): 107-134.

Williamson, Emma. *Domestic Violence and Health. The Response of the Medical Profession*. Bristol: The Policy Press, 2000.

Young, D. *The Economic Implications of Domestic Violence in Greater Glasgow*. University of York: Unpublished MSc thesis, 1995.

Zubin, David A. and Lynne E. Hewitt. "The Deictic Center: A Theory of Deixis in Narrative." In *Deixis in Narrative. A Cognitive Science Perspective*, edited by Judith F. Duchan, Gail A. Bruder and Lynne E. Hewitt, 129-155. Hillsdale, NJ: Lawrence Erlbaum, 1995.

Note on Contributor

Jarmila Mildorf completed her PhD in sociolinguistics at the University of Aberdeen (Scotland) in 2002. She is now lecturer of English linguistics and literature at the University of Stuttgart (Germany).

Treating Wellness: How Clown Doctors Help to Humanize Health Care and Promote Good Health[1]

Bernie Warren

1. Introduction

As the first-born son in a Jewish medical family I was expected to follow in my grandfather's footsteps and become a Physician. Needless to say, I did not follow the path chosen for me by my family. Nevertheless all my life I have been involved in some aspect of healing and/or health promotion. Much of my professional work has concerned the use of drama with people who, by illness, accident of birth, or social circumstances have in some way been disempowered or disenfranchised, to help them in some way to overcome their individual challenges.

I grew up in a household, where dinner conversation often focused on medical topics, remember we were Jewish and our family has its fair share of neurotics and hypochondriacs. My Poppa (my mother's father) was a doctor. He qualified in 1922 and practiced medicine until his death in 1966. He was a modest man, never sought glory or the 'limelight' but 'notable' and learned doctors (including the Queen's personal physician) often sought his advice on a variety of medical matters. He lived his life by the proverb, "a cheerful heart does good like a medicine" and his obituary stressed that he had "a good bedside manner and a fine sense of humour." He used humour as part of his act. For him it came naturally, he had a gift and he used it to make patients smile or laugh.

My Poppa was not unique. Like so many other 'old time' family doctors he believed that bedside manner was more than half the healing process. Something, many would argue that modern western technological medicine has forgotten. From my grandfather I learned for myself the value of laughter. As I grew up I began to realize that one of the few skills I have is that I can make people laugh and that humour, most notably physical humour, transcends language. One result of this was that I started to research the role of humour in healing and health care and in particular the work of clowns in hospitals.

2. Laughter: The Best Medicine?

Throughout history laughter has helped to unite people, create social unrest or simply make people feel better. More than this, a simple smile can do wonders to change a person's mood. While the actual connection between laughter and healing is rather sketchy; a great deal has been written in academic journals and the lay press (by people such as

William Fry, David McClelland, Henri Rubinstein, Norman Cousins) about how humour and the resulting laughter can have positive physiological and psychological effects on body systems. The research suggests that laughter helps to: reduce muscular tension; stimulate secretions which encourage coughing and expulsion of "toxins"; increase production of Immunoglobulins ("chemicals" which help to fight infection); stimulate increased oxygenation of the blood supply, giving more energy to "cope" with illnesses and their medical treatments; release endorphins to help cope with pain. The researchers often go on to suggest that effects associated with laughter may exert a positive influence on the body's ability to recover from illness, disease, surgery etc.

3. Clowns in Hospitals: A Brief History

> You shall this twelve-month term from day to day
> Visit the speechless sick, and still converse
> With groaning wretches; and your task shall be,
> With all the fierce endeavor of your wit,
> To force the pained impotent to smile.[2]

While clown doctoring is a relatively new profession, scholarly works are full of examples of fools, clowns and other performers working in hospital settings since Antiquity. For example, it's believed that the hospital of Hippocrates, on the Greek Island of Kos, maintained constant troupes of players and clowns in the quadrangle, as the doctors of the day believed that mood influenced healing, "an early fool at Henry IV's twelfth century court founded St. Bartholomew's Hospital."[3] In more modern times "The Fratellini Brothers," a famous clown trio, probably began the current tradition of clowns visiting children in hospitals. While there were many precursors the tradition of professional clowns being employed as part of a health care team began in 1986.

In 1986 Karen Ridd, a solo performer (*Robo*), who was also a child life specialist initiated an experimental project in Winnipeg Children's Hospital in Canada. This became Winnipeg's Therapeutic Clown program. Almost simultaneously, Michael Christensen (*Dr. Stubbs*), along with Jeff Gordon (*disorderly Gordoon*) first set foot in a hospital. Their groundbreaking work led to the first clown doctor program and to the formation of the *Big Apple Circus Clown Care Unit* (hereafter CCU) in New York. Interestingly enough neither knew about the other's work and to this day, as far as I know, they have never met one another! Both programs are alive and well. They have expanded and acted as catalysts for many programs around the world and represent two major approaches to the way clowns work in hospitals; the solo therapeutic clown and clown doctors who work in pairs. I should add that there are other models of practice for clowns working in hospitals. For example, some clowns are also clergy, “Clowns for Christ,” others are simply “entertainers,” either as volunteers or on a semi-professional basis, while still others are doctors who use humour as part of their medical practice. Currently hundreds of professional clown doctors are employed in hospitals and health care settings in at least a dozen different countries around the world (including Canada, Britain, France, Brazil, Austria, Germany, Italy, Switzerland, Spain and The States).

4. What is a Clown Doctor?

A clown doctor is a specially trained professional artist who works in a hospital or health care facility. They are *not* simply entertainers but rather integral components of the health care delivery process. Clown doctors do not practice medicine. They are the latest in a long line of mirth makers who help to heal not through diagnosis and therapy but rather through humour and by sharing the gift of laughter. As such contemporary clown doctors are probably closer in their philosophy to clown healers such as certain “shaman” in Southeast Asia or Pueblo, Hopi and other Native American cultures, where clowns are often identified as the most powerful healers.

Clown Doctors:

- Work in pairs (dubbed a “clown marriage”); wear a white coat, a red nose and minimal make up.

- Combine interpersonal and communication skills with improvisational performance (e.g. lazzi [pratfalls, comic business], mime, music, movement/dance, poetry, juggling, magic, storytelling).

- They are usually called “Doctor” (e.g. *Dr. Haven’t-a-clue*, *Dr. Figzit*) have a unique personality and name, often identified by a distinctive trademark connected to that name (e.g. *Dr. Twinkle-Toes*’ yellow taffeta tutu).

- While some clowns have highly developed specialized skills such as juggling, and magic (particularly true of American clowns), most clown doctors carry minimal props and work by improvising with whoever or whatever is in the room (known as “empty pocket clowning”).

- Clown doctors are verbal, use music and song extensively and communicate using gesture, sound and language ranging from silence and simple gesture through to loud and gregarious dialogue, as each situation demands.

- They play in a wide range of 'styles' – from the use of quiet 'meditative' music or sitting quietly at a bedside; to creating carnival-like processions that spread music and mirth wherever they trail; through to loud, boisterous and anarchic productions of Shakespeare's plays or Tchaichovsky's ballets that involve anyone in close proximity at the time (patients, family, nurses, doctors, etc.).

- They focus as much on the family members and health care workers as on the patient.

- In addition to all of their other skills many clown doctors are able to communicate in more than one language. This ability to communicate in more than one language is sometimes a great asset as wards in urban hospitals are often multi-cultural and multi-lingual environments.

5. A Word or Two About Clown Marriages

Clown doctors come in all shapes and sizes. They are all different. But the good ones share a certain genetic bonding. They have common core skills, sensitivities and attributes. The best ones have the ability to: listen actively, and fully; communicate through words, music or even through the "inspired" use of silence; see the "one door" they can open for a child (or adult); and as a clown "character" they are, or say, something "unique."

As mentioned before they work in pairs and these partnerships are usually called "clown marriages," a term coined by Caroline Simonds and Kim Winslow (*Dr. Lune*), when they worked together on the Big Apple Circus Clown Care Unit. An important point, however, is that clown marriages are not defined by conventional gender pairings but rather they are cemented by the chemistry of the relationship: by energies and sensibilities and by complementary skills and rhythms of the performers, irrespective of whether they are a man or a woman.

In the partnership usually one performer plays a "white" clown, the other an "Auguste." In very simple terms white clowns are a rational voice of reason, the orderly decision-maker while Augustes are fun loving impulsive and often "trouble makers." Each exerts an influence on the other. While the white Clown may think they are the "Boss," in charge of the situation, the Auguste often controls events through their actions. Generally the Auguste has more "fun," and so clowns who habitually play this role are often reluctant to give it up.

In April 1999, I was invited to be a presenter at the first World Symposium on Culture, Health and the Arts held in Manchester, England. It was here that I first encountered the work of Caroline Simonds, AKA *Dr. Giraffe*, and the work of the clown doctors of "Le Rire Medecin." I was immediately fascinated. The work seemed to bring together all of the things that I have been interested in my whole life. After that first meeting, I made several trips to France where I shadowed the clowns and took notes in the hospitals, followed by long hours discussing how and what Caroline and "Le Rire Medecin" do and why they are successful. So in July 2001, nearly 15 years after I began my academic quest into the role of humour in health and using a model developed by "Le Rire Medecin," I began "Fools For Health," my own clown doctor company in Windsor, Ontario, Canada.

"Fools For Health" delivers programs in three Windsor Hospitals to adults and children, involves a university, and other community partners working together to design, deliver and evaluate site-specific clown doctor programs as an integral part of the health care process for children and adults; conducts research into the effects of clown doctor programs not only on patients, family and staff but also on health care delivery; is committed to promoting community awareness about the role of humour in health care and to developing an institute to provide the first university-affiliated professional training program for clown doctors.

6. What is the Value of a Smile?

"Fools for Health" clown doctor program has been working as a member of our interdisciplinary team on inpatient rehabilitation for approximately one year. During this time we have seen a definite value to clown doctors being with patients or families, caregivers and staff.

Patients have commented that the clown doctors made them work harder in therapy, almost in a competitive sense, and also that they allow them to have a bit of normalcy to their lives, for a few moments. When clown doctors are near, smiles are everywhere. There is an infusion of endorphins into the air. Staff sing with them, react with them and if needed are quiet with them.

Now is the time for the "value of a smile" to be evaluated on inpatient rehabilitation. By participating in this research, areas can be identified where clown doctors actually make a difference.[4] While there are still obstacles to overcome (and every now and again a colleague who could do without us) every indicator, both qualitative and quantitative, suggests tremendous positive effects of having clown doctors as part of the rehab team. More importantly, almost all the patients and their families (as well as hospital staff and administrators) are not only very happy having clowns in the hospital but also very impressed with "results."

However we are now entering a new phase where some clear data, especially empirical data, is needed to support the overwhelming belief that the work clown doctors do, with patients, family and staff, does make a difference. My colleague Dr. Pam McAuslan and I are currently trying to make sense of the anecdotal data, to develop appropriate quantitative instruments to collect "hard" data to convince the "naysayers."

We are hopeful that in a year's time we will have more empirical evidence to balance the wealth of anecdotal evidence and that this will help to substantiate the work of clown doctors not only in Windsor but also in other parts of the world. In the meantime let me tell you a story or two...

7. Let's Start at the Very Beginning

After two weeks of intensive training, the clown doctors first entered the in-patient rehabilitation ward on the afternoon of Friday the 13th.

As soon as they entered the ward, they started to sing up and down the halls as they went. People started quietly coming out of their rooms wondering what was going on. The clowns circled the ward and ... *stop*! They finished their song and they looked at me in "panic." "What do we do now?" I suggest they "huddle" (get together and talk it through) and split into pairs and go in opposite directions. They went into all the rooms, even room 9! (We had been warned *not* to go into this room, so we didn't. However, 40 minutes into the controlled chaos an urgent request comes from Room 9, "Why aren't you visiting US?" Our "gag order" was instantly lifted!) It is obvious just from the change in noise levels and "energy" even from our first initial entries that this is going to work. Bernice the unit manager is ecstatic. She plays with the clowns. *Dr. Fifi & Dr. Twinkle-Toes* using a blood pressure cuff and inspired lunacy, perform a 'squeakotomy' on Bernice's leg. A crowd has gathered in wheelchairs and is laughing at the mayhem.

Meanwhile *Dr. Ops & Dr. Poops* have made three depressed Caballeros' day. The three came wheeling down the hall laughing out loud. I ask Bernice later if this was usual? She let me know this was anything but! Usually these three just sat around and "moaned." The moment when *Ops & Poops* walk into a room where a woman has had a tracheostomy, they start singing "You are my sunshine" and the woman put her hand over her incision and "sings" along, taps her feet and is animated! We later found out that this woman was still singing and laughing long after the clowns left. Later on in the program, she still loved the clowns singing "You are my sunshine" to her and could often be seen late in the evening wheeling herself around the ward 'singing' the song to herself long after the clowns had left.

Through the use of music, interactive dances and general playfulness, the clown doctors of "Fools for Health" help patients and their families take their mind off the illness, reduce anxiety in young children awaiting surgery (sometimes even accompanying them from the waiting room to the operating room), and brighten the mood of nurses, doctors and other health care staff.

In the year or so since this information was collected, our research already suggests our clown doctors help to increase satisfaction with rehabilitation programs (based on Outcome Surveys), reduce the need for pain and anti-depression medication, and reduce the overall length of stay in the hospital.

In addition, clown doctors work with speech and language pathologists, physiotherapists and occupational therapists to develop clown interactions that encourage patients with a tracheostomy or aphasia to speak (e.g. singing songs, telling interactive stories, or simply encouraging patients to blow paper windmills or balloons) or extend the range of motion for stroke and aphasia patients (e.g. singing higher and higher as patient lifts his/her leg, encouraging patient to kick a rubber chicken, creating an imaginative journey as clowns accompany patients in their daily routines).

Recently while Caroline Simonds was visiting "Fools For Health" she interviewed patients immediately after the clown doctors had visited them. One patient in Complex Continuing Care Barbara had the following comment:[5]

> We should have the clowns here more often. I have a lot of fun with them. They bring sunshine and laughter. They put a smile on your face and it lasts the rest of the day and when you think of them (the clowns) it (the smile) comes back. They leave good feelings behind.[6]

8. The Importance of Being a Team Member

Before beginning, the clowns always ask the nurses which children are treated for pain. In return, health care teams encourage us to provide information on what we observe during our meetings with patients in pain. Very often, doctors will ask us our opinion to help evaluate the pain. Above all, we want to work together.[7]

All reputable clown doctor programs have some form of daily check-in before visiting patients. In Winnipeg, where David Langdon is employed as a child-life specialist, on clown days he simply refers to a cardex system used by all child life specialists. In Paris and in Windsor the clowns usually meet with a charge nurse and where needed other members of the medical team. These meetings provide clowns with information about the patients on a day to day basis and provide the staff with the opportunity to make requests about who needs a visit and perhaps what sort of intervention is being asked for from the clowns.

Many programs also have some form of check out where clown doctors share any important information with the health care staff on a daily basis either verbally or through some form of communication log. In some programs there is also a structured time for health care staff to give feedback about the clown's work, behaviour and noise levels. This is important because sometimes what may be beneficial for a patient and their family may seem "disruptive" to members of the health care team who are trying to do their job. In addition to a daily check-in, some programs participate in team meetings. David Langdon, in his child-life role, is a de facto member of childcare meetings.

In Windsor, the clowns on the in-patient rehabilitation unit attend all inter-disciplinary team meetings where patients' weekly progress is viewed from the perspective of all the doctors, nurses, therapists, and other health care professionals who work with them. These meetings provide a time for clowns both to gain and share information. The clown doctors also have regular weekly meetings with a liaison person from all the therapeutic areas. However, as one clown points out, "I'll get all this information about a patient" (but) "when I'm in clown I completely forget what I was told." It must be noted that clowns often know salient information not cerebrally but "in their bones."

As I have been seeing on a regular basis choices made for a patient in clown are directly related to the patient's treatment program as discussed in rounds, or even on the fly in the hallway with a nurse. However, clowns when complimented on their planning look blank and make it clear that any connection was subconscious. However, this "mindlessness" rather than being seen as a weakness is one of the reasons why the clowns are successful.

In addition to these structured information gathering and sharing sessions, there are also many ad hoc meetings on the wards between clowns and health care staff where information is shared. This may range from a brief notification concerning a patient's health, a request to leave a patient alone, through to a need for a clown to visit a particular room. This sharing on the fly is often essential. It is important to develop a ritual or routine by which this information sharing may occur. This can range from a brief word whispered in a clown's ear as they pass, to a request for a "noses down" [8] moment alone.

Besides finding ways of sharing information on the fly it is most important that when necessary the health care staff have a way to "shoo away" clowns, a simple signal that lets the clowns know they are not wanted. This helps prevent misunderstandings where a family member or a patient invites the clowns in to the room to play at a time when a health care worker is trying to carry out a delicate procedure or begin a difficult discussion.

Finally, and perhaps most importantly, significant learning occurs when clowns go "inclownito"[9] to join health care staff for lunch or coffee. Once the clowns have been accepted as members of the "health care family" it is important to build in times to simply "hang out" with colleagues and discuss stuff NOT related to the patients or the hospital. For in these moments of shared repose are developed irrevocable bonds of trust that often act as catalysts for the sharing of information more easily and at a deeper clinical level.

It is a two way street, for health care professionals are probably the next greatest source of clowns' informal learning. The information gained may also be the most significant. Many anecdotal stories bear witness to how clowns have learned to deal with weighty topics such as the death of a child to more light-hearted advice concerning how to cope with hospital smells, especially those of faces and urine. Information is gained from colleagues in different ways, some more formal than others are.

"Hey pay attention to me, *I'm the one who's sick!"*[10]

The key thing overall is that the clown has to learn to be fully attentive. The French clowns refer to this as "listening with all antennas up." To be successful and to continue to grow a clown doctor must be a "creative detective." They have to learn to not go in with a set agenda but must be ready, willing and able to listen to any and every clue they are given.

When I was visiting Paul Hooson (*Doc Willikers*) in Vancouver, Doc was playing with a young girl who has cancer. Using a standard lazzi of a "squeakotomy," he was placing and removing a squeak from parts of the girl's body. However, this young girl had other ideas as to how to use the squeaker! She used it like a television remote allowing the clown to speak or be mute, at her discretion. After leaving the room Paul said: "I'd never have thought of that but I'm sure she will want to play this game again." The child was clearly telling us that she needed to be in control. She had been stuck in a hospital, poked and prodded and given "foul concoctions" probably often against her will, the squeeker helped her gain a measure of control.

Also the gift of laughter allows the patient, and all involved with them, to see that they are much more than their illness. They enable patients to take responsibility for themselves in something as simple as deciding whether or not to laugh at the clown doctor at their bedside. Often information is freely given to a clown that either puts the patient's behaviour in a new light or gives ideas about how to approach the patient or a family member.

Many clowns talk about how sometimes the patient will share information that is *not* contained anywhere in patient records! For example clowns in Windsor working with a patient who had had a tracheostomy and was being taught how to speak again found out that she loved to sing and had a large repertoire of songs. Or they will find ways of getting the patients to be compliant, to cooperate with their treatment that no one else can do. For example one day a 90 year old man in rehabilitation simply refused to go downstairs to his physiotherapy sessions. So the clowns brought physiotherapy to his bedside. Working alongside his therapist we persuaded him to do his physiotherapy with us in the hallways on the ward. Apparently this was the first time he had agreed to do his physiotherapy for almost a week. The clown can then share this with other members of the health care team. This has added benefits as it increases the interactions and informal learning with the health care team. They may not always be able to make sense or make use of the information immediately. It may take some time and perhaps discussion with other members of the health care team to process how best to incorporate this new knowledge into their work. However, the point stands that if you have switched off your receiver you won't hear the incoming message!

9. The Power of Saying Sorry

"I am sorry (je m'excuse, mi scuzi)"

Few people ever say these three little words in a hospital and I have rarely heard it. However, clowns say it all the time. Their mere entrance into a room reveals their own brand of blatant social imperfection, verbal ineptness and physical blundering. So what's better or funnier than to say, "I'm sorry," especially when nothing has fallen, broken or even happened yet? It is our calling card.

When a doctor has just announced a child's imminent death to his or her parents, I wonder if he has added, "I'm sorry" to his painful explication. Can he say that? It is so damn heavy. Doctors, too, need to cope and survive. In an oncology ward, they must announce hundreds of difficult things year round and nothing except experience usually prepares them for these challenging tasks. Constantly saying they were sorry for an illness or even their failure to cure it would probably be the rocky road to suicide or chronic depression. But when he feels the need (usually instinctively), the clown can take it on himself to "play" with the notion of apology; thus helping the medical staff.[11]

10. Clown Doctors as Scapegoats

Clown doctors serve many purposes within a hospital. One of the most important is, that from time to time they act as 'scapegoats' for the sick children, their families and even for the medical staff who work with them. Unfortunately this task, like making people laugh, has probably always been part of a clown or fool's job description!

At times the patients, their parents or one or more of the hospital staff (sometimes all of them together) feel the need to collect their "sins and misfortunes" and bind them upon some unfortunate. They do not have far to look for a scapegoat, for at these times the clown doctor is easy prey. They make too much noise. They are not always 100% sensitive to a nurse or doctor's mood (swing) and their irreverence can disrupt medical routines.

Like the court fools, jesters and clowns who preceded them clown doctors seem to serve no useful purpose and are easily expendable. So why not project your fears, failings and general unhappiness on these "mirth makers." At these moments, the clown's value as a meaningful element in the continuing wellness of the individuals and the community is forgotten.

We are back in ancient times and the clown is not a human being but rather a goat to be sacrificed. However, unlike their ancient ancestors, the clown doctor like the Festival Fool of the Sword Dance can be resurrected. For when they have served their purpose as a "whipping boy," their status within the hospital community is not only restored but may be raised if the community or individual, like the wise "king," recognizes the value of the scapegoat to his own health and sanity.

11. Fools Bearing Gifts ... How Clowns Help in the Healing Process

> *"We treat wellness."*[12]
> *"To find a solution, the first thing to be done is to recognize the true problem."*[13]

While clown doctors often keep extensive notes, they do not make a medical diagnosis or write up a medical case history (although the best of them are well informed about these). This is the domain of the physician or surgeon who prescribes a "suitable course of treatment or intervention" (e.g. surgical procedure, medicines etc.). Rather they create their own clown "prescription," one that does not focus on the patient's limitations. As Ami Hattab, *Dr. Balthazar* puts it, "doctors, nurses and other therapists work with the parts of the patient that are 'sick', clown doctors work with everything else."

In a recent interview Caroline Simonds made the following points: during the course of a medical evaluation, clowns can transform the examining room, which then becomes less terrifying for the child. They allow moments of relief, rest from the tension that surrounds an examination. Children relax when clowns make music, make bubbles or play with puppets, which can make the consultation a little more pleasant, and can allow the doctor to more easily approach a withdrawn child; interactions between clowns and children can facilitate the observation of the child's physical and emotional behaviour. Clowns help the health care givers to relax and laugh, which shows the children another side of them. The clowns presence let the doctors see another side of their patients: that of a child full of life, not that of a medical case, of a tumour or of a statistic.

There are other ways that the clowns help the health care team. In France at least one "Professor"[14] sees the clown doctor's function in relation to the needs of the medical staff. This Professor acknowledged the wonderful contribution the clown doctors provide for the life and health of the patients and their families. However, he also emphasized the role the clown doctors play in shaking up the staff. As he puts it: "The day you cannot bother us ... is the day you must leave…"

By creating noise and processions, and by disturbing the oh so serious business of healing clown doctors force the medical staff to confront the patients and themselves as human beings. The laughter is infectious but it is not always welcome. Sometimes, complaints that it is too loud or inappropriate may even be legitimate. However, this Professor believes that having clown doctors on the treatment team helps the team members do their own job more humanely, and arguably more effectively. For if the nurse or doctor takes a genuine interest in that person as a human being, the likelihood is the patient will place more faith in and be more compliant with the treatment being suggested by the medical team. In so doing the clown doctor does not only humanize but may also increase the success of the medical treatment itself.

This is being backed up by the research currently underway in Windsor. After a rocky first few days of trying to accommodate to the noise and commotion, members of the therapy team are openly applauding the clown doctors' successes and commenting on how they help improve the work of the team as a whole. One day the clowns were doing a "clown recital": an interactive weekly session that lasts about half an hour uses a free form improvised blend of music and shtick[15] and indirectly incorporates what the clowns have seen in therapy sessions and heard in rounds.

On this day I overheard the physiotherapists comment: "Look at that ... they're doing therapy and the patients are enjoying it..." " ... I'd have never thought of that... but I'm going to incorporate it in what I do..."

Sometimes clowns also teach hospital administrators and program managers about human dignity and the needs of patients. Debra Kaufman of the CCU recalls one instance, when they were able to help managers adapt better to suit the needs of the children they serve:

> ...after we did our first surgical escort, for a child who begged us to come with him. We went down and we waited in the surgery waiting area with this child and we were looking around going ... you have this kid in here with all these moaning adults who are drugged and children were not pre-sedated so they were totally awake and all the adults who are coming in are drooling and moaning and we said why are you doing this ... that's not fair to the children, and they went... DUH! And within two months, they had separated an area for children, re-decorated it, and separated it totally from the adults. And they did the same thing in radiation; they made a separate playroom. And it's only because we came down and went, '…you want to put them down here?'

In France on a children's ward Caroline Simonds noted the following:

> I would see the clowns coming from afar and start observing and recording: the noise level before they come in, what kind of activity is going on, were the people having conversations, how loud it was.
>
> ...one thing that I noticed consistently was that people talk louder after the clowns leave and people talk more to the kids, they talk more to each other... Or a child instead of playing by himself in bed, he'd play with his mom. More interactive play...

In Windsor at the end of one particularly long and dreary rounds, the team was discussing a patient who could not be motivated to participate in her therapy program. At this point Crystal Brennan, *Dr. Opera*, told the group that the clowns hadn't been having the same problems: "All you have to do to get her to participate is to show her your knickers."... at which point the unit manager turned to the Senior Consultant[16] and asked if he would flash his underwear the next time he worked with the patient. As frivolous as this moment may appear it did awaken the team to a problem. As Einstein suggested "insanity is constantly repeating the same actions expecting a different result." Clown doctors because they can step outside the constraints of hospital policies and procedure, like the Lords of

Misrule that they are, can do what is needed, not simply what is allowed. For as improvisers they must "accept the gift" and look for solutions, *not* the problems"!

Clown doctors do not forget the illness but work with those parts of the individual that are healthy. They help educate parents and the rest of the medical team to the fact that the patient is not simply their illness. In doing this, the patient, their family and the medical team who are helping make them healthy again are all able to see beyond the medical problem. In this way clown doctors give everyone a gift of sight.

Notes

[1] Some of the material contained in this chapter is to be found in my previously published work, notably Bernie Warren, "Fools for Health: Introducing Clown Doctors to Windsor Hospitals," in *Creating a Theatre in your Classroom and Community,* 2nd Edition (Captus University Publications).

[2] Rosaline speaking to Berowne *Love's Labor's Lost* Act V sc. ii (RIVERSIDE SHAKESPEARE).

[3] Quoted in John Doran, *A History of Court Fools.*

[4] Bernice Markham, Manager In-patient Rehabilitation Unit, Letter to the Research Ethics Board, Windsor Regional Hospital.

[5] Barbara has had a stroke and is on a long-term care ward for people requiring continuing rehabilitation and nursing care.

[6] Quote collected by Caroline Simonds from Barbara, (a Patient in Long Term Continuing Complex Care) 17th June 2002 *immediately* after *Dr. Twinkle-Toes* and *Dr. Figzit* (two "Fools For Health" clown doctors) had left a room.

[7] Simonds Caroline, *Pain and Laughter.*

[8] Clowns who wear a red nose can simply step out of character by taking off or lowering the nose (attached by elastic behind the neck).

[9] Inclownito is a term used to describe when, as part of their work, a clown communicates or interacts as them self with hospital personnel and occasionally patients' family.

[10] Eight year old boy with three polite brothers at his side (quote courtesy of research conducted by Caroline Simonds).

[11] Caroline Simonds, unpublished notes.

[12] Kim Wimslow, Big Apple circus Clown Care Unit, circa 1989.

[13] Richard in Terry Goodkind, *Soul of the Fire.*

[14] The French use this term for a medical doctor who heads a unit.

[15] "Schtick" is a word used by performers to describe any prepared or unscripted improvisational interactions between them or between them and an audience. It conveys slightly more than the Commedia Dell'Arte term "Lazzi," which describes repeatable 'set pieces' of physical business.

[16] I am using this term to denote the unit's senior medical specialist.

Bibliography

Fry, William F. "The Physiologic Effects of Humor, Mirth, and Laughter." *Journal of the American Medical Association*, 267 (1992): 1857-1858.

Martin, Rod A. "Humor, Laughter, and Physical Health: Methodological Issues and Research Findings." *Psychological Bulletin*, 127 (2001): 504-519.

Oppenheim, Daniel, Caroline Simonds, and Olivier Hartmann. "Clowning on Children's Wards." *Lancet*, 350 (1997): 1838-1840.

Simonds, Caroline, and Bernie Warren. *Le Rire Medecin: Journal du docteur girafe*. Paris: Albin Michael, 2001.

Spitzer, Peter. *A Study of the Overseas-Based Clown Doctor Programs and their Impact on the Health Care System.* Report to the Winston Churchill Memorial Trust of Australia, 2002.

Towsen, John H. *Clowns*. New York: Hawthorn, 1976.

Van Blerkom, and Linda Miller. "Clown Doctors: Shaman Healers of Western Medicine." *Medical Anthropology Quarterly*, 9 (1995): 462-475.

Warren, Bernie. "Knowing Laughter: What do Clown-Doctors Know and How do they Learn to do What they do?" New Approaches to Life Long Learning (SSHRC GRANT), Final Report, 2001.

Warren, Bernie. "Fools for Health: Introducing Clown-Doctors to Windsor Hospitals." In *Creating a Theatre in your Classroom and Community*, edited by Bernie Warren, 225-246. North York: Captus University Publications, 2002.

Warren, Bernie, and Pamela McAuslan. "What is the Value of a Smile? An Investigation of the Role of Clown-Doctors Working on an In-Patient Rehabilitation Unit." *Interim Research Paper* Windsor, Canda, 2002.

Welsford, Enid. *The Fool: His Social and Literary History*. 1935. Reprint. London: Faber and Faber, 1968.

Note on Contributor

Bernie Warren, Ph.D. is a teacher, researcher and professional clown-doctor. He holds the position of professor in the school of dramatic art at the University of Windsor, where he teaches on drama in the education and community program. He is also director of the 'Fools for Health' clown doctor programs.

The Medical Humanist: A Pilot Program in the Cancer Center Setting

Celia E. Bandman, Bernard M. Bandman, Patricia A. Barr, and Letha E. Mills

Humanism in the practice of medicine is not a new concept. It has been discussed, written about in professional journals, taught in medical schools and offered as part of continuing education for doctors and other caregivers. As early as 1927, Dr Francis Peabody wrote, "The art of medicine and the science of medicine are not antagonistic but supplementary to one another."[1] Dr Lewis Thomas, a physician and former President of Memorial Sloan Kettering Hospital in New York City, is one of many authors who has described the gulf between scientists and humanists. He said,

> The 'two cultures controversy of several decades back has quieted down some, but it is still with us, still unsettled because of the polarized views ... At one edge, the humanists are set up as knowing and wanting to know very little about science and even less about the human meaning of contemporary science. On the other side, scientists are served up as a bright illiterate lot, well-read in nothing except science.[2]

As essential as cutting edge clinical science is for the practice of good medicine, it has become overly identified as the definition of best care for the patient. The human component is often viewed as being of lesser value in the doctor/patient communication despite the studies which show that listening to, and expressing empathy with, patients can reduce some clinical symptoms and increase compliance. [3]

There are three models that have been developed to improve doctor/patient communication which all focus on the role of empathy. One model exposes medical students to the humanities and addresses the issue of empathy within their training.[4-6] Dr Howard Spiro has observed,

> First and second year [medical] students are eager for the bridge between the world of doctor and the world of patient. We call it a meeting place or crossroad. Sadly, by the third and fourth year those students are not interested in the humanities as experienced by stories or anecdotes. They value science far more and they are pressed for time.[7]

Another model encourages the practicing doctor to imagine or write an alternative narrative,[8-10] while yet another model encourages doctors to be sensitive to and express their own emotions.[11-13] In all models the medical professional is asked to do more at a time when medical school curricula are expanding to include new fields and the doctor in the medical system is dealing with ever increasing pressures. These models recognize the value of understanding the doctor's and patient's experience and seek to enhance doctor/patient communication, but none of them addresses the relationship of doctor and patient in real time.

1. The Medical Humanist Model

We have designed a new model for bridging the 'two cultures', whether characterized as the art and science of medicine or the humanities and science of medicine. The model incorporates six core beliefs: The untreated side effect of a serious illness for both doctor and patient is uncertainty;[14] language and metaphor shape experience;[15-16] doctors' language as characterized in the patient's chart creates a narrative that shapes the doctor's experience of the patient's illness;[17] patients at diagnosis first experience their bodies as separate from self and later experience their bodies in illness through suffering and loss of function;[18] the narrative that patients use to describe their experience is qualitatively different than that used by doctors;[19] and the differences in language used and understood by doctors and patients impede doctor/patient communication which has been recognized as an important component of best care.[20] The new model incorporates a medical humanist in the daily care of patients.

> To care for the sick in a morally responsible manner, the doctor must delve into the patients experience, imagine the patients future, integrate thought and feeling, and with the patient, co-author the next chapter in a life story whose story-line had been interrupted by illness. For this literary skills are needed, skills of close reading – a feel for pathos, a discriminating ear, a discerning eye, an analogical imagination, a way with words...[21]

The medical humanist model has been evolving over four years. Initially, an advocacy group and private practice oncologist jointly funded a part-time patient advocate. It soon became evident that it was not advocacy in the traditional sense that was needed but, rather, support for both doctor and patient. In October of 2001, The Institute of Medical Humanism, Inc. was founded in Bennington, Vermont. One of its missions is the promotion of the medical humanist in practice model. The Institute created a job description for a medical humanist and joined with Southwestern Vermont Health Care, a regional hospital, in a collaboration to produce a replicable model and extend the use of humanism throughout the healthcare system. A significant commitment to incorporate a medical humanist and the humanities into the care of patients has been made.

On behalf of the Institute for Medical Humanism a doctor, writer, patient advocate and clinical psychologist developed the medical humanist model. Each has played an important role in the evolution of the model within the cancer center setting.

2. Medical Humanist

The medical humanist is a writer and not a medical professional. A review of her work described her as a poet who writes stories. Her function is not clinical. She speaks no medical language. "The poet's function is to speak of the encounter."[22] She is not to be confused with either a medical social worker or case manager, both of whom bring external resources to the patient. The medical humanist relates directly to the patient and presents the opportunity for discovery, creativity, and deeper insight through the window of the humanities. This process draws on the patient's inner resources. The medical humanist listens carefully and bears witness to the patient's narrative/description about his/her cancer experience. She is skilled at recognizing stories from the lived world of illness and documenting them for the patient's health care team. In doing so she validates the patients' experience, enhances doctors' understanding of the patient's view and improves doctor/patient communication. The medical humanist becomes an interpreter for the doctor and an escort for the patient in the new and unfamiliar world of illness. The medical humanist provides increased opportunities to acknowledge the uncertainties involved in illness for both doctor and patient. She serves as a bridge between the "two cultures" of humanities and science.

The medical humanist works directly with patients who are newly diagnosed, whom have recurrent disease or who are in the end stage of life. By necessity, she also works with the families of those patients. The medical humanist also participates in Cancer Center staff meetings, tumor board, and hospice educational programs. She is a member of the *Task Force on Breast Cancer Quality Improvement* and the *Task Force to Improve the Care Of the Dying Patient*. She also provides consultation services to nurses on the hospital oncology service, radiologists responsible for cancer screening and the staff of the long-term care facility where many oncology patients spend a period of time. In addition, the medical humanist provides patients the opportunity to write either individually or with a bi-monthly writing group. Studies have shown that reframing the illness experience through writing can be transformative[22] and reduces side effects of treatment.[24] The importance of listening to the language and story of the patient's in-illness experience is being brought to the patient, doctor, health care system and the community.

3. The Doctor

The doctor has been practicing oncology for 22 years. Nineteen of those years were spent practicing academic medicine. She has published widely, and has trained interns and residents. She moved into private practice in the hope that she would have more time to spend with patients. Moving from an academic center to private practice changed the demands but did not lessen them. The doctor plays a role in promoting the medical humanist in practice model and articulating the problems from her perspective. She has said,

> "So much of what we do as doctors is about language. We have a special language to match our specialized knowledge. The more we speak in this language the more comfortable it becomes. The language we use influences our thinking. Medical language separates us from others. It also forces us to limit and objectify our impressions of our patients. This process can limit our vision."

She continued,

> "In her search for the right words as a writer, the medical humanist has developed acute powers of observation. She often hears the question lurking underneath. Patients are often able to speak of their concerns to her without fear of offending a doctor they depend on. A medical humanist provides skilled listening. She can help doctors script difficult conversations. She quotes Emily Dickinson to remind doctors to 'Tell all the truth, but tell it slant – The truth must dazzle gradually – Or every man be blind.'"[25-26]

The major obstacle to integration in the health care team from the physician perspective has been in keeping the boundary clear between counseling and skilled listening. The medical humanist has to report to the health care providers what the patient is hearing without offering counseling to the patient. This takes skill and understanding on the part of both the health care team and the medical humanist but can be done with time and experience.

4. Patient Advocate

The patient advocate, a woman with advanced metastatic disease, has focused on the needs of the population she represents. She has opened her journals, served as reporter, and exposed her fear and vulnerability in a way that has informed both the medical humanist and doctor. She brings her own sensitivity to the language used during medical encounters to the development of the model.

5. Clinical Psychologist

The psychologist brings 14 years of work in this oncology practice to the project. Throughout his tenure with the practice, he has been a referral resource for patients and their families undergoing unusual stress and has facilitated support groups. He provides supervision for the medical humanist in her direct work with patients. He has been an advocate for the incorporation of the medical humanist in the practice because of his belief that fear, vulnerability and uncertainty are normal responses to diagnosis. The psychologist also facilitates Balint groups for all the providers in the practice as another way of acknowledging the normal emotional challenges they face.[27] Doctors need to be released from the requirement to always be in control and to be free to learn from their uniquely intimate exposure to the uncertainty of the human condition. If they are able to do this, doctor/patient communication becomes an opportunity for personal growth for both parties.[28]

6. Medical Humanist's Notes from The Field

The medical humanist makes contact with the new patient prior to his/her first appointment with the doctor. This becomes the opportunity for the medical humanist to introduce herself as his/her escort into unknown territory where the language is foreign and the outcome is uncertain. Often the patient provides cues about their own perspective on diagnosis in early conversations.

The patient verbalizes, "You hear the word cancer and your whole world is turned upside down." The medical humanist uses metaphor as a way of moving from the known to the unknown and says, "Most of us come into the world head first." The patient replies, "Are you likening a diagnosis of cancer to a birth?" "I am," she says and tells him the word "cancer" first kills us with its name because we have allowed it to become synonymous with death. It is not a death sentence but rather one word in a sentence.

The word is difficult to hear and to say. One patient asks the medical humanist if there is a protocol for notifying family and friends that you have been diagnosed with cancer. The medical humanist admits there is not. "Do you think e-mail is an acceptable form?" the patient asks. The medical humanist tells her it could be one of the prescribed forms. It is a form of writing. E-mail allows you the time to compose your thoughts, to construct the actual message you want to send and to connect with another. The person receiving your message has time to think about what it is you have said and how to respond. E-mail protects you from seeing someone's initial response to hearing the word "cancer."

The patient is looking out the window when he says, "If only I had been more religious – prayed more I wouldn't have gotten cancer." The medical humanist brings the words of the poet W.H. Auden to the patient as an opportunity to reframe his belief. From memory she says, "To pray is to pay attention to something or someone other than oneself. Whenever a man so concentrates his attention on a landscape, a poem, a geometrical problem, an idol or the True God – that they completely forget their own ego and desires, he is praying …"[29] The patient's response is one of relief, "So maybe I've prayed more than I think."

Doctors often request assistance when they have explained something and the patient still says he doesn't understand.[30] It is easy to forget that bad news is not heard in complete sentences. The medical humanist can often discover the source of misunderstanding and translate the patient's cues so that misunderstandings are clarified.[31] Often the patients want information to which they can relate their own experience of illness rather than the medical description. The medical humanist has helped the doctor to see that collapsed veins are not a medical crisis – they are a personal crisis – symbolizing failure and being worn out, worn thin and collapsed by treatment.

Many patients seek alternative care providers. Often they are seeking assurance that cure is possible. While some reject traditional care altogether, many others do not tell their doctors about the alternatives they are using.[32] In a number of cases, alternative treatments used by a patient are not discussed during visits with the doctor but are discussed with the medical humanist. One patient is a nationally known artist in her sixties. Throughout her treatment, she has continued to work in her studio. Her energy is now limited as are her options for treatment. The medical humanist goes in to talk with her while she's being treated. In her lap is a book: it's unopened, and the title advertises "A Beautiful Life." The medical humanist asks her, "What are you reading?" The patient replies, "It's a book written by a woman who also has Stage IV ovarian cancer who says she's alive fourteen years after her diagnosis because she adheres to a strict macrobiotic diet." She describes, in detail, how she has to prepare what it is she is allowed to eat. "The vegetables," she says, "must be indigenous to the area." It is at that moment that the patient realizes that she could spend her energy on food preparation and adjust to a new diet in an effort to stave off death or she could spend time in her studio and use her art to live.

The medical humanist finds another patient scanning the bookshelves in the cancer center library. He had been diagnosed with multiple myeloma and was post bone marrow transplant. She asks if she can help him find something. “Someone suggested that I consult a healer. Do you have a directory of healers?” he asks. “Healers,” the medical humanist says, “come in unexpected places. Be cautious of leaflets that offer the promise of cure. What exactly are you looking for?” He answers, “My old self back.” He had worked in construction and found himself physically weakened by treatment. Using his former occupation as the metaphor, we talked about how he could reconstruct his life. The medical humanist offered to speak with his doctor about having him work with a physical therapist to regain his strength in an attempt to get his “old self back.” Six weeks later the doctor received a progress note from the physical therapist reporting that he was getting stronger, had increased the weights he used and had begun walking on the treadmill.

Humor can also be a tool of the medical humanist. She overhears a patient who has just walked into a full waiting room announcing, “I don’t want to be here.” She responds, “Anyone who wants to be here, raise your hand.” The open laughter creates a climate in which patients begin to exchange stories. Another patient asked the question “How do I live one day at a time?” Crouched down next to the patient while looking up at him, the medical humanist does not quote Robert Frost, Soren Kierkegaard or a Zen master. In this instance, with the patient’s voice in mind, she quotes the wisdom of her 83-year-old mother who advises, “Don’t buy green bananas.”

As a member of *The Task Force to Improve the Care Of the Dying Patient*, the medical humanist asks if the name doesn’t belie the task. “Shouldn’t we be thinking about how to help patients live until they take their last breath?”

The medical humanist regularly visits patients on the hospital oncology service. She was in the room when a dying patient had to decide whether or not to be intubated. Intubation would prolong her life so that she might see her daughter who had not yet arrived from Chicago. However, it would prevent her from being able to speak. The patient voiced her overriding concern, “But there are things I need to say to her…” There was a feeling of urgency in the room for the doctor who needed to begin medical intervention and the mother who wanted to see and speak to her daughter for what would be the last time. The tools of a medical humanist, who is a writer, are a paper and pen. “Tell me what you want to say to your daughter, I will write it down in your own words for her.” The patient spoke; the medical humanist wrote, as the anesthesiologist and surgeon prepared to intubate her. When the daughter arrived, they used the written words to have a meaningful dialogue.

Following the death of three patients in one week the medical humanist sent an e-mail to the nurses and case manager at the hospital to acknowledge the extraordinary care they provided and to recognize their loss. She began her message with an epigram, "The Dyings have been too deep for me, and before I raise my heart from one, another has come"[33] and ends with "I will report to the *Task Force Working to Improve the Care of the Dying Patient* how you helped each patient live until they took their last breath. It is a privilege to work with each of you."

At Christmas, the medical humanist chose to show her gratitude to surgeons in whose hands we put our lives. She decided on a gift of hand cream to which she attached an Emily Dickinson poem. "Surgeons must be very careful / When they take the knife! / Underneath their fine incisions / Stirs the Culprit – *Life!*"[34] In several of the thank you notes to the medical humanist, the surgeons acknowledged the poem as the real gift.

In another effort to bridge the humanities and medicine, the medical humanist has worked with a professional curator and a local foundation to introduce abstract art into the cancer center. "Human life itself may be almost pure chaos, but the work of the artist is to take these handfuls of confusion and disparate things that seem to be irreconcilable, and put them together in a frame to give them some kind of shape and meaning."[35] One of the doctors in the practice came to the medical humanist to ask, "What am I supposed to say to patients who say they don't like abstract art?" "Ask them why they don't like it," the medical humanist encouraged. The doctor reported, "They said they don't understand it." "Great!" she exclaimed. "Tell them it's sort of like cancer… you don't like it and you don't understand it… and it will open up the conversation about what it means for him or her to have cancer!" And it did. On another day, the medical humanist noticed an oncology nurse sitting in a treatment chair. "What are you doing?" she inquired. "I'm sitting here looking at this painting, trying to see what the patient told me they saw in the painting," the nurse replied. "That's exactly what I intended with this exhibit," the medical humanist explained, "for all of us to see the experience through the patient's eyes."

Both examples show what the medical humanist intended with these exhibits. She wanted to provide opportunities for discovery, creativity, and deeper insight into the human condition, with the intention of relaxing barriers and opening doors for improved communication among patients, doctors, and nurses.

7. Conclusion

An oncologist, clinical psychologist, patient advocate, and writer have worked in collaboration with a regional medical center to implement a new program aimed at improving doctor-patient communication. This program puts a writer/medical humanist into the oncology practice on a daily basis working directly with providers, patients, their families, and other hospital staff in real time. The writer/medical humanist brings to her work a keen sense of observation, empathetic listening skills, and access to the humanities. Patients feel cared for and doctors and patients report increased satisfaction with doctor/patient communication. The medical humanist is only slowly being accepted throughout the system because a lack of any credentials in medical training has been perceived as a barrier to acceptance. It is important to keep skilled listening separate from counseling, so integration into the health care team remains tentative at times. The role of the clinical psychologist in clarifying the difference has been important to everyone developing the model. A great deal has been learned within the oncology practice and much of it can be applied in the care of patients with other chronic illnesses. The expansion of this program will require research that documents its outcomes. The assurance that the medical humanist program can be systematized and replicable is far from complete. Further research is necessary to assess the impact that the medical humanist has on doctors and patients but to date, anecdotal evidence suggests both have judged the program a success. Replication of the model will require training of additional medical humanists as well as doctors who will welcome them into their practices.

Notes

[1] Francis W. Peabody, "The Care of the Patient," *Journal of the American Medical Association* 88 (1927): 877-82; reprinted 252 (1984): 813-818.

[2] Lewis Thomas, "On Matters of Doubt" in *Late Night Thoughts on Listening to Mahler's Ninth Symphony* (New York: Viking Press, 1980), 156-157.

[3] Wendy Levinson et al., "A Study of Patient Clues and Physician Responses in Primary Care and Surgical Settings," *Journal of the American Medical Association* 284 (2000): 1021-1027.

[4] William T. Merkel et al., "Teaching Humanistic and Psychosocial Aspects of Care: Current Practices and Attitudes," *Journal of General Internal Medicine* 5 (1990): 34-41.

[5] W. T. Branch et al., "Teaching Medicine as A Human Experience: A Patient-Doctor Relationship Course for Faculty and First-Year Medical Students," *Annals of Internal Medicine* 114 (1991): 482-489.

[6] Robert M. Arnold et al., "The Humanities, Humanistic Behavior and The Humane Physician: A Cautionary Note," *Annals of Internal Medicine* 106 (1987): 313-318.

[7] Howard M. Spiro, "What Is Empathy And Can It Be Taught?" *Annals of Internal Medicine* 116 (1992): 843-846.

[8] Abraham Verghese, "The Physician as Storyteller," *Annals of Internal Medicine* 135 (2001): 1012-1017.
[9] William J. Donnelly, "Righting the Medical Record: Transforming Chronicle Into Story," *Journal of the American Medical Association* 260 (1988): 823-825.
[10] Rita Charon, "The Narrative Road to Empathy," in *Empathy and the Power of Medicine*, ed. Howard M. Spiro (New Haven: Yale University Press, 1993), 147-159.
[11] Ronald M. Epstein, "Mindful Practice," *Journal of the American Medical Association* 282 (1999): 833-839.
[12] Dennis H. Novack et al., "Calibrating the Physician, Personal Awareness and Effective Patient Care: Working Group on Promoting Physician Personal Awareness, American Academy on Physician and Patient," *Journal of the American Medical Association* 278 (1997): 502-509.
[13] Schwartz Center Rounds Program, Kenneth B. Schwartz Center.
[14] Timothy E. Quill and Anthony L. Suchman, "Uncertainty and Control: Learning to Live with Medicine's Limitations," *Humane Medicine* 9 (1993): 109-120.
[15] George Lakoff and Mark Johnson, *Metaphors We Live By* (Chicago: University of Chicago Press, 1980).
[16] Stephen S. Pearce, *Flash of Insight: Metaphor and Narrative in Therapy* (Boston: Allyn and Bacon, 1996).
[17] Katheryn Montgomery Hunter, *Doctors' Stories: The Narrative Structure of Medical Knowledge* (Princeton, NJ: Princeton University Press, 1991).
[18] S. Kay Toombs, "The Meaning of Illness: A Phenomenological Account of the Differences of Physician and Patient," *Philosophy of Medicine* 42 (1992).
[19] Quill and Suchman, 109-20.
[20] Robert C. Smith and Ruth B. Hoppe, "The Patient's Story: Integrating the Patient and Physician-Centered Approaches to Interviewing," *Annals of Internal Medicine* 115 (1991):470-477.
[21] Ronald Carson, "Teaching Ethics in the Context of Medical Humanities," *Journal of Medical Ethics* 20(4) (1994): 235-8.
[22] Maxine W. Kumin, *Always Beginning: Essays on a Life in Poetry* (Port Townsend, Washington: Copper Canyon Press, 2000).
[23] James W. Pennebaker, "Telling Stories: The Health Benefits of Narrative," *Literature and Medicine* 19 (2001): 3-18.
[24] Joshua M. Smyth et al., "Effects of Writing about Stressful Experiences on Symptom Reduction in Patients with Asthma or Rheumatoid Arthritis: a Randomized Trial," *JAMA* 281 (1991):1304-1309.
[25] Thomas H. Johnson, ed. *The Complete Poems of Emily Dickinson* (New York: Little, Brown and Company, 1961), 506.

[26] Letha Mills, Talk Presented at Brown University Medical School, January, 1999.
[27] John Salinsky, "Balint Groups: History, Aims and Method," *American Balint Society*. 1997. <http://familymed.musc.edu/balint/overview.html> (4 December 2000).
[28] Quill and Suchman, 109-120
[29] W.H. Auden, *A Certain World: Nature of Prayer* (New York: Viking Press, 1970).
[30] Eduardo Bruera et al., "Treatment Decisions for Breast Carcinoma," *Cancer* 94 (2002): 2076-2080.
[31] Levinson et al., 1021-1027.
[32] Anne Hunsaker Hawkins, "Restoring The Patient's Voice: The Case of Gilda Radner," *Yale Journal of Biology and Medicine* 65 (1992): 173-181.
[33] Howard M. Spiro et al., *Facing Death: Where Culture, Religion and Medicine Meet* (New Haven: Yale University Press, 1996).
[34] Johnson, ed., 506.
[35] George Plimpton, ed. *Women Writers at Work* (2nd series) Paris Review (New York: Random House, 1968).

Bibliography

Arnold, Robert M., Gail J. Povar, and Joel D Howell. "The Humanities, Humanistic Behavior and The Humane Physician: A Cautionary Note." *Annals of Internal Medicine* 106 (1987): 313-318.

Auden, W.H. *A Certain World: "Nature of Prayer*". New York: Viking Press, 1970.

Branch, W.T., R.A. Arky, B. Woo, J.D. Stoekle, D.B. Levy and W.C. Taylor. "Teaching Medicine as a Human Experience: A Patient-Doctor Relationship Course for Faculty and First-Year Medical Students." *Annals of Internal Medicine* 114 (1991): 482-489.

Bruera, Eduardo, J.S. Willey, P.J. Lynn and M. Rosales. "Treatment Decisions for Breast Carcinoma." *Cancer* 94 (2002): 2076-2080.

Carson, Ronald. "Teaching Ethics In The Context Of Medical Humanities." *Journal of Medical Ethics* 20 (4) (1994): 235-8.

Charon, Rita. "The Narrative Road To Empathy." In *Empathy and the Power of Medicine*, edited by Howard M. Spiro, 147-159. New Haven: Yale University Press, 1993.

Donnelly, William J. "Righting the Medical Record: Transforming Chronicle into Story." *Journal of the American Medical Association* 260 (1988): 823-825.

Epstein, Ronald M. "Mindful Practice." *Journal of the American Medical Association* 282 (1999): 833-839.

Hawkins, Anne Hunsaker . "Restoring The Patient's Voice: The Case Of Gilda Radner" *Yale Journal of Biology and Medicine* 65 (1992): 173-181.

Hunter, Katheryn Montgomery. *Doctors' Stories: The Narrative Structure of Medical Knowledge.* Princeton, NJ: Princeton University Press, 1991.

Johnson, Thomas H., ed. *The Complete Poems of Emily Dickinson*. New York: Little, Brown and Company, 1961.

Kumin, Maxine W. *Always Beginning: Essays on a Life in Poetry*. Port Townsend, WA: Copper Canyon Press, 2000.

Lakoff, George and Mark Johnson. *Metaphors We Live By*. Chicago: University of Chicago Press, 1980.

Levinson, Wendy, Rita Gorwara-Bhat, and Jennifer Lamb. "A Study of Patient Clues and Physician Responses in Primary Care and Surgical Settings". *Journal of the American Medical Association* 284 (2000): 1021-1027.

Merkel, William T., Ronald B. Margolis, and Robert C. Smith. "Teaching Humanistic and Psychosocial Aspects of Care: Current Practices and Attitudes." *Journal of General Internal Medicine* 5 (1990): 34-41.

Mills, Letha. Talk Presented at Brown University Medical School, January, 1999.

Novack, Dennis H., Anthony L. Suchman, William Clark, Ronald M. Epstein, Eva Najberg, and Craig Kaplan. "Calibrating The Physician, Personal Awareness And Effective Patient Care: Working Group On Promoting Physician Personal Awareness, American Academy on Physician and Patient." *Journal of the American Medical Association* 278 (1997): 502-509.

Peabody, Francis W. "The Care of the Patient." *Journal of the American Medical Association* 88 (1927): 877-82; reprinted 252 (1984): 813-818.

Pearce, Stephen S. *Flash of Insight: Metaphor And Narrative In Therapy*. Boston: Allyn and Bacon, 1996.

Pennebaker, James W. "Telling Stories: The Health Benefits Of Narrative." *Literature and Medicine* 19 (2001): 3-18.

Plimpton, George, ed. *Women Writers at Work.* (2nd series) Paris Review. New York: Random House, 1968.

Quill, Timothy E. and Anthony L. Suchman, "Uncertainty And Control: Learning To Live With Medicine's Limitations." *Humane Medicine* 9 (1993):109-120.

Salinsky, John. Balint Groups: History, Aims and Method. American Balint Society. 1997. <http://familymed.musc.edu/balint/overview.html> (4 December 2000).

Schwartz Center, Kenneth B. Schwartz Center Rounds Program.

Smith, Robert C. and Ruth B. Hoppe. "The Patient's Story: Integrating The Patient And Physician-Centered Approaches to Interviewing." *Annals of Internal Medicine* 115 (1991): 470-477.

Smyth, Joshua M., "Effects of Writing about Stressful Experiences on Symptom Reduction in Patients with Asthma or Rheumatoid Arthritis: A Randomized Trial." *Journal of the American Medical Association* 281 (1991): 1304-1309.

Spiro, Howard M., ed. *Empathy and the Power of Medicine*. New Haven: Yale University Press, 1993.

Spiro, Howard M., Mary McCrea Curnen, and Lee Palmer Wandel. *Facing Death: Where Culture, Religion and Medicine Meet*. New Haven: Yale University Press, 1996.

Spiro, Howard M. "What Is Empathy And Can It Be Taught?," *Annals of Internal Medicine* 116 (1992): 843-846.

Thomas, Lewis. "On Matters of Doubt" in *Late Night Thoughts on Listening to Mahler's Ninth Symphony*. New York: Viking Press, 1980.

Toombs, S. Kay. "The Meaning Of Illness: A Phenomenological Account Of The Differences Of Physician And Patient". *Philosophy of Medicine* 42 (1992).

Verghese, Abraham. "The Physician as Storyteller," *Annals of Internal Medicine* 135 (2001): 1012-1017.

Note on Contributors

Bernard M. Bandman, PhD, is a clinical psychologist at Southwestern Vermont Regional Cancer Center in Bennington, Vermont. He is a co-founder of the Institute of Medical Humanism whose mission is to improve doctor/patient communication. The Institute's model incorporates a medical humanist, a writer, into day-to-day medical practice to bridge the differences between the languages of medicine and the patient's lived world of illness. The model is now being expanded to other medical practices that care for patients with chronic illness.

Celia Bandman, is a published writer who works as a medical humanist at Southwestern Vermont Regional Cancer Center and is a co-founder of the Institute of Medical Humanism. Ms. Bandman has developed a writing program for patients. It is a new genre; the genre of the patient's voice, which communicates what he or she understands and feels about their diagnoses and how they are coping with the effects of chronic illness. This is included in their medical record.

Patricia Barr (1950-2003), an attorney, patient advocate, health policy advisor and a co-founder of the Institute of Medical Humanism used her personal cancer experience to inform her work for the benefit of a larger population. In 2003, she was posthumously awarded *The Genetic Alliance Art of Advocacy Award* for her work on the Secretary of Health and Human Services Advisory Committee on Genetic Testing.

Letha E. Mills, M.D. is a practicing hematologist/oncologist and medical director at Southwestern Vermont Regional Cancer Center in Bennington, Vermont. Prior to joining the Cancer Center staff she was at Dartmouth Hitchcock Medical Center where she trained interns and residents. She has published 74 documents including articles, book chapters, abstracts and written numerous clinical trials. She is interested in medical humanism, palliative care and improving care for women with breast cancer.

Acknowledgments

The authors would like to acknowledge the support of the staff of SVHC Oncology Associates, Southwestern Vermont Health Care Corporation and Anne Conklin Gatling.

Part 4

Making Sense of Living with Illness

Theoretical Perspectives of Health and Understandings of Living Well with Chronic Illness

Susan L. Mills

1. Introduction

Researchers have spent considerable effort developing knowledge of the ways individuals respond, and live with illness, and studies reveal considerable diversity in the way individuals adapt on a day-to-day basis. [1,2] It is apparent that some individuals integrate illnesses into their lives in a way that may enable them to have a good life, or live well as evidenced by a wide variety of findings of positive[3] (or favourable) responses, and experiences. These findings present interesting paradoxes in relation to more common understandings of illness as a life long burden of suffering, and pain,[4] and in relation to considerable societal effort to prevent disease, and find cures.[5] As such, living well with chronic illness presents an intriguing area of inquiry.

Within this developing body of knowledge, understandings of living well with chronic illness are influenced by theoretical perspectives of health, and related concepts that provide frameworks for conceptualizing positive notions of a good life. Studies investigating chronic illness experiences are situated in particular theoretical perspectives of illness that, by and large, define ways of understanding how illness experiences are shaped and created. Understandings of living well with illness are necessarily situated within these theoretical frameworks, and particular constructions of chronic illness. However, theoretical ideas on health are intertwined with perspectives of illness,[6] and provide frameworks for conceptualizing, and making sense of what it means to have a good life or live well with chronic illness. Since theoretical perspectives are not always explicitly acknowledged or considered in the interpretation of data, and development of chronic illness knowledge,[7] it is useful to reflect on how perspectives of health may be shaping our understanding of living well with illness.

This paper explores some of these theoretical perspectives of health and the ways in which they may be influencing developing knowledge. I begin with an overview of some of positive illness findings emerging in diverse bodies of research, and outline major understandings of living well presented in the literature. Then, I review some of the major theoretical perspectives of health (and related concepts) articulated in the health, and social science literature, and discuss how these ideas are shaping our current thinking about, and knowledge of, living well with chronic illness. For purposes of this paper, 'chronic illness' is defined as a way of living with, or experiencing, a biomedically diagnosed disease that is incurable, dynamic, and continuous across an individual's lifespan.[8] 'Living well' with chronic illness is used as a working term to represent a favourable way of living with illness, or a good life that is described in the health and social science literature using different concepts and terminology.

2. Findings Related to Living Well with Chronic Illness and Current Understandings

Favourable outcomes, and experiences of illness are becoming common in the literature.[9,10,11] They emerge in research using a range of theoretical perspectives (positivistic, interpretive etc.), analytical foci (e.g. psychological, behavioural, social), methods (e.g. quantitative, and qualitative), and research questions (e.g. What is the quality of life of chronically ill populations?; What are the psychological benefits of living with chronic stress?; What are the lived experiences of chronic illness?) but all document aspects of chronic illness that clearly differ from those of pain, suffering, loss, disability, and social isolation.[12-13] Findings are found in studies exploring living with chronic illness in a general sense[14] or in research explicitly addressing positive representations of illness (e.g. benefit-finding,[15] doing well,[16] health within illness,[17] positive narratives,[18] positive life experiences[19]), and they are described within a number of different research frameworks as optimal levels of health outcomes, psychological benefits, certain kinds of illness phenomena, and specific types of narratives. Living well experiences are also outlined in the lay literature through autobiographical accounts.

Researchers investigating the psychosocial effects of chronic illness in quantifiable terms (i.e., using health outcome measures) have found that some chronically ill and/or disabled individuals perceive themselves to have high levels of functioning, well-being and/or quality of life,[20] and these findings are also supported in qualitative research where, for example, Albrecht and Devlieger found 54.3% of persons with severe disabilities (e.g. arthritis, multiple sclerosis, diabetes, paralysis, head injury, mental illnesses) felt they had good or excellent quality of life.[21] Research has also found that some individuals perceive themselves as healthy in the presence of chronic illness and/or disability.[22]

Additional evidence of positive illness findings is found in the field of positive psychology. Within this body of research, studies on the positive outcomes of stress, and coping have found evidence of positive affect in individuals experiencing chronic stress[23] as well as evidence of other types of positive outcomes such as stress-related growth, positive personal changes, meaning-making, benefit-finding, and crisis growth.[24] For instance, a number of perceived benefits such as strengthening of personal relationships, favourable changes in personality such as greater patience, courage, empathy, and changing of life priorities, and personal goals have been articulated by individuals with a wide range of major medical conditions.[25] These types of findings are supported by research on life crisis, and growth where researchers have identified enhanced social resources (e.g. stronger relationships with family and friends, new support networks); enhanced personal resources (e.g. cognitive, and intellectual differentiation, self-reliance, empathy, altruism, changes in priorities, and values); and the development of new coping skills (e.g. cognitive coping skills, problem solving skills as three types of positive outcomes) as major types of positive responses to crisis situations.[26]

Research exploring the subjective experience of illness from the perspective of individuals living with long term conditions also identifies favourable illness findings. In fact, results from a recent meta-synthesis of these qualitative studies suggest that this type of research has shifted its focus in the last decade to "uncovering those aspects of chronic illness that are healthy, transformative, and positive."[27] Positive illness phenomena described in the literature include finding connections with others, growth, transformation, expanding consciousness, transcendence, finding meaning or purpose in life, and feeling healthy.[28] In addition to these types of findings that relate favourable experiences to psychological phenomena such as change and transformation, other research has found that behavioural aspects such as the performance of social roles and functions, and participating in desired activities are also related to positive illness experiences.[29]

Findings also emerge in narrative research, particularly in descriptions of heroic narratives (illness stories that progressively move towards personally valued goals),[30] restitution narratives (illness stories that emphasize positive outcomes, and ideas of health), and quest narratives (illness stories where individuals search for alternative ways of being ill such as finding meaning, and transcendence through their illness experience).[31,32] For example, Robinson's investigations into the narratives of individuals with multiple sclerosis have revealed that some individuals have more positive, and optimistic approaches to living with chronic illness.[33,34] In addition to narrative stories, autobiographical accounts provide another important source of positive illness experiences outside of the research context.[35] These life stories often articulate a view of overcoming the adversities, and challenges of chronic illness to find new meaning, and perspectives of life (e.g. living in the moment, finding increased capacity to enjoy life etc.)[36] and often suggest that spiritual, intellectual, and emotional capacities are enhanced rather than diminished by long term conditions.[37] Some even imply that life can be transformed for the better by disease.[38]

These diverse findings reflect a range of understandings of what living well with chronic illness entails, and represent different research paradigms (positivistic, interpretive etc.) and purposes. Positivistic research has developed conceptual notions related to a good life that can be quantified, and measured in chronically ill populations with the intent of assessing the impacts of chronic illness on individuals' lives, describing the characteristics of specific illness populations, and/or determining differences between groups of individuals. Measures of functional ability, well-being and quality of life represent well-accepted, population-based ideas, or standards of what is considered important in living with illness. In chronic illness research, quality of life is often described as the optimum level of "mental, physical, role and social functioning, including relationships and perceptions of health, fitness, life satisfaction and well-being"[39] and represents an individual's combined perceptions of functional ability, health status, and well-being as well as perceptions of overall health.[40] This body of research conceptualizes living well with illness as being able to function in society and partake in desired activities, experiencing pleasant emotions and moods, and/or achieving a global sense of satisfaction or happiness in life, and often sets the standard for the optimal life with illness in relation to both particular types of feelings, and daily behaviours or functions.

In contrast, interpretive approaches have used insider[41] or subjective illness knowledge to gain insights into the complexities of living with chronic illness, to identify important themes and patterns, as well as variation and diversity in individualized understandings. Within this research, some studies have documented positive illness phenomena cited earlier (e.g. growth, transformation, transcendence etc.) as well as other characteristics that seem associated with positive illness experiences, such as being in control,[42] having mastery over disease/life,[43] having positive attitudes/thinking,[44] and functional concepts such as doing things you want to do,[45] being active,[46] and fulfilling social roles.[47] Much of this research is focused on understanding individuals' favourable responses to illness in relation to psychological phenomena but the diversity of terminology and concepts used to describe findings in these qualitative studies makes it difficult to determine the inter-relatedness of concepts both within and across studies,[48,49] and has created a body of knowledge related to living well with chronic illness that is confusing and elusive.[50] Some authors acknowledge the inter-relationships between the themes in their studies,[51] or between their study and other work in the field,[52] but on the whole researchers place emphasis on describing the phenomenon of interest rather than interpreting their findings in relation to the broader context of knowledge.[53] Although it is difficult to get a clear understanding of major patterns, and themes involved in living well from insider research, this research suggests that a large number of psychological, and behavioural phenomena are associated with a more favourable life with illness.

As noted, positivistic, and interpretive research present different frameworks for studying chronic illness that influence how we conceptualize living a good life, or well in the context of illness. However, theoretical perspectives of health (and related concepts) in the health, and social science literature present a number of important views of what it means to have a good life that also influence these areas of research, and our understandings of living well with illness.

3. Theoretical Perspectives of Health and Related Concepts

Numerous authors have put forth ideas on what it means to have a good life, most notably in relation to understandings of health, and related concepts. These perspectives of health hold different assumptions about the nature of the health-illness relationship, and although understandings of health and illness/disease cannot conceptually co-exist in some theories, many of the health related ideas have been influential in chronic illness research. A review of some of the major theories originating in medicine, nursing, psychology and sociology provides insights into some of the major ideas that seem to be shaping how understandings of living well are developing in the literature. These include the biomedical, World Health Organization (WHO), adaptation, wellness, humanist, developmental, and functional perspectives of health.[54]

In the biomedical sciences, health has traditionally represented freedom from disease, disability and physiological abnormalities[55] and is represented by a body with physiological integrity.[56] This understanding has shaped biomedical practice and research and has been influential in discourse on health and illness in the social sciences,[57] and in chronic illness research.[58] It is based on biologic (or disease) theory,[59] and ideas from philosophical traditions in Greek medicine such as Decartes' (1596-1650) dualistic and mechanistic interpretation of the human body,[60] and reductionism.[61] The biomedical perspective of health was expanded by the World Health Organization (WHO) who defined health as a "state of complete physical, mental and social well-being, not merely the absence of disease or infirmity."[62] This interpretation constructed health as a positive and enhancing experience above, and beyond the absence of disease, and placed human health in a broader social context.[63] Since its publication, the WHO's model of health has become the most widely accepted understanding in the Western world,[64] and many other theoretical perspectives of health have been developed in response to this view.

In opposition to the WHO perspective, Rene Dubos, a microbiologist and experimental pathologist, presented an adaptational view of health that moved beyond the absence of disease and an ideal state of well-being to an understanding of a whole person interacting with their physical and social environment.[65] He argued that "health is not an ideal state of well-being achieved through the complete elimination of disease but a modus vivendi enabling imperfect men to achieve a rewarding and not too painful existence while they cope with an imperfect world."[66]

Health is the ability of an individual to maintain a flexible two-way interaction with the environment (conceptualized as the physical and social realms as well as man's perceptual and conceptual worlds).[67] An individual adjusts his biological and social responses to cope with the environment but also changes the environment to meet his needs. Dubos developed his ideas using systems theory,[68] and although he did not deny the functioning of physiological mechanisms in the process of adaptation, the emphasis was clearly placed on psychological, social and cultural dimensions.[69]

Around the same time, Halbert Dunn, a physician and statistician, introduced the concept of high level wellness as an interpretation of the WHO's notion of 'complete physical, mental and social well-being.'[70] He defined it as an "integrated method of functioning which is oriented toward maximizing the potential of which the individual is capable within the environment where he is functioning."[71] From his perspective, mind, body and spirit of human beings are an interrelated and interdependent whole, and individuals continually move towards higher and higher levels of functioning. This dynamic and continually changing process is dependent upon an open ended and ever expanding environment that challenges individuals to live at their full potential. In recent years the concept of wellness has become synonymous with a specific type of lifestyle aimed towards disease prevention, health promotion and a future state of holistic health.[72,73] Although a variety of interpretations of wellness have been articulated since the publication of Dunn's original work, many of them define the concept as the complete integration of an individual's physical, social, mental, emotional and spiritual dimensions that is achieved via a reciprocal communication process between individuals and their environments.[74] In addition, they often place a strong role on individual responsibility by arguing that the ability to achieve wellness resides within the individual.[75] Dunn viewed high level wellness as an approach to disease prevention but more recent interpretations of wellness do not preclude disease or illness.[76]

Within psychology, another important health theory developed within a humanist framework. Abraham Maslow viewed health as a process of self-actualization, defined as "experiencing fully, vividly, selflessly, with full concentration, and total absorption," and he conceptualized it as both an end state, as well as a "process of actualizing one's potentialities at any time."[77] Self-actualization is a holistic experience that focuses on the inner world of an individual, and is a latent self-development ability within all individuals.[78-80] Disease (or illness) can impede or prevent the process of self-actualization given that optimal physiological functioning is one of the first steps along the journey.[81] But others have interpreted the pool of ideas associated with the humanist perspective of health in such a way that disease, illness and health can co-exist.[82]

Another important view of health is represented in the development model created in nursing science by authors such as Rogers, Newman, Pender, and Parse. Rogers[83] is attributed with developing the original idea of a developmental, and transformative understanding of health but it is also described in terms of expanding consciousness and self-actualization.[84] Newman presents a synthesized view of health and illness whereby illness allows for patterns of expanding consciousness to emerge that are manifestations of health.[85] Pender also supports an unitary perspective of health and illness but describes the developmental process in self-actualizing terms.[86] According to Parse, health is a dynamic concept that is not defined by societal norms but rather individually created and defined. Health also varies over time and under different circumstances.[87] It is a process of unfolding that occurs regardless of an individual's health-illness condition, and is "co-created through human-environment interaction."[88-89] Although there are some distinct differences in the developmental conceptualizations of health, most assume that health is represented by the dynamic whole of life experience (not the physiological integrity of the human body); that health is not on a linear continuum with illness; and that there is no single understanding of health shared by everyone.[90]

Outside of the health science domain, a very different but important conceptualization of health emerged in medical sociology through the work of Talcott Parsons who sought to understand the structures and functions of the social system, and to define health and illness in the context of social role structure and control.[91-92] He built his ideas upon the systems theory from physiology and biology as well as the structural functionalism tradition in anthropology, to relate the health and illness of an individual to the broader social context. Parsons defined health as "the state of optimum capacity of an individual for the effective performance of the roles and tasks for which he has been socialized."[93]

4. Influence of Understandings of Health on Developing Knowledge of Living Well with Chronic Illness.

These theoretical perspectives of health (biomedical, WHO, adaptation, wellness, humanist, developmental, and functional) provide a number of different lenses through which to view, and interpret what living well with chronic illness represents. The biomedical model focuses on the physiological level, and constructs favourable responses to illness in relation to survival, disease remission and/or lack of symptoms. The WHO understanding broadens the focus from the physical level to include the mental and social dimensions of experience, and promotes an understanding that equates positive and enhancing experiences of chronic illness with ideas of mental and social well-being. This view is extended by the humanist model that promotes the idea of self-actualization as the desired goal in life, and the wellness perspective that constructs health as the complete integration and functioning of an individual's mind, body and soul in relation to his/her environment. The emphasis on mental processes is also supported within the developmental model where favourable illness experiences are represented by transformation, expanding consciousness and/or self-actualization phenomena that occur through human-environment interaction, and are individually created and defined. Other health theories such as the adaptation and functional perspectives place greater emphasis on the relationship between an individual, and their environment or broader society. These theoretical frameworks can be seen to view living well with chronic illness as a life where one achieves flexible adaptation or maximum functioning in society through the performance of appropriate social roles and behaviours.

In reflecting on current research, it is evident that different theoretical perspectives of health dominate in different fields of research. For example, in positivistic research, the conceptual ideas inherent in measures of function, well-being, and quality of life derive, in part, from functional, and adaptation views of health where someone is healthy if they are able to physically, psychologically, and socially function in their environment, and do things that they need and want to do, and from the WHO perspective where health is a complete sense of well-being.[94-96] This is in contrast to interpretive research, where insider studies on favourable illness experiences, largely centred in nursing science, place greater emphasis on developmental and humanistic perspectives[97] in addition to functional and adaptational views.[98] Evidence of the influence of these perspectives of health is found in some authors' explicit descriptions of theoretical frameworks used in their study, and can also be implicitly inferred from the focus of inquiry, and language of findings.

The challenge of having particular interpretations of the 'good life' dominate studies, particularly in interpretive research, is that it leads to a greater emphasis being placed on particular types of positive illness phenomena to the exclusion of other interpretations, and the development of a complete, and integrated understanding. If, for example, we look at living well experiences through the developmental health lens, and see it as being a process of psychological transformation, we may fail to consider other dimensions of the experience such as personality changes, inter-personal relationships, values, beliefs etc. that may also be very important aspects of living well experiences. Emphasis on particular theoretical perspectives of health by particular disciplines and/or fields of research develops specific types of knowledge that provide insights on particular aspects of the experience but does not promote an in-depth, integrated understanding of living well experiences.

In addition, understandings of living well expressed in both applied concepts, and interpretive findings, are largely centred at the individual level. This may be partially explained by the fact that the theoretical perspectives of health that are influential in chronic illness research are largely related to the domain of life that concerns an individual's physical condition, well-being, and/or ability to function in a changing environment (or a stable society).[99] Chronic illness experience is recognized as a complex, and multi-faceted phenomenon that extends through all aspects of life and yet, there is a limited understanding of living well in relation to social, and cultural domains.[100-101] Consequently, knowledge is developing on living well with chronic illness in relation to how an individual feels and/or functions in their life, rather than in relation to all life dimensions.

5. Conclusion

In conclusion, there are enough indications of positive illness findings across diverse bodies of literature to strongly suggest that living well with chronic illness is a legitimate, and important topic for research inquiry. This paper has identified some important theoretical perspectives of health that seem to be influencing knowledge development in this field and has outlined some of the ways that they are being used in research that may be limiting our ability to develop a more complete, multi-dimensional view of what living well represents at physical, psychological, behavioural, spiritual, social and cultural levels. Researchers need to become more conscious of the particular theoretical orientations of health that are shaping studies, and findings, and to place more emphasis on considering sociocultural understandings of a good life, in relation to more psychological, and behavioural interpretations. More interdisciplinary research is needed that can build on existing knowledge generated in different fields of study, and use multi-theoretical understandings of health to create a more in-depth, and integrated understanding. Advancing knowledge on living well will not only create deeper insights into this type of experience, but will also serve to extend our understanding of the complexities of living with chronic illness.

Notes

[1] Michael Bury, "The Sociology of Chronic Illness: A Review of Research and Prospects," *Sociology of Health and Illness* 13, no. 4 (1991): 451-468.
[2] Michael P. Kelly and David Field, "Conceptualising Chronic Illness," in *Sociological Perspectives on Health, Illness and Health Care*, ed. David Field and Shelley Taylor, (London: Blackwell Science, 1998), 3-20.
[3] These experiences are framed in 'positive' or favourable terms to reflect the general way these types of experiences are described, and interpreted in relation to other types of illness phenomenon
[4] Elizabeth Lindsey, "Health within Illness: Experiences of the Chronically Ill/disabled," (Ph.D. diss., University of Victoria, 1993).

[5] Susan Wendell, "Panel: Narrative and Ethics," in *Narrative of Disease, Disability and Trauma: An Interdisciplinary Conference*, (Vancouver: University of British Columbia, 2002), 52.
[6] Alan Radley, *Making Sense of Illness: The Social Psychology of Health and Disease* (London: Sage Publications Ltd., 1994).
[7] Sally Thorne, Barbara Paterson, Sonia Acorn, Connie Canam, Gloria Joachim and Carol Jillings, "Chronic Illness Experience: Insights From a Metastudy," *Qualitative Health Research* 12, no. 4 (2002): 437-452.
[8] Curtin, Mary and Ilene M. Lubkin, "What is Chronicity?" in *Chronic Illness: Impact and Interventions*, ed. Ilene. M. Lubkin, (Boston: Jones & Bartlett, 1990).
[9] Arthur Frank, *The Wounded Storyteller: Body, Illness, and Ethics* (Chicago: University of Chicago Press, 1995).
[10] Ian Robinson, "Personal Narratives, Social Careers and Medical Courses: Analysing Life Trajectories in Autobiographies of People With Multiple Sclerosis," *Social Science and Medicine* 30, no. 11 (1990): 1173-1186.
[11] Sally Thorne and Barbara Paterson, "Shifting Images of Chronic Illness," *Image: Journal of Nursing Scholarship* 30, no. 2 (1998): 173-178.
[12] See, for example, Karen Anderson, L.A. Bradley, L.D. Young, L.K. McDaniel and C.M. Wise, "Rheumatoid Arthritis: Review of Psychological Factors Related to Etiology, Effects, and Treatment," *Psychological Bulletin* 92, no. 2 (1985): 358-387; Kathy Charmaz, "Loss of Self: a Fundamental Form of Suffering in the Chronically Ill," *Sociology of Health and Illness* 5 (1983): 168-195; Kathy Charmaz, "Struggling for a Self: Identity Levels of the Chronically Ill," in *Research in the Sociology of Health Care: A Research Annual, the Experience and Management of Chronic Illness*, ed. J. Roth and P. Conrad. (Greenwich, Connecticut: JAI Press Inc., 1987); Kathy Charmaz. *Good Days, Bad Days: The Self in Control, Illness and Time* (New Brunswick, NJ: Rutgers University Press, 1991); H.M. Craig and J.E. Edwards, "Adaptation in Chronic Illness: An Eclectic Model for Nurses," *Journal of Advanced Nursing* 8, no. 5 (1983): 397-404.
[13] Recognition that some individuals have positive illness responses/experiences that suggest they may live well with chronic illness does not negate the extensive literature documenting challenging, and often painful impacts of living with serious long term disease. But these types of findings do challenge the view that chronic illness is only comprised of difficult impacts and phenomena in all individuals, and forces us to reconceptualize chronic illness as a more multi-facted and complex experience.
[14] See, for example, Susan R. Michael, "Integrating Chronic Illness into One's Life: A Phenomenological Inquiry," *Journal of Holistic Nursing* 14, no. 3 (1996): 251-267; and Robinson, 10.

[15] See, for example, Glenn Affleck and Howard Tennen, "Construing Benefits From Adversity: Adaptational Significance and Dispositional Underpinnings," *Journal of Personality* 64 (1996): 899-922; and Howard Tennen and Glenn Affleck, "Finding Benefits in Adversity," in *Coping: The Psychology of What Works*, ed. C. R. Snyder, (New York: Oxford University Press, 1999), 279-304.

[16] See, for example, Judy Kendall, Barbara Gloerson, Patricia Gray, Susan McConnell, Jennifer Turner and Judith West, "Doing Well With AIDS: Three Case Illustrations," *Archives of Psychiatric Nursing* 3, no. 3 (1989): 159-165.

[17] See, for example, Lindsey, 4; and Susan Moch, "Health Within the Experience of Breast Cancer," *Journal of Advanced Nursing* 15 (1990): 1426-1435.

[18] See, for example, Ian Robinson, "Exceptional People? Understanding Medical and Social Explanations of 'Abnormal Responses' to Illness," (Paper presented to the *European Society of Medical Sociology*, Zaberg, Sept. 1988).

[19] See, for example, Jenny M. Young and Paule McNicoll, "Against All Odds: Positive Life Experiences of People With Advanced Amyotrophic Lateral Sclerosis," *Health and Social Work* 23, no. 1 (1998): 35-43.

[20] Gregory K. Brown, Kenneth A. Wallston and Perry M. Nicassio, "Social Support and Depression in Rheumatoid Arthritis: A One Year Prospective Study," *Journal of Applied Social Psychology* 19 (1989): 1164-1181.

[21] Gary L. Albrecht and Patrick J. Devlieger, "The Disability Paradox: High Quality of Life Against all Odds," *Social Science and Medicine*, 48 (1999): 977-988.

[22] See, for example, Health and Welfare Canada, *The Active Health Report: Perspective on Canada's Health Promotion Survey (*Ottawa: Minister of Supply and Services Canada, 1987); and Alexa K. Stuifbergen, Heather A. Becker, Karrie Ingalsbe and Dolores Sands, "Perceptions of Health Among Adults With Disabilities," *Health Values* 14, no. 2 (1990): 18-26.

[23] See, for example, Susan Folkman, "Positive Meaningful Events and Coping in the Context of HIV/AIDS," in *Coping With Chronic Stress*, ed. Benjamin. H. Gottlieb, (New York: Plenum Press, 1997), 293-314.

[24] Mark A. Somerfield and Robert R. McCrae, "Stress and Coping Research: Methodological Challenges, Theoretical Advances, and Clinical Applications," *American Psychologist* 55, no. 6 (2000): 620-625.

[25] See, for example, Affleck and Tennen, 15; and Tennen and Affleck, 15.

[26] See, for example, Charles J. Holahan, Rudolf H. Moos and Jeanne A. Schaefer, "Coping, stress resistance and growth: conceptualizing adaptive functioning," in *Handbook of Coping, Theory, Research, and Applications*, ed. Moshe Zeidner and Norman Endler, (John Wiley and Sons Inc., 1996), 24-43; and Jeanne A. Schaefer and Rudolf H. Moos,

"Life Crises and Personal Growth," in *Personal Coping: Theory, Research, Application*, ed. Bruce. N. Carpenter, (Westport, CT: Praeger, 1992), 149-170.

[27] Thorne and Paterson, 175.

[28] See, for example, Cynthia Baker and Phyllis N. Stern, "Finding Meaning in Chronic Illness As the Key to Self-Care," *Canadian Journal of Nursing Research* 25 (1996): 23-36; Charmaz, 12; Doris Coward, "The Lived Experience of Self-Transcendence in Women with Advanced Breast Cancer," *Nursing Science Quarterly* 3, no. 4 (1990): 162-169; Betsy L. Fife, "The Conceptualisation of Meaning in Illness," *Social Science and Medicine* 38, no. 2 (1994): 309-316; Priscilla LeMone, "Transforming: Patterns of Sexual Function in Adults with Insulin Dependant Diabetes Mellitus," (Ph.D. diss., University of Alabama, 1991); Elizabeth Lindsey, "Health Within Illness: Experiences of Chronically Ill/Disabled People *Journal of Advanced Nursing* 24 (1996): 465-462; Maxine E. Loomis and Diana Conco, "Patients' Perceptions of Health, Chronic Illness, and Nursing Diagnosis," *Nursing Research* 2, no. 4 (1991): 162-170; Carol McWilliam, Moira Stewart, Judith Belle Brown, Kathryn Desai and Patricia Coderre, "Creating Health With Chronic Illness," *Advances in Nursing Science* 18, no. 3 (1996): 1-15; Susan Moch, "Health Within Illness: Conceptual Evolution and Practice Possibilities," *Advances in Nursing Science* 11, no. 4 (1989): 23-31; Barbara Paterson, Sally Thorne, John Crawford and Michel Tarko, "Living With Diabetes as a Transformational Experience," *Qualitative Health Research* 9, 6 (1999): 786-802; Karen M. Schaefer, "Women Living in Paradox: Loss and Discovery in Chronic Illness," *Holist Nursing Practice* 9, 3 (1995): 63-74.

[29] See, for example, Loomis and Conco, 28; McWilliam et al., 28; and Stuifbergen et al., 22.

[30] Robinson, 10.

[31] Frank, 9.

[32] Arthur Kleinman and Don Seeman, "Personal Experience of Illness," in *Handbook of Social Studies in Health and Medicine*, ed. Gary. L Albrecht. (London: Sage Publications, 2000), 230-242.

[33] Robinson, 10.

[34] Robinson, 18.

[35] See, for example, Kat Duff. *The Alchemy of Illness*. (New York: Random House Inc, 1993); and Robert L. Yocum. *My Adventure with Lupus: Living with a Chronic Illness* (Glendale, CA: Griffin Publishing, 1995).

[36] Wendell, 5.

[37] Mary A. Ruffing-Rahal, "Well-Being and Chronicity: Being Singular Rather Than Sick," *Health Values*, 9, no. 5 (1985): 17-22.

[38] Wendell, 5.

[39] Ann Bowling, *Measuring Disease: A Review of Disease-Specific Quality of Life Measurement Scales* (Buckingham: Open University Press, 1995), 3.
[40] Ian McDowell and Claire Newell, *Measuring Health: A Guide to Rating Scales and Questionnaires.* 2nd ed. (New York: Oxford University Press, 1996).
[41] Chronic illness research is often differentiated by 'insider' and 'outsider' perspectives. As Conrad summarizes, " an insider's perspective typically focuses directly and explicitly on the subjective experience of living with, and in that " an insider's perspective typically focuses directly and explicitly on the subjective experience of living with, and in spite of illness", and uses inductive approaches to focus on the perspectives of ill individuals. This is in contrast to outsider approaches to research that conceptualize illness from outside the experience, disregarding the subjective reality of the individual, and takes a deductive approach to addressing medical or social questions. See Peter Conrad, "The experience of illness: recent and new directions," in *Research in the Sociology of Health Care, vol.6*, ed. J.A. Roth and P. Conrad (Greenwich, Connecticut: JAI Press Inc., 1987); and Peter Conrad, "Qualitative Research on Chronic Illness: A Commentary on Method and Conceptual Development," *Social Science and Medicine* 30, no. 11 (1990): 1259.
[42] See, for example, Michael, 14.
[43] See, for example, Kendall et al., 16.
[44] See, for example, Barbara Gloerson, Judy Kendall, Patricia Gray, Susan McConnell, Jennifer Turner and Judith West Lewkowicz, "The Phenomena of Doing Well in People with AIDS," *Western Journal of Nursing Research*, 15, no.1 (1993): 44-54 and Kendall et al., 16.
[45] See, for example, Loomis and Conco, 28; and McWilliam et al., 28.
[46] See, for example, Gloerson et al., 44.
[47] See, for example, Marjorie Kagawa-Singer, "Redefining Health: Living With Cancer," *Social Science and Medicine* 37, no. 3 (1993): 295-304.
[48] Lindsey, 4.
[49] Thorne and Paterson, 11.
[50] Sally Thorne and Barbara Paterson, "Two Decades of Insider Research: What We Know and Don't Know About Chronic Illness Experience," *Annual Review of Nursing Research* (2000).
[51] See, for example, Lindsey, 28; and Paterson et al., 28.
[52] See, for example, Julie Barroso, "Focusing on living: Attitudinal approaches of long-term survivors of AIDS," *Issues in Mental Health Nursing*, 17 (1996): 395-407; Fife, 28; and Paterson et al., 28.
[53] Thorne and Paterson, 50.
[54] There are a large number of other theories and models of health in the literature but many of them provide an explanatory framework for exploring the determinants of health rather than providing a conceptualization or definition of health. The perspectives of health

reviewed in this paper have been chosen because they seem to play an important role in shaping chronic illness research.
[55] Bowling, 39.
[56] Kagawa-Singer, 47.
[57] Jane Odgen, "The Rhetoric and Reality of Psychological Theories of Health," *Journal of Health Psychology* 2, no. 1 (1997): 21-29.
[58] Sally Wellard, "Constructions of Chronic Illness," *International Journal of Nursing Studies* 35 (1998): 49-55.
[59] George L. Engel, "The Need for a New Medical Model: A Challenge for Biomedicine," *Science* 196, no. 4286 (1977): 129-136.
[60] Maare E. Tamm, "Models of Health and Disease," *British Journal of Medicine Psychology* 66 (1993): 213-228.
[61] Engel, 59.
[62] World Health Organization, "Constitution of the World Health Organization," *Chronicle of the World Health Organization* 1, no. 1/2 (1947): 29.
[63] James S. Larson, "The World Health Organization's Definition of Health: Social Versus Spiritual Health," *Social Indicators Research* 38, no. 2 (1996): 181-192.
[64] McDowell and Newell, 40.
[65] Judith A. Smith, *The Idea of Health: Implication for the Nursing Professional* (Columbia, New York: Teachers College Press, 1983).
[66] Rene Dubos, "Determinants of Health and Disease," in *Man, Medicine, and Environment*, ed. Rene Dubos, (New York: Mentor Books, New American Library, 1968), 32.
[67] Rene Dubos, *Mirage of Health: Utopias, Progress, and Biological Change* (Garden City, New York: Anchor Books, 1961).
[68] Ludwig von Bertalanffy, *General System Theory* (New York: George Braziller, 1968).
[69] Rene Dubos, *Man Adapting* (New Haven: Yale University Press, 1965).
[70] Halbert L. Dunn, "High-level Wellness: A Collection of Twenty-nine Short Talks on Different Aspects of the Theme 'High-level Wellness for Man and Society'," (Arlington, VA: R. W. Beatty Co., 1961).
[71] Ibid., 4.
[72] Donald B. Ardell, "The History and Future of Wellness," *Health Values* 9, no. 6 (1985): 37-56.
[73] James S. Larson, *The Measurement of Health: Concepts and Indicators* (Westport, Connecticut: Greenwood Press, 1991).
[74] See, for example, Ardell, 72; Jerold S. Greenberg, "Health and Wellness: A Conceptual Differentiation," *Journal of School Health* 55, no. 10 (1985): 403-406; and Gwyn C. Jones and Allie C. Kilpatrick, "Wellness Theory: A Discussion and Application to Clients With Disabilities," *Families in Society: The Journal of Contemporary Human Services* 77, no. 5 (1996): 259-268.
[75] Ardell, 72.

[76] See, for example, Ruth Davidhizar and Ruth Shearer, "Helping the Client With Chronic Disability Achieve High-Level Wellness," *Rehabilitation Nursing* 22, no. 3 (1997): 131-134; and Kathleen D. Mullen, "Wellness: the Missing Concept in Health Promotion Programming for Adults," *Health Values* 10, no. 3 (1986): 34-37.
[77] Abraham H. Maslow, *The Farther Reaches of Human Nature* (New York, NY: Viking Press, 1971), 45-47.
[78] Ibid.
[79] Tamm, 60.
[80] David Seedhouse, *Health: The Foundation for Achievement* (Brisbane: John Wiley & Sons, 1986).
[81] Smith, 65.
[82] Seedhouse, 80.
[83] Martha E. Rogers, *An Introduction to the Theoretical Basis of Nursing.* (Philadephia: E. A. Davis, 1970).
[84] Margaret A. Newman, "Health Conceptualizations," *Annual Review of Nursing Research* 9 (1991): 221-243.
[85] Margaret A. Newman, *Health as Expanding Consciousness* (St. Louis, MS: Mosby, 1986).
[86] Nola Pender, "Expressing Health Through Lifestyle Patterns," *Nursing Science Quarterly* 3 (1990): 115-122.
[87] Rosemarie R. Parse, *Man-Living-Health: A Theory of Nursing* (New York: Wiley, 1981).
[88] Ibid.
[89] Rosemarie R. Parse, "Health: a Personal Commitment," *Nursing Science Quarterly* 3 (1990): 136-140.
[90] Lindsey, 4.
[91] Talcot, Parson, *The Social System* (Glencoe, Illinois: The Free Press, 1951).
[92] Talcot Parson, "Definitions of Health and Illness in the Light of American Values and Social Structure," in *Patients, Physicians, and Illness*, ed. Gartly. E. Jaco (Glencoe, Illinois: The Free Press, 1958), 165-187.
[93] Ibid., 176.
[94] Bowling, 39.
[95] Harold Hansluwka, "Measuring the Health of Populations, Indicators and Interpretations," *Social Science and Medicine* 20, no. 12 (1985): 1207-1224.
[96] McDowell and Newell, 40.
[97] See, for example, Coward, 28; Coward, Doris D. and Frances Marcus Lewis, "The Lived Experience of Self-Transcendence in Gay Men with AIDS," *Oncology Nursing Forum* 20, no. 9 (1993): 1363-1368 and Lindsey, 28.
[98] See, for example, Loomis and Conco, 28; and McWilliam et al., 28.

[99] Irving Rootman and John Raeburn, "The Concept of Health," in Health Promotion in Canada: Provincial, National & International Perspectives, ed. Ann Pederson, Michel O'Neill and Irving Rootman, (Toronto: W.B. Saunders Canada, 1994), 56-71.
[100] Juliet M. Corbin and Anselm Strauss, *Unending Work and Care: Managing Chronic Illness at Home* (San Francisco: Jossey-Bass Publishers, 1988).
[101] Ariela Royer, *Life with Chronic Illness: Social and Psychological Dimensions* (Westport, Connecticut: Praceger, 1998).

Bibliography

Affleck, Glenn and Howard Tennen. "Construing Benefits From Adversity: Adaptational Significance and Dispositional Underpinnings." *Journal of Personality* 64 (1996): 899-922.

Albrecht, Gary L. and Patrick J. Devlieger. „The Disability Paradox: High Quality of Life Against all Odds." *Social Science and Medicine*, 48 (1999): 977-988.

Anderson, Karen, L.A. Bradley, L.D. Young, L.K. McDaniel and C.M. Wise. "Rheumatoid Arthritis: Review of Psychological Factors Related to Etiology, Effects, and Treatment." *Psychological Bulletin* 92, no. 2 (1985): 358-387.

Ardell, Donald B. "The History and Future of Wellness." *Health Values* 9, no. 6 (1985): 37-56.

Baker, Cynthia and Phyllis N. Stern. "Finding Meaning in Chronic Illness As the Key to Self-Care." *Canadian Journal of Nursing Research* 25 (1996): 23-36.

Barroso, Julie. "Focusing on Living: Attitudinal Approaches of Long-term Survivors of AIDS." *Issues in Mental Health Nursing*, 17 (1996): 395-407.

Bowling, Ann. *Measuring Disease: A Review of Disease-Specific Quality of Life Measurement Scales*. Buckingham: Open University Press, 1995.

Brown, Gregory K., Kenneth A. Wallston and Perry M. Nicassio. "Social Support and Depression in Rheumatoid Arthritis: A One Year Prospective Study." *Journal of Applied Social Psychology* 19 (1989): 1164-1181.

Bury, Michael. "The Sociology of Chronic Illness: a Review of Research and Prospects." *Sociology of Health and Illness* 13, no. 4 (1991): 451-468.

Charmaz, Kathy. "Loss of Self: a Fundamental Form of Suffering in the Chronically Ill." *Sociology of Health and Illness* 5 (1983): 168-195.

Charmaz, Kathy. "Struggling for a Self: Identity Levels of the Chronically Ill." In *Research in the Sociology of Health Care: A Research Annual, the Experience and Management of Chronic Illness*, edited by J. Roth and P. Conrad. Greenwich, Connecticut: JAI Press Inc., 1987.

Charmaz, Kathy. *Good Days, Bad Days: The Self in Control, Illness and Time*. New Brunswick, NJ: Rutgers University Press, 1991.

Conrad, Peter. "The Experience of Illness: Recent and New Directions." In *Research in the Sociology of Health Care, vol.6*, edited by. J. A Roth and P. Conrad. Greenwich, Connecticut: JAI Press Inc., 1987.

Conrad, Peter. "Qualitative Research on Chronic Illness: A Commentary on Method and Conceptual Development." *Social Science and Medicine* 30, no. 11 (1990): 1257-1263.

Corbin, Juliet M. and Anselm Strauss. *Unending Work and Care: Managing Chronic Illness at Home.* San Francisco: Jossey-Bass Publishers, 1988.

Coward, Doris. "The Lived Experience of Self-Transcendence in Women With Advanced Breast Cancer." *Nursing Science Quarterly* 3, no. 4 (1990): 162-169.

Coward, Doris D. and Frances Marcus Lewis. "The Lived Experience of Self-Transcendence in Gay Men with AIDS." *Oncology Nursing Forum* 20, no. 9 (1993): 1363-1368.

Craig, H.M. and J.E. Edwards. "Adaptation in Chronic Illness: An Eclectic Model for Nurses." *Journal of Advanced Nursing* 8, no. 5 (1983): 397-404.

Curtin, Mary and Ilene M. Lubkin. "What is Chronicity?" In *Chronic Illness: Impact and Interventions*, edited by Ilene M. Lubkin. Boston: Jones & Bartlett, 1990.

Davidhizar, Ruth and Ruth Shearer. "Helping the Client With Chronic Disability Achieve High-Level Wellness." *Rehabilitation Nursing* 22, no. 3 (1997): 131-134.

Dubos, Rene. *Mirage of Health: Utopias, Progress, and Biological Change.* Garden City, New York: Anchor Books, 1961.

Dubos, Rene. *Man Adapting*. New Haven: Yale University Press, 1965.

Dubos, Rene. "Determinants of Health and Disease." In *Man, Medicine, and Environment*, edited by Rene Dubos, 32. New York: Mentor Books, New American Library, 1968.

Duff, Kat. *The Alchemy of Illness*. New York: Random House Inc, 1993.

Dunn, Halbert L. *High-level Wellness: A Collection of Twenty-nine Short Talks on Different Aspects of the Theme "High-level Wellness for Man and Society."* Arlington, VA: R. W. Beatty Co., 1961.

Engel, George L. "The Need for a New Medical Model: A Challenge for Biomedicine." *Science* 196, no. 4286 (1977): 129-136.

Fife, Betsy L. "The Conceptualisation of Meaning in Illness." *Social Science and Medicine* 38, no. 2 (1994): 309-316.

Folkman, Susan. "Positive Meaningful Events and Coping in the Context of HIV/AIDS." In *Coping With Chronic Stress*, edited by Benjamin. H. Gottlieb, 293-314. New York: Plenum Press, 1997.

Frank, Arthur. *The Wounded Storyteller: Body, Illness, and Ethics*. Chicago: University of Chicago Press, 1995.

Gloerson, Barbara, Judy Kendall, Patricia Gray, Susan McConnell, Jennifer Turner and Judith West Lewkowicz. "The Phenomena of Doing Well in People with AIDS." *Western Journal of Nursing Research*, 15, no.1 (1993: 44-54.

Greenberg, Jerrold S. "Health and Wellness: A Conceptual Differentiation." *Journal of School Health* 55, no. 10 (1985): 403-406.

Hansluwka, Harald. "Measuring the Health of Populations, Indicators and Interpretations." *Social Science and Medicine* 20, no. 12 (1985): 1207-1224.

Health and Welfare Canada. *The Active Health Report: Perspective on Canada's Health Promotion Survey.* Ottawa: Minister of Supply and Services Canada, 1987.

Holahan, Charles J., Rudolf H. Moos and Jeanne A. Schaefer. "Coping, Stress Resistance and Growth: Conceptualizing Adaptive Functioning." In *Handbook of Coping, Theory, Research, and Applications*, edited by

Moshe Zeidner and Norman Endler, 24-43. John Wiley and Sons Inc., 1996.

Jones, Gwyn C. and Allie C. Kilpatrick. "Wellness Theory: A Discussion and Application to Clients With Disabilities." *Families in Society: The Journal of Contemporary Human Services* 77, no. 5 (1996): 259-268.

Kagawa-Singer, Marjorie. "Redefining Health: Living With Cancer." *Social Science and Medicine* 37, no. 3 (1993): 295-304.

Kelly, Michael P. and David Field. "Conceptualising Chronic Illness." In *Sociological Perspectives on Health, Illness and Health Care*, edited by David. Field and Shelley. Taylor, 3-20. London: Blackwell Science, 1998.

Kendall, Judy, Barbara Gloerson, Patricia Gray, Susan McConnell, Jennifer Turner and Judith West. "Doing Well With AIDS: Three Case Illustrations." *Archives of Psychiatric Nursing* 3, no. 3 (1989): 159-165.

Kleinman, Arthur and Don Seeman. "Personal Experience of Illness." In *Handbook of Social Studies in Health and Medicine*, edited by Gary. L Albrecht, 230-242. London: SAGE Publications, 2000.

Larson, James S. *The Measurement of Health: Concepts and Indicators.* Westport, Connecticut: Greenwood Press, 1991.

Larson, James S. "The World Health Organization's Definition of Health: Social Versus Spiritual Health." *Social Indicators Research* 38, no. 2 (1996): 181-192.

LeMone, Priscilla. "Transforming: Patterns of Sexual Function in Adults with Insulin Dependant Diabetes Mellitus." Ph.D. diss., University of Alabama, 1991.

Lindsey, Elizabeth. "Health within Illness: Experiences of the Chronically Ill/disabled." Ph.D. diss., University of Victoria, 1993.

Lindsey, Elizabeth. "Health Within Illness: Experiences of Chronically Ill/Disabled People." *Journal of Advanced Nursing* 24 (1996): 465-462.

Loomis, Maxine E. and Diana Conco. "Patients' Perceptions of Health, Chronic Illness, and Nursing Diagnosis." *Nursing Research* 2, no. 4 (1991): 162-170.

Maslow, Abraham H. *The Farther Reaches of Human Nature.* New York, NY: Viking Press, 1971.

McDowell, Ian and Claire Newell. *Measuring Health: A Guide to Rating Scales and Questionnaires.* 2nd ed. New York: Oxford University Press, 1996.

McWilliam, Carol, Moira Stewart, Judith Belle Brown, Kathryn Desai and Patricia Coderre. "Creating Health With Chronic Illness." *Advances in Nursing Science* 18, no. 3 (1996): 1-15.

Michael, Susan R. "Integrating Chronic Illness into One's Life: A Phenomenological Inquiry." *Journal of Holistic Nursing* 14, no. 3 (1996): 251-267.

Moch, Susan. "Health Within the Experience of Breast Cancer." *Journal of Advanced Nursing* 15 (1990): 1426-1435.

Moch, Susan. "Health Within Illness: Conceptual Evolution and Practice Possibilities." *Advances in Nursing Science* 11, no. 4 (1989): 23-31.

Mullen, Kathleen D. "Wellness: the Missing Concept in Health Promotion Programming for Adults." *Health Values* 10, no. 3 (1986): 34-37.

Newman, Margaret A. *Health as Expanding Consciousness.* St. Luious, MS: Mosby, 1986.

Newman, Margaret A. "Health Conceptualizations." *Annual Review of Nursing Research* 9 (1991): 221-243.

Odgen, Jane. "The Rhetoric and Reality of Psychological Theories of Health." *Journal of Health Psychology* 2, no. 1 (1997): 21-29.

Parse, Rosemarie R. "Health: A Personal Commitment." *Nursing Science Quarterly* 3 (1990): 136-140.

Parse, Rosemarie R. *Man-living-health: A Theory of Nursing.* New York: Wiley, 1981.

Parson, Talcot. "Definitions of Health and Illness in the Light of American Values and Social Structure." In *Patients, Physicians, and Illness*, edited by Gartly. E. Jaco, 165-187. Glencoe, Illinois: The Free Press, 1958.

Parson, Talcot. *The Social System.* Glencoe, Illinois: The Free Press, 1951.

Paterson, Barbara, Sally Thorne, John Crawford and Michel Tarko. "Living With Diabetes as a Transformational Experience." *Qualitative Health Research* 9, no. 6 (1999): 786-802.

Pender, Nola. "Expressing Health Through Lifestyle Patterns." *Nursing Science Quarterly* 3 (1990): 115-122.

Radley, Alan. *Making Sense of Illness: The Social Psychology of Health and Disease*. London: Sage Publications Ltd., 1994.

Robinson, Ian. "Exceptional People? Understanding Medical and Social Explanations of 'Abnormal Responses' to Illness." Paper presented to the *European Society of Medical Sociology*, Zaberg, Sept. 1988.

Robinson, Ian. "Personal Narratives, Social Careers and Medical Courses: Analysing Life Trajectories in Autobiographies of People With Multiple Sclerosis." *Social Science and Medicine* 30, no. 11 (1990): 1173-1186.

Rogers, Martha E. *An Introduction to the Theoretical Basis of Nursing*. Philadephia: E. A. Davis, 1970.

Rootman, Irving and John Raeburn. "The Concept of Health." In *Health Promotion in Canada: Provincial, National & International Perspectives*, edited by Ann Pederson, Michel O'Neill and Irving Rootman, 56-71, Toronto: W.B. Saunders Canada, 1994.

Royer, Ariela. *Life with Chronic Illness: Social and Psychological Dimensions*. Westport, Connecticut: Praceger, 1998.

Ruffing-Rahal, Mary A. "Well-Being and Chronicity: Being Singular Rather Than Sick." *Health Values*, 9, no. 5 (1985): 17-22.

Schaefer, Jeanne A. and Rudolf H. Moos. "Life Crises and Personal Growth." In *Personal Coping: Theory, Research, Application*, edited by Bruce. N. Carpenter, 149-170. Westport, CT: Praeger, 1992.

Schaefer, Karen M. "Women Living in Paradox: Loss and Discovery in Chronic Illness." *Holist Nursing Practice* 9, no. 3 (1995): 63-74.

Seedhouse, David. *Health: The Foundation for Achievement*. Brisbane: John Wiley & Sons, 1986.

Smith, Judith A. *The Idea of Health: Implication for the Nursing Professional*. Columbia, New York: Teachers College Press, 1983.

Somerfield, Mark A. and Robert R. McCrae. "Stress and Coping Research: Methodological Challenges, Theoretical Advances, and Clinical Applications." *American Psychologist* 55, no. 6 (2000): 620-625.

Stuifbergen, Alexa K., Heather A. Becker, Karrie Ingalsbe and Dolores Sands. "Perceptions of Health Among Adults With Disabilities." *Health Values* 14, no. 2 (1990): 18-26.

Tamm, Maare E. "Models of Health and Disease." *British Journal of Medicine Psychology* 66 (1993): 213-228.

Tennen, Howard and Glenn Affleck. "Finding Benefits in Adversity." In *Coping: The Psychology of What Works*, edited by C.R. Snyder, 279-304. New York: Oxford University Press, 1999.

Thorne, Sally, Barbara Paterson, Sonia Acorn, Connie Canam, Gloria Joachim and Carol Jillings. "Chronic Illness Experience: Insights From a Metastudy." *Qualitative Health Research* 12, no. 4 (2002): 437-452.

Thorne, Sally E. and Barbara Paterson. "Shifting Images of Chronic Illness." *Image: Journal of Nursing Scholarship* 30, no. 2 (1998): 173-178.

Thorne, Sally E. and Barbara Paterson. "Two Decades of Insider Research: What We Know and Don't Know About Chronic Illness Experience," *Annual Review of Nursing Research* (2000).

von Bertalanffy, Ludwig. *General System Theory.* New York: George Braziller, 1968.

Wellard, Sally. "Constructions of Chronic Illness." *International Journal of Nursing Studies* 35 (1998): 49-55.

Wendell, Susan. "Panel: Narrative and Ethics." In *Narrative of Disease, Disability and Trauma: An Interdisciplinary Conference*, 52. Vancouver: University of British Columbia, 2002.

World Health Organization. "Constitution of the World Health Organization." *Chronicle of the World Health Organization* 1, no. 1/2 (1947): 29-43.

Yocum, Robert L. *My Adventure with Lupus: Living with a Chronic Illness*. Glendale, CA: Griffin Publishing, 1995.

Young, Jenny M. and Paule McNicoll. "Against All Odds: Positive Life Experiences of People With Advanced Amyotrophic Lateral Sclerosis." *Health and Social Work* 23, no. 1 (1998): 35-43.

Note on Contributor

Susan Mills is a PhD candidate in the Individual Interdisciplinary Studies Graduate Program, Institute of Health Promotion Research at the University of British Columbia, Vancouver, Canada.

Acknowledgements

The author wishes to acknowledge the financial support of the Canadian Institutes of Health Research and the British Columbia Health Research Foundation.

Ethical Issues in Narrative Research in Palliative Care

Jane Appleton

This chapter explores some of the ethical issues encountered in a research study which used narrative approaches to access patient's experiences of life-threatening illness. The research sought to answer the question: 'What is the experience of living with a life-threatening illness like and what effect does it have on a person's life?' Narrative interviews with patients diagnosed with advanced disease were conducted to investigate their experiences of life-threatening illness, this exposed particular ethical concerns related to confidentiality, gate-keeping of research participants, the relationship between the participants and myself as researcher, participants experiencing distress within the interview and the ownership of the story. Ethical challenges, which arose as a result of this study, are reflected upon and debated not with respect to solutions, rather to raise these as worthy of greater debate and to illustrate the complexity of research ethics within a palliative care context. Examples from the research study are used throughout to illustrate some of the difficulties encountered. The aim of this chapter therefore is to highlight some of the practical, methodological and ethical issues of conducting this research. The chapter concludes that the ethical dilemmas raised in narrative research require a different approach to more traditional research ethics, it is suggested that traditional assumptions like confidentiality are re-examined.

1. Introduction

In this chapter I examine some of the ethical dilemmas raised by a study which aimed to capture the experience of life-threatening illness. In the context of this research palliative care is taken to mean maximising a person's quality of life in the face of life threatening illness. The impetus for the study came from my practice experience, as a palliative care nurse and lecturer, where I commonly hear peoples' illness stories. I have been particularly struck by the eagerness with which these stories are expressed; despite I suspect having been recounted many times before. The impulse to construct personal illness narratives is strong and compulsive, particularly at the end of life. My own experience of illness and childbirth and seeing how that experience was documented on the computer screen at my general practitioner's caused me to reflect on the power and dominance of the medical narrative, which becomes the 'official story of the illness' and is 'trump' over other narratives.[1] In addition, I was interested in the narrative pedagogy from a teaching and learning perspective in my role as a lecturer.[2] Capturing patients' illness narratives appears therefore to offer a rich resource for education and practice. Furthermore, I have an interest in reading autobiographical and biographical accounts of illness and life-threatening disease. These accounts give you access to experiences you have no personal experience of and insights into what that experience might be like; in addition they are a valuable means of health care professionals understanding the patient's perspective of illness.

2. Background to the Study

The research study on which this chapter is based explored illness using a Heideggerian phenomenological approach to elicit the lived experience of life-threatening illness with a palliative care population. It took place between December 2001 and early 2002 in the form of in-depth narrative interviews with palliative care patients attending a specialist palliative care centre in the United Kingdom (U.K.). The participants all had advanced disease, prominently cancer, however a minority were living with non-malignant causes of life-threatening illness, such as heart disease. Qualitative methods were used to invite participants to narrate their personal experiences of illness and to explore the meaning of that experience. Unstructured narrative interviews were conducted with six participants if they were willing to tell their illness story and to have the interview tape-recorded. The resulting data were interpreted using hermeneutics and narrative analysis techniques suggested by Polkinghorne.[3] Individual biographical narratives were written for each participant and discussed in relation to the similarities, differences and what could be learned from the accounts. Analysis of the data revealed that stories of life-threatening illness are dominated by the bio-medical discourse of illness. However, counter-narratives were identified relating to relationships, independence and thinking about death; participants renegotiated their identity and life priorities in relation to being ill. In addition, the patient narratives challenged the espoused values of palliative care in that they presented a picture of living with life-threatening illness which is at odds with the principles of palliative care. The study therefore raised issues about the philosophy of palliative care as it is experienced by patients in contrast to professionals, in terms of meaning.

The starting point for many research projects is the research ethics approval process, which seeks to safeguard the interests of research participants and researchers and to promote ethically sensitive research. This process, in the UK, commonly takes place 'behind closed doors' without the researcher present. Discipline-specific ethical guidelines such as the British Sociological Association, Royal College of Nursing and the British Psychological Society (BPS 1996) underpin the work of ethics committees.[4] Research ethics focuses on how well research participants are treated and tends to assume that participants will be untouched or unchanged by the experience of taking part, either positively or negatively. The experience of gaining ethical approval for this study in itself raised some difficult challenges. My experience of that approval process was a 'tick box' approach to ethics, where the emphasis was to gain ethical approval for the study, rather than to promote ethical practitioners who could engage in debate about the difficult issues raised. This chapter argues that research conducted with dying people needs to be mindful of the ethical challenges involved, it needs to creatively consider and debate these issues rather than to use a 'one size fits all' approach. Research ethics tends to focus on the four principles approach of autonomy, beneficence, non-malficence and justice. However these principles are in themselves problematic, in that they may be in conflict with each other, be subjective and culturally bound. It appears that there are certain assumptions underpinning research ethics generally and the research approval process in particular. Firstly, that dying people are a vulnerable group, who should not take part in research and that many health and social care professionals see it as their role to protect patients from researchers at the end of life. Secondly, that it is in the participant's best interests to remain anonymous and for confidentiality to be maintained in research. Finally, that the participant will be untouched or unchanged by the experience of taking part in a research study. These assumptions will now be discussed in light of my experience using examples from the study.

3. Research Involving Dying People

The notion of vulnerability suggests that certain groups within society require additional protection in terms of research due to their powerlessness or susceptibility to being exploited or degraded, children are one group who are frequently referred to as vulnerable. In addition, the issue of vulnerability is closely linked to research which is of a sensitive nature or relates to personal experiences. There has been considerable debate within the palliative care literature regarding whether vulnerable groups should participate in research and indeed if the dying are to be considered vulnerable.[5] For example, de Raeve has argued that "strong moral grounds exist for objecting to research in the field of palliative care" on the grounds that dying people are a vulnerable group.[6] However, this viewpoint has received much criticism in palliative care, on the grounds that it is "paternalistic, devaluing and disrespectful," as it does not give dying people the opportunity to decide for themselves whether or not to participate in a research study.[7] Indeed, it can be argued that it is unethical not to undertake research on palliative care populations as neglecting this area of research may result in unresolved pain, symptoms managed by treatments and practices which are ineffective, with a dubious evidence base, or practices which are even harmful to patients and families. It has been argued that palliative care patients should only be involved in research if they personally will derive some direct benefit.[8] Others have argued that patients receiving palliative care often wish to participate in research even if they themselves will not benefit directly from the work.[9] The reasons this client group participate in research tend to be altruistic, understanding that personal benefit might be absent or limited, however wanting to be part of something after they have died or to give something back to society, feeling indebted to the health care team or wanting to help others following in their footsteps. Furthermore, dying people may not view themselves as dying and vulnerable, rather they may consider themselves as ill and going to die.

4. Gaining Access to Research Participants

Gaining access to research participants is an important ethical aspect of any research project however it is commonly given little attention within research reports. According to Alty and Rodham this is particularly problematic when undertaking research of a sensitive nature, such as with people who are dying.[10] Gaining access to potential participants via a third party is common practice to prevent coercion. However, this makes the researcher dependent on others and reliant on them to progess the research project. The decision to take part in a research study is personal and individual, however, there maybe common factors in terms of motivation. I asked participants prior to signing the consent form, why they wished to take part in the study. Several thought that it might help future patients or help health care professionals to understand the patient's perspective better. One patient was encouraged to do so by her family as it was thought to be a way to 'give something back.' Conversely, some families may discourage participation, as time spent in research is precious time not spent with them. Motivation to take part in research is therefore complex and requires time and understanding on the part of the researcher. One participant said that she had hoped to write a book about her experiences, but had 'left it too late' and now she did not have the energy to do so, taking part in the research was seen as an alternative to writing the book. Prior to the interview, when I was answering potential participants questions about the research one patient cautiously asked what type of questions I would ask in the interview. I replied that I didn't have a list of questions but was more interested in her story of the illness experience. I said that I saw my role as prompting her to tell her story, rather than asking lots of questions.

It is common practice in qualitative research to access participants via gate-keepers. Indeed it is viewed as good practice for researchers to access via gate-keepers rather than to approach potential participants directly, and this is supported in ethical guidelines cited earlier. However, the notion of gate-keeping has fairly negative connotations in terms of language. A gate-keeper, in research terms, refers to individuals who are in a position to permit or not access to others for the purpose of research, commonly for interview. Besides being a third party or an intermediary between researchers and participants, gate-keeping has also come to mean preventing that access. Gate-keeping of research participants has been described as not presenting the research project or selectively presenting the project thus, potential participants are denied the opportunity to take part, or, presenting the research in such a way as to discourage potential participants from taking part. This situation has been widely documented in research generally and in palliative care in particular.[11] Rose found in a study exploring informal caring in palliative care that health and social care professionals acted as gate-keepers to potential participants by not referring patients to the researcher and adopting a protectionist approach, despite the espoused values of palliative care regarding patient decision-making and autonomy. It seems that sometimes professionals make the decision that research would be 'too much' or a burden to potential participants and do not inform them about the study. The burden of participating in research is however an important consideration, in palliative care populations fatigue is a common and distressing symptom. Some practical strategies to manage potential fatigue might be considered by researchers, for example, where the interview will take place, journey time to be interviewed, scheduling the interview in the morning or being mindful about the length of the interview and encouraging participants to determine when they wish to finish.

Gate-keeping by health care professionals was experienced in this study, despite the inclusion criteria of anyone willing to tell their story and be tape-recorded, practitioners were commonly rejecting potential participants on my behalf, they were selective on the basis of who in their view 'had a good story to tell,' was 'articulate,' 'interesting' or who would 'benefit' from the experience of the interview, in terms of it being viewed as cathartic to talk about the illness experience. What made a story 'good' was not entirely clear. However, it appeared that judgements were being made about who might be a 'suitable' interviewee. Some health care professionals saw their role as protecting patients from the burden of research, others as deciding which stories were best told and which were best not told. This raises questions about the ethical issues of treating dying people differently and paternalistically, by taking decisions on behalf of consenting adults, rather than enabling people to decide for themselves. In addition, gate-keeping and the issues associated with it, highlight the power differentials between potential participants, researcher and professionals, in the practice of gate-keeping the power of one group is exercised over another. Early discussions took place with two teams working in a specialist palliative care unit to introduce the research and seek their support as gate-keepers to potential participants. One team of health care professionals referred no patients to me as being interested in taking part in the research. This was in stark contrast to the other team who had many patients who were very keen to take part. It seemed there was a different approach to research generally and paternalistic practice in the former team while the latter team appeared open to research and happy for patients to decide for themselves if they wanted to take part.

5. Informed Consent

Process consent has been advocated by Beaver et al. as a means of renegotiating consent throughout the research process rather than as a 'one off' procedure, where consent is not revisited once participants have agreed to take part.[12] Consent, in this study, was continually sought with the participants each time contact was made. Gaining access was not a one off activity but the result of on-going negotiation between the participant and myself. Repeated attempts were made to give people opportunities to withdraw from the research, however none of the participants chose to do so. One potential participant who had discussed the research with me and arranged a time for the interview however died at home prior to the interview taking place the following week. Process consent is especially important in longitudinal research and research involving people with palliative care needs as a person's condition may change rapidly. I never assumed that because a person had consented to take part that they would still feel the same a week later.

True informed consent or informed choice is problematic, particularly in qualitative research using narrative approaches, when it is not clear what is being consented to prior to the event, in this case the interview. Indeed, participants do not necessarily know in advance what will take place within the interview, how much they will self-disclose or how intimate and personal the data will be is unknown when people consent to be involved.[13] Do people make rational decisions to self-disclose in research interviews or is it more a situation that evolves due to the safe environment created or the rapport developed with the researcher? It may well be difficult to forecast, with any accuracy what will happen in a research interview, thus consent becomes a continuously negotiated process. The idea of forewarning participants about the possible intimate nature of interviews is therefore difficult. Hollway and Jefferson suggest that people's decision to take part in a research study had more to do with how they perceived the researchers, than the information they gave to people about the study or any forewarnings.[14] Miller and Bell highlight this dilemma and suggest that the true nature of consent may only become clear at the end of a study.[15] In some qualitative research, the researcher revisits participants and asks them to read transcripts for accuracy, or to comment on the researcher's interpretation of the data to authenticate it; this was rejected in this study for methodological and ethical reasons. It was decided that this would not be an appropriate course of action in this research for two reasons. Firstly, stories are told for particular reasons and shaped accordingly; therefore they change according to the context and over time. The story is already authentic since it was constructed by the storyteller. To aspire to authenticity is therefore misplaced, as it assumes one version and one truth rather than multiple truths. Secondly, from an ethical viewpoint it was not considered feasible to return transcripts to the participants as it was anticipated that they may not be well enough or may have already died, given the timescales involved and that this would have been too intrusive.

6. Confidentiality and Anonymity

The issue of confidentiality and anonymity is closely related to issues of consent and access and will now be discussed. The right to confidentiality and anonymity is generally considered to be a 'good thing' in terms of research ethics. Indeed, its importance is highlighted by several authors.[16] It is the right of individuals not to have their personal and private information disclosed. Agreeing to confidentiality and anonymity are ways that researchers protect their participants' right to privacy. However, the experience of undertaking this research suggests that it is more complex to achieve in practice and may not necessarily be desired by participants themselves.

Confidentiality in research suggests that any information obtained about individuals in the course of the study should be utilised in a secure way to protect the anonymity of participants. Maintaining a participant's confidentiality, by protecting a person's identity is generally considered to be a good thing in health care research, particular emphasis is placed on this in the process of ethical approval. It appears that the maintenance of confidentiality is a universal requirement proposed in various ethical codes and guidelines of our professional organisations, for example, the British Sociological Association, Royal College of Nursing and the British Psychological Society and the research ethics committee reviews.[17] However, it may not always be in the best interests of participants to remain anonymous. Having your story attached to you personally and being identified as the person who has lived through the illness experience appeared to be particularly important for participants. Stories told by participants in this study were unique, thus, using pseudonyms and changing biographical data to try to preserve a person's anonymity proved inadequate to maintain confidentiality. Changing further details pertaining to a person's story changed the essence of the story itself. What makes a story unparalleled amongst other accounts of illness? In particular, the assurance of confidentiality may not be in the best interests of participants. It results in decontextualising and standandardising of the interview and emphasises the power differential between the researcher and participants. Participant's stories are reduced to an anonymous mass rather than linked to them as individuals. Anonymity is particularly difficult to achieve in qualitative research where there is reliance on small sample sizes and direct quotes are used in research reports.

A recent exception in the UK where participants have been identified is the Database of Individual Patient Experience (DIPEx), where multimedia video clips are used on a website with patients talking about their illness experiences.[18] Clearly these people can be identified; their anonymity and confidentiality not imposed or insisted upon by ethics committees. It raises the question, have these participants been harmed in any way by this process or should it always be assumed that to remain anonymous is preferable? It could be suggested therefore that it would be good practice in narrative research to ask participants to decide for themselves if they wish to remain anonymous. Barnard et al., in a study of palliative care patients in Canada, point out that participants would probably recognise themselves within their research report however much effort was made to disguise their identity, and that close friends, family and the care team may also be able to identify the person.[19] Furthermore, in Barnard et al.'s study, participants wished to be identified in the published research and book and were disappointed that the stories they told about their lives, in particular the end of their life, would not bear their name. Some participants viewed the research as a last chance to make an impact or to leave something tangible, their written story, after their death. It could be argued that true confidentiality cannot be maintained in qualitative research as a range of direct quotes are commonly used in the final report and researchers do not maintain control over how direct quotes are used once published, thus it is difficult to be sure that you have consent for all future uses of the quotes. Moreover, participants may change their minds regarding their wish or not for anonymity. Furthermore, there is little guidance for researchers regarding how to manage consent and confidentiality after a person's death.[20]

7. Ownership of the Story

During the course of the research I was concerned by the question of whose story was being recorded in the research process. Was this my story of someone else's illness experience or their story told through me? Was I speaking for others or seeing stories through my own lenses? Was I telling stories of other people's lives or constructing stories for others? Whose voice was represented in the story? Would participants feel that the stories were true to their experience of illness? These questions were ones which I found particularly challenging throughout the research.

How could I be sure that I had understood correctly and been true to the experience? Any story which I tell, I do so through my past experiences, history, culture, gender, belief systems and values. In Heideggerian phenomenological research it is accepted that the researcher will not only influence the data collection and analysis, but the whole research process. In addition, it was accepted that the context of the enquiry was crucial to the findings of the research. A reflective diary was kept during the entire project which proved helpful particularly during the analysis of the data and in terms of the contextual issues and my changing perceptions. A section from my reflective diary reveals my concerns with narrative ownership:

> I am concerned that I need to be true to the participant's stories and to represent them as they would themselves. I recognise that as a researcher involved in phenomenological research I have an impact on the whole research process and that I will see these stories through my own lenses yet I still feel uncomfortable about speaking for others.

The issue of who owns the research participant's story and perhaps the more central issue of whose story is actually being told is a key concern in narrative research. When there is so much personal investment in the account, when one's whole identity is tied up with the story it becomes an ethical and methodological dilemma for researchers. Some authors highlight the possible difficulties for narrative researchers when participants are unhappy with the researcher's account of their story.[21] It is possible that participants might feel betrayed by the researcher if they consider the researcher has misrepresented their story in some way. However, the approach taken by narrative researchers is different to that taken by the individual who tells their life story or the story of a specific experience like illness. Narrative researchers while being interested in the individual and their story are also interested in the wider social context of the experience, in my case life-threatening illness. It is therefore commonly agreed that narrative researchers need to accept some ownership and maintain authority and control over the narratives in their research. Given this position, the ethical dilemma is to manage this control in an ethical way so that participants are not exploited or disempowered as a result of the research. These issues are complex and warrant further exploration so that research participants feel that their voice has been heard when they take part in a research study.

8. Relationship between Participant and Researcher

There is a constant tension between the role of being a researcher and a professional practitioner. We are unable to leave one aspect of ourselves at the interview door; I for instance, remain a palliative care nurse undertaking research. The atmosphere created by the researcher in order to put participants at ease and to encourage self-disclosure draws on interpersonal skills developed in practice and relies on an ability to create a rapport with the participant. The nature of that rapport and how it is achieved requires further exploration by qualitative researchers. In research we use ourselves therapeutically to 'invite intimacy' to promote stories of a private and intimate nature, the success of the interview itself, for the researcher, may depend on hearing something personal and/or intimate.[22] This situation invites participants to narrate experiences to us as researchers, who become temporary confidantes and/or 'friends.' Duncombe and Jessop describe this as akin to 'faking friendship' to create the context for self-disclosure by being friendly and informal.[23] The ethical issues raised by this are considerable, for example, how we respond to someone in a research encounter whom we dislike or would not be drawn to in a social situation. When participants say things in the course of a research interview like 'I have never told anyone else that before.' Do we, as researchers, take this as a compliment or does it concern us? Power differentials or disparity between participants and researchers presents a dilemma that requires the responsible use of the researcher's power. What happens when for whatever reason rapport is not established between the participant and the researcher? Can we assume that self-disclosure and openness does not happen? Supposing we feel that we have established a rapport with an interviewee and they have disclosed their intimate feelings and experiences it may still feel unsatisfying or intrusive from the researchers' point of view. After one such interview for example, I felt guilty that the participant had used their clearly limited time being interviewed.

Alty and Rodham highlight the difficulties of 'hearing too much off the record' during the course of qualitative research interview, when a researcher is asked by a participant not to include certain aspect of the story or participants might add or embellish the story after the tape recorder has been turned off.[24] This situation did not arise in my research, however one similar situation did cause a dilemma. On several occasions when I went to meet a potential participant to talk about the study and answer any questions they might have, they began to tell me their story there and then, at the point when I was ready to make an interview date and talk about consent. This may have been influenced by the situation these people were in, related to the uncertainty of their future even in the short term.

Duncombe and Jessop describe a situation of meeting a research participant two years after an interview and being embraced in the street as if by an old friend, an apparent demonstration of over-familiarity and friendship resulting from 'faking friendship.'[25] This situation is perhaps more likely to occur in longitudinal research when the participant/researcher relationship develops over time. The reverse of this situation is also possible, of participants 'faking friendship' to please the researcher or to try to give the researcher what they need for the purpose of the research. During the data collection period of the research I sometimes met participants I had interviewed in previous weeks. I felt that there was a link between us, due to the time we had spent together, and the sharing and self-disclosure which had taken place. However, I never felt uncomfortable or that my boundaries were unclear. I was concerned to know how these people were and what had happened since the interview. Subsequent conversations frequently involved acknowledging their deteriorating condition.

9. Distress in Research Interviews

The issue of participants becoming distressed in research interviews is important to consider from an ethical point of view as it is commonly linked to the notion of causing harm. Parkes in his guidelines for conducting ethical bereavement research highlights the possibility of an interviewee becoming distressed during the course of an interview.[26] Becoming upset or distressed is not uncommon in palliative care and bereavement research. Indeed, Aranda in discussing her palliative care research says that:

> Almost all of those visited cried or become distressed at sometime during the session, yet continued to express a willingness to participate. An inexperienced researcher, or one unused to working with dying people, may have fled at this point and decided that the study entailed too significant a risk of harm for the participants.[27]

Participants may express emotions during a research interview and it could be suggested that the interview 'puts' participants in a distressed state. An alternative interpretation might be that individuals are merely expressing what they are feeling and it is not as a result of the interview itself. Participants were more likely to be distressed by coping with dying rather than by actually talking about it. The question of under what circumstances one would stop an interview is also important to consider from an ethical viewpoint. This case example from my research illustrates this difficult aspect of research interviewing.

Annie was a 44 year old woman diagnosed with advanced breast cancer, she was a wheelchair user, and had difficulties talking and expressing herself due to neurological disease, however her competence was not in doubt. She was keen to take part in the research and to tell her illness story. As a researcher I was concerned that I would not be able to understand her speech or be able to transcribe the dialogue from the tapes. However, the story proved to be one of the most moving and insightful of the interviews undertaken. It was reminiscent of Frank's chaos narrative[28] when Annie said "I thought I would get better but it's been like a downward slope … I think it can't get any worse, then it does."

Annie's suffering was implicit within the illness narrative and difficult to hear as the listener. When she became upset during the interview, I asked her 'shall I stop the tape now?' However she clearly indicated that she did not wish to stop the tape or terminate the interview at that point. In response I acknowledged the distress and sadness she expressed about her illness and listened to her story. It was clear that for Annie to tell her story had taken considerable time and effort on her part, I wanted to respect this and value the effort she was making to be part of the research. This, not uncommon example from my research, highlighted that despite showing emotion and feeling upset participants may not necessarily want to discontinue the interview or withdraw from the research. It seemed to me Annie was upset and distressed at her situation, not distressed by talking about it.

Davies et al. discuss the experience of a study involving severely ill people with incurable brain tumours, they suggest that the majority of people interviewed found positive benefits to being involved. However, for a minority of people, the interviews were thought to have caused distress.[29] In narrative interviewing there is no list of questions. The interviewee has control over what aspects of their illness they wish to talk about or indeed the focus the interview takes. Sensitive research might therefore be better adopting an unstructured approach to interviewing where the participants define the areas of concern rather than the researchers.

10. The Boundary between Research and Therapeutic Relationships

The research interview itself, in this study, was not designed specially to be therapeutic. However, it is possible that this type of research when conducted in an ethical manner will have positive therapeutic effects. For example, to talk and actually verbalise a difficult experience may in itself be helpful to people. It may be that the boundary between research and therapy is not entirely distinct; several participants said informally that it had been good for them to tell their story and to have someone listen attentively to them, particularly someone outside the family and the care team, who they would probably not see again. Rosenblatt, in a paper exploring the ethical issues related to bereavement research, states:

> I am not a therapist. However, I am strongly inclined to provide appropriately human support to anyone with whom I interact. I have no qualms about moving outside the frame of research interactions to speak to someone's

> pain or confusion. Depending on what the person I am interviewing seems to think appropriate, I can offer sympathy, cry with him or her, talk about experiences of my own that are similar, or acknowledge the person's pain. I do not see that as crossing a line into therapy.[30]

Rosenblatt sees this as entirely consistent with bereavement research guidelines which state that the needs of participants must take priority over the needs of the research study.[31] The boundary between research and therapy is particularly difficult when as a practitioner one is used to working with people experiencing loss and emotions are commonly expressed. I found the non-directive style of narrative interviewing difficult as in a similar practice situation I would have responded differently, perhaps exploring issues more, or maybe challenging the patient's ideas. In the research interviews I tended to listen more and mainly ask questions to make sure I had understood the meaning. There are links here with the previous section, which considered the relationship between the participant and researcher in terms of the lengths researchers go to in order to develop rapport with participants. For some participants a research interview may be one of the few occasions they have to talk at length about their concerns, feelings and perceptions of the illness and the impact that it has had on their life. Researchers engaged in this type of research need to be in a position to refer on, or be able to know where and how a participant might gain further support after the research is finished. At the end of each interview it is good practice to check out with participants if there is anything further they wish to discuss and have the contact details of someone who can be contacted for additional support. This is recommended for all participants, regardless of whether or not they were upset during the interview, as it is possible that thinking about the interview afterwards could provoke emotions or distress later.

11. Conclusion

This chapter is based on a research study with people with palliative care needs who narrated their experiences of life-threatening illness; it captures the attempt to conduct ethically sensitive research in a palliative care population and the dilemmas raised as a result of this. The ethical challenges encountered during the course of this study were difficult and included amongst others the issues of confidentiality, gate-keeping of research participants, the relationship between the researcher and the participant and narrative ownership. Although these represent the ethical dilemmas encountered in this research, with dying people, there are many other ethical issues in qualitative research than those I have discussed here. Whilst it has not been the aim of this chapter to produce a comprehensive review of the ethical dilemmas which might occur, I hope that drawing attention to these issues, which are not always viewed as problematic, that ethical debate will be promoted and it will encourage others to consider these issues. These examples and reflections are given from the research to illustrate points and to identify strategies which maybe helpful. However, it is also accepted that there may be no straightforward or simple answer to these problems. It appears to be a feature of qualitative research to continually wonder if one is doing the right thing and to question if one is behaving in an ethically sensitive manner. To achieve this aim researchers need to reflect on their research practice and to be self-critical of all decisions made. In addition, more researchers need to engage in the process of writing about some of the difficulties experienced while actually doing qualitative research as frequently these difficulties relate to ethical dilemmas which are not well documented in health care research.

It has been suggested within this chapter that certain assumptions underpinning research ethics require greater debate particularly in narrative research, for example, the assumption that confidentiality is always in the best interests of participants or that participants always desire it, requires further debate, within the literature and at the ethics approval stage. It is suggested that research ethics requires a rethink in terms of traditional research ethics, more of a partnership approach to research is required, rather than viewing people as passive participants in research projects. Current ethical guidelines are at best problematic and, at worst, misguided as they fail to take account of the real world of qualitative research and the dilemmas facing researchers. In conclusion, undertaking qualitative research and becoming an ethically responsible researcher is a difficult and challenging endeavour in which frequently more questions are raised than answered.

Notes

[1] A.W. Frank, *The Wounded Storyteller: Body, Illness, and Ethics* (London: The University of Chicago Press, 1995).

[2] S. Aranda, and A.Street, "From Individual to Group: Use of Narratives in a Participatory Research Process," *Journal of Advanced Nursing*, 33, 6 (2001): 784-790.

[3] D.E. Polkinghorne, *Narrative Knowing and the Human Sciences* (New York: State University of New York Press, 1988) and Polkinghorne, "Narrative Configuration in Qualitative Analysis," in J. Amos Hatch and R. Wisniewski, eds., *Life History and Narrative* (London: The Falmer Press, 1995).

[4] British Sociological Association (BSA), *Statement of Ethical Practice* (Mountjoy Research Centre: Durham, 1996); Royal College of Nursing (RCN), *Research Ethics: Standards of Care* (London: Royal College of

Nursing, 1998) and British Psychological Society (BPS), *Code of Conduct: Ethical Principles and Guidelines* (Leicester: BPS Press, 1996).

[5] S. Aranda, "Conducting Research with the Dying: Ethical Considerations and Experience," *International Journal of Palliative* Nursing, 1,1 (1995): 41-7; B. Mount et al., "Ethical Issues in Palliative Care Research Revisited," *Palliative Medicine* 9 (1995): 165-170; and L. de Raeve, "Ethical Issues in Palliative Care Research," *Palliative Medicine* 8 (4), (1994): 298-305.

[6] L. de Raeve, "Ethical Issues in Palliative Care Research," *Palliative Medicine* 8 (4), (1994): 298.

[7] B. Mount et al., "Ethical Issues in Palliative Care Research Revisited," *Palliative Medicine* 9 (1995): 165.

[8] See, for example, K. Beaver et al., "Conducting Research with the Terminally Ill: Challenges and Considerations," *International Journal of Palliative Nursing*, 5, 1 (1999): 13-17.

[9] See, for example, R.G. Twycross and G. Dunn, *Research in Palliative Care: The Pursuit of Reliable Knowledge.* Occasional Paper 5 (London: National Council for Hospice and Specialist Palliative Care Services, 1994).

[10] A. Alty and K. Rodham, "Pearls, Pith and Provocation: The Ouch! Factor: Problems in Conducting Sensitive Research," *Qualitative Health Research*, 8, 2 (1998): 275-282.

[11] For example, K. Rose, "Gaining Access to Potential Research Participants," *Professional Nurse* 15, 7 (2000): 465-467.

[12] Beaver et al., "Conducting Research with the Terminally Ill."

[13] W. Hollway and T. Jefferson, "The Ethics of Researching Psychosocial Subjects," in *Doing Qualitative Research Differently: Free Association, Narrative and the Interview Method* (London: Sage Publications, 2000), 83-103.

[14] Ibid.

[15] T. Miller and L. Bell, "Consenting to What? Issues of Access, Gate-keeping and ''Informed' Consent," in M. Mauthner et al., *Ethics in Qualitative Research* (London: Sage Publications, 2002), 53-69.

[16] See, for example, C.M. Parkes, "Guidelines for Conducting Ethical Bereavement Research," *Death Studies* 19 (1995): 171-181.

[17] British Sociological Association (1996), Royal College of Nursing (1998) and the British Psychological Society (1996).

[18] A. Herxheimer et al., "Database of Patient's Experiences (DIPEx): a Multi-media Approach to Sharing Experiences and Information," *The Lancet* 355 (2000): 1540-43.

[19] D. Barnard et al., *Crossing Over: Narratives of Palliative Care* (Oxford: Oxford University Press, 2000).

[20] J. Lawton, "Gaining and Maintaining Consent: Ethical Concerns Raised in a Study of Dying Patients," *Qualitative Health Research*, 11, 5 (2001): 639-705.
[21] W.E. Smythe. and M.J. Murray, "Owning the Story: Ethical Considerations in Narrative Research," *Ethics and Behavior* 10, 4 (2000): 324.
[22] M. Birch and T. Miller, "Inviting Intimacy: the Interview as Therapeutic Opportunity," *International Journal of Social Research Methodology* 3, 3, (2000): 189-202.
[23] J. Duncombe and J. Jessop, "'Doing Rapport' and the Ethics of 'Faking Friendship'," in M. Mauthner et al., *Ethics in Qualitative Research* (London: Sage Publications, 2002), 107-22.
[24] Alty and Rodham (1998).
[25] Duncombe and Jessop, "'Doing Rapport' and the Ethics of 'Faking Friendship.'"
[26] Parkes, "Guidelines for Conducting Ethical Bereavement Research."
[27] Aranda, "Conducting Research with the Dying: Ethical Considerations and Experience," 44.
[28] Frank, *The Wounded Storyteller*.
[29] E.A. Davies et al., "Do Research Interviews Cause Distress or Interfere in Management?" *Journal of the Royal College of Physicians of London* 32, 5 (1998): 406-411.
[30] P.C. Rosenblatt, "Ethics of Qualitative Interviewing with Grieving Families," *Death Studies* 19 (1995), 149.
[31] Parkes, "Guidelines for Conducting Ethical Bereavement Research."

Bibliography

Alty, A. and K. Rodham. "Pearls, Pith and Provocation: The Ouch! Factor: Problems in Conducting Sensitive Research." *Qualitative Health Research*, 8, 2 (1998): 275-282.

Aranda, S. "Conducting Research with the Dying: Ethical Considerations and Experience." *International Journal of Palliative* Nursing, 1,1 (1995): 41-7.

Aranda, S. and A. Street. "From Individual to Group: Use of Narratives in a Participatory Research Process." *Journal of Advanced Nursing*, 33, 6 (2001): 784-790.

Barnard, D., A. Towers, P. Boston, Y. Lambrinidou. *Crossing Over: Narratives of Palliative Care*. Oxford: Oxford University Press, 2000.

Beaver, K., K. Luker, and S. Woods. "Conducting Research with the Terminally Ill: Challenges and Considerations." *International Journal of Palliative Nursing*, 5, 1 (1999): 13-17.

Birch, M. and T. Miller. "Inviting Intimacy: The Interview as Therapeutic Opportunity." *International Journal of Social Research Methodology* 3, 3, (2000): 189-202.

British Psychological Society (BPS). *Code of Conduct: Ethical Principles and Guidelines*. Leicester: BPS Press, 1996.

British Sociological Association (BSA). *Statement of Ethical Practice* Mountjoy Research Centre: Durham, 1996.

Davies, E. A., S. Hall, C. Clarke, M. Bannon, M., and A. Hopkins. "Do Research Interviews Cause Distress or Interfere in Management?" *Journal of the Royal College of Physicians of London* 32, 5 (1998): 406-411.

de Raeve, L. "Ethical Issues in Palliative Care Research." *Palliative Medicine* 8 (4), (1994): 298-305.

Duncombe, J. and J. Jessop. "'Doing Rapport' and the Ethics of 'Faking Friendship'." In M. Mauthner, M. Birch, J. Jessop, and T. Miller, *Ethics in Qualitative Research*, 107-22. London: Sage Publications, 2002.

Frank, A. W. *The Wounded Storyteller: Body, Illness, and Ethics*. London: The University of Chicago Press, 1995.

Herxheimer, A., A. McPherson, R. Miller, S. Shepperd, J. Yaphe, and S. Ziebland. "Database of Patient's Experiences (DIPEx): a Multi-media Approach to Sharing Experiences and Information." *The Lancet* 355 (2000): 1540-43.

Hollway, W. and T. Jefferson. "The Ethics of Researching Psychosocial Subjects." In *Doing Qualitative Research Differently: Free Association, Narrative and the Interview Method*, 83-103. London: Sage Publications, 2000.

Lawton, J. "Gaining and Maintaining Consent: Ethical Concerns Raised in a Study of Dying Patients." *Qualitative Health Research*, 11, 5 (2001): 639-705.

Miller, T and L. Bell. "Consenting to What? Issues of Access, Gate-keeping and ''Informed' Consent." In Mauthner, M. Birch, J. Jessop, and

T. Miller, *Ethics in Qualitative Research*, 53-69. London: Sage Publications, 2002.

Mount, B., R. Cohen, N. MacDonald, E. Bruera, and D.J. Dudgeon. “Ethical Issues in Palliative Care Research Revisited.” *Palliative Medicine* 9 (1995): 165-170.

Parkes, C.M. “Guidelines for Conducting Ethical Bereavement Research.” *Death Studies* 19 (1995): 171-181.

Polkinghorne, D. E. *Narrative Knowing and the Human Sciences.* New York: State University of New York Press, 1988.

Polkinghorne, D. E. “Narrative Configuration in Qualitative Analysis.” In J. Amos Hatch and R. Wisniewski, eds., *Life History and Narrative* London: The Falmer Press, 1995.

Royal College of Nursing. *Research Ethics: Standards of Care.* London: Royal College of Nursing, 1998.

Rose, K. “Gaining Access to Potential Research Participants.” *Professional Nurse* 15, 7 (2000): 465-467.

Rosenblatt, P.C. “Ethics of Qualitative Interviewing with Grieving Families.” *Death Studies* 19 (1995): 139-155.

Smythe, W. E. and M.J. Murray. “Owning the Story: Ethical Considerations in Narrative Research.” *Ethics and Behavior* 10, 4 (2000): 311-336.

Twycross, R.G and G. Dunn. *Research in Palliative Care: The Pursuit of Reliable Knowledge.* Occasional Paper 5, London: National Council for Hospice and Specialist Palliative Care Services, 1994.

Note on Contributor

Jane Appleton is the programme leader for palliative care, Oxford Brookes University, UK.

Post-Cancer Distress in Some Cancer Survivors: Well-being, Self-determination Theory and a Downward Cycle

Emma-Jane Sayers and Miles Little

1. Introduction

For five years, we have been examining the narratives of cancer survivors, whom we define as people who are living apparently free of cancer at any time after treatment.[1] Our interviews have been biographical in style, addressing the generic question "How did you come to be where you are today?" Prompts have been kept to a minimum, and interviewers have adopted the stance of empathic witnesses. We have been impressed by the way that narrators, under these circumstances, convey the mixed nature of the survival experience. There is a particular kind of narrative that is told by about 25% of survivors, in which the darker side predominates.[2] This narrative tells of a downward cycle of events and self-perceptions occurring at some stage after the end of treatment, in which self-confidence and self-esteem diminish, self-efficacy contracts, close relationships are strained or disrupted, and a mood of sadness, anxiety and a sense of loss dominate affect. In this paper we offer an account of one such narrative, examine it in the context of other narratives, and suggest that theories of well-being and self-determination theory (SDT) provide a rich explanation of the forces behind the downward cycle.

2. Plan of the Paper

The index narrative is that of one of us (E-JS), reflecting on the events and experiences that followed her diagnosis of Hodgkin's disease at age 20. It appears here as a much condensed abstract of a long narrative. Other narratives, generated by our own research, and published stories are used to illustrate the process of the downward cycle. We examine the phenomenology of survival, drawing on our own previous work. Then we use self-determination theory to explain how the downward cycle is initiated and perpetuated. Finally, we comment on ways in which the cycle may be broken. Throughout, we use qualitative methods. We attempt to validate our hypotheses by both introspection, a process of comparing theory to personal experience, and extrospection, a process of objectifying and generalising from a number of individual accounts. We have generated our own data using grounded theory,[3] and we routinely test our conclusions in workshops and seminars directed to survivors affected by the work we do.

3. Emma's story

I was 20 years old when my Hodgkin's disease was diagnosed, a Law student in a stable relationship. My academic results were good, and I was enjoying my Law course.

Chemotherapy was pretty bad, but I got through it safely, and at 6 months was given good news that the disease seemed to be cured. My specialist told me that I had a 90% chance of permanent cure.

I was weary but a bit euphoric. I went back to university, and joined CanYA, a support group for young adults affected by cancer. I joined CanYA's committee and became a support person, advising others with problems similar to mine. I felt fatigued, but was happy to be involved in doing useful things with my cancer experience.

After a year or so, however, things started to go wrong. I lost my motivation to do Law, and suffered panic attacks before exams. I still managed to pass (just), but felt I couldn't cope with the stress, and deferred.

I also found myself less interested in telling the story of my illness to newly diagnosed cancer patients, and to groups of nurses and other students. I found more satisfaction in working with a research group that was trying to understand problems that they'd identified among long-term cancer survivors.

Despite this renewed interest, I felt fatigued and unsure of the direction that I might take in life. My confusion and lack of motivation upset my parents, and that made me feel guilty. Then my partner left me under very distressing circumstances. My work remained important, but often [it] was hard to preserve perspective and focus. I couldn't explain, to myself or others, just what was wrong. I felt hesitant to start anything, in case I somehow failed. I'd lost the drive to complete my Law degree; I was no longer sure that I could go on helping people newly diagnosed with cancer; my partner had left me; and it was even a battle to do the research and teaching that I loved.

This was the worst stage of my life, worse than diagnosis and treatment. Over a very miserable Christmas break, I talked and thought about my aspirations and my abilities, and decided to make

> adjustments, to concentrate on those things I could do and wanted to do.
> I came back to the research group, and set out to identify myself with education and support for people who have survived cancer. I have established an identity in the field, and as an advocate for cancer services and better representation of cancer voices in policy making. I have recovered some of my old energy. There's a long way to go, but I look forward to each day's work, I've gone back to dancing, and I've finished my Law degree. There's some purpose to my life again. It's taken more than six years to reach this point.

4. Other Accounts

Emma's narrative finds counterparts in narratives given to us by many survivors. Ann, a former nurse and business-woman who had both large bowel and breast cancer, and Danny, an actor and script-writer who had large bowel cancer, for example, both speak of the near-euphoria of finishing treatment, and the initial enthusiasm for incorporating the cancer into their new lives by entering the world of cancer support and advocacy, and by speaking publicly about their experiences. Then, both also tell of a dreadful let-down between one and two years after treatment, when meaning vanished from life, the drive to do familiar things seemed to dwindle and vanish, relationships were strained, and fatigue and sadness dominated the experience of life. Survivors who tell this story speak of a downward cycle of mood and achievement, in which sadness, diminution in achievement, and alienation reinforce one another, to produce a state of what we call *post-cancer distress* (PCD), where 'distress' implies a kind of unfixed anxiety generated (in part) by consciousness of a frail and uninterpretable existence.

It is hard to estimate the frequency of significant PCD and the downward cycle. We do not believe that structured questionnaires allow sufficient trust and relationship to develop between interviewees and interviewers for an accurate estimate of prevalence. Much of the trouble reported by narrators in our research emerged late in the interview (at about one hour), when survivors felt enough trust to report on intimate matters. In thirteen interviews, six narrators emphasised the difficulties of the survival experience, and four of the six reported major life disruptions and persistent distress that illustrate the phenomena and effects of the downward cycle.

The patients, from our original study, whose narratives we have drawn from in this paper are:

1. Bill, aged 74, self-employed businessman, colorectal cancer, with a colostomy, 76 months after treatment.
2. Lynn, aged 57, former nurse, colorectal cancer, permanent ileostomy, 30 months after treatment.
3. Helen, aged 40, housewife, colorectal cancer, no stoma, 48 months after treatment.
4. Jean, aged 71, housewife, colorectal cancer, no stoma, 6 months after treatment.
5. Mark, aged 39, warehouseman, colorectal cancer, no stoma, 20 months after treatment. Sharon, Mark's wife, was interviewed with Mark.
6. Anna, aged 20, university student, liver cancer, 6 years after treatment.

There is a tendency in popular literature to emphasise the positive dimensions of cancer survival.[4] There are, however, some personal accounts of the negative aspects and the cumulative effects of the downward cycle. We draw particularly on autobiographical accounts by Samantha Miles[5] and Evan Handler,[6] both of whom have had bone-marrow transplants for leukaemia.

5. Organizing the Accounts

We can group descriptions of the negative experiences under the following headings:

A. Loss of continuity – body and mental life.
B. Loss of life plan.
C. Loss of life meaning.
D. Loss of comfortable ignorance.
E. Existential insecurity.
F. Loss of significant relatedness – alienation
G. Fatigue.
H. Sense of ageing.
I. Achievement/aspiration mismatch.
J. Loss of 'future memory'.
K. Guilt, accountability, debt.

A. Loss of Continuity – Body and Mental Life

Cancer illnesses profoundly disrupt life. Cancer occurs *in* the body, mysteriously, and beyond the body's control. It may also produce changes to the body that impair its functions. Bill, for example, has a colostomy that restricts his social life:

> But I wasn't prepared for a) the trauma that I would have to go through, the surgical trauma, and b) the restrictions it placed on my life afterwards … The restrictions I am talking about are physical restrictions. Right? For instance, I don't go swimming … For fear of infection … I can't dance. I can't play any sport. I can't play any sport whatsoever, right? Ah, and these are the sort of restrictions I have got on my life. You know, I used to love my swimming. I used to love playing golf. I used to love playing table tennis. All those sort of things. Even at that age. I've been used to it all my life. This is what –maybe they didn't even think it was - and I am not being critical of Dr. K— or H— or anybody else. Maybe they just didn't realise that that was such an importance part of person's life.

Bill registers his sense of anger at having lost the continuity of his physical, embodied life, but also his subjective sense of enjoyment of important recreational activities.

B. Loss of Life Plan

Bill also remarks on the changes brought about to his ability to plan the rest of his life. Deprived of his favourite recreations, he has only his work to fill his future:

> I just live for the day. I go to work officially twenty hours a week. [Pause.] I've got no future plans whatsoever so far as my business is concerned. It would - I know if I was to give it away I wouldn't last a month … At the moment I have got nothing else better, right? There has got to be a day sometime sooner or later, I have got to walk out of that. But to what, I don't know. What the alternative is, I don't know.

C. Loss of Life Meaning

In the same vein, Bill perceives that his life has been so robbed of meaning by cancer and its aftermath that death might have been a better option than 'cure':

> And on reflection I think maybe, maybe, maybe with what's happened with my restricted life-style *since* -

> maybe I shouldn't have had it. Maybe I should have said "No, let's go and die and be done with it."

D. Loss of Comfortable Ignorance

The experience of cancer brings uncomfortable insights into the fragility of life and the vulnerability of the body. Most of us are aware of our mortality, but that awareness has no daily currency, unless we have an extreme, life threatening experience. Helen notes the radical change in her perceptions of what is important in her life:

> Just little things like that that you think, they're not important. I mean, if I wake up alive that's what's important to me now.

Evan Handler, recovered from leukaemia and a bone-marrow transplant, writes of an episode in which he walks off the stage during a performance because the lead actor's arrogance and unpleasantness suddenly become too much to bear:

> I realised that, compared to where I had been in my life, this was a meaningless engagement. The stakes – money, honour, reputation – while seemingly enormous, were really about pride, and had very little to do with one's ability to exist. The distinction I was able to make at last, was the difference between forces that are annoying and those that pose a real threat.[7]

This walk-out threatens Handler's career, but he is proud to have taken the step.

E. Existential Insecurity

This loss of comfortable ignorance leads to existential insecurity, a state in which symptoms, events and remarks provoke concerns about cancer and death. Helen is speaking again:

> I worry about if I am going to live, you know, tomorrow. I don't worry about things nearly as much as I used to worry about things. I suppose when I got out of hospital it was on my mind all the time, like I'd think about it twenty-four hours a day at first. You know what I mean? Now, still probably a day doesn't go by that I don't think about it once … You think – I suppose when

> I heard about it, I thought – you think of cancer, *death*. I mean you just think of dying, you don't think of the people that recover … I mean anything I get, if I get a headache or if I get a backache, I think oh God it's gone to your liver … or anything I get you associate it, I just think of cancer straight away.

Handler writes:

> While I try to continually remind myself to live each day as if it might be my last one, the knowledge that every day could be my last makes me too sad to enjoy them.[8]

F. Loss of Significant Relatedness – Alienation

These kinds of insight and existential tensions are not easy to talk about, nor easy to convey to others, however close they may be. Furthermore, most 'normal' people want to avoid talking about issues of mortality and bodily frailty. The difficulty of framing in speech and the unwillingness to hear the story combine to disrupt friendships. Helen sums up the sense of alienation:

> No, not that many people talk about it with me. I suppose they think, well, they don't want to. Unless I bring it up, which I don't a lot. I mean, you have to go for my test, I think – I usually stress out at the time for a week, and thinking, you know, what they are going to see? But most people don't want to talk about it.

Anna, who developed liver cancer at age 13 years, returned to school after her chemotherapy and surgery, to find that she viewed her school-friends differently:

> If you have been away from school for a long time, and have been through something that 99.9% of the kids at school wouldn't even dream about, you just, it's just natural to feel like you having nothing in common any more. Because just the whole perception of life changes when you have gone through something like that, and it was really hard for them to adjust to me coming back being as different as I was, as well, and I think the friends of people like me need a lot of support as well, because they aren't told anything. I mean the family is told, and the family has the duty of telling the friends,

> but they really don't know what's going on, and what to do if I get sick at school or something like that, so it was really hard going back to school

Alienation may lead to changes in various kinds of relationship. Mark and Sharon speak about friendships, and Sharon says:

> …we lost a hell of a lot of friends through this.
> Mark: Well we have lost all our friends.
> Sharon: Simply because ... probably because they don't know what to say. And it is easier to stay away… But then obviously they weren't real close friends. We have got a dozen close friends that have stuck by us through thick and thin. And they have been really, really good… And they understand the whole lot. And they have just been very, very supportive, haven't they [looks to Mark]

Sharon also point out that family relationships may be stressed:

> His, Mark's family, apart from one brother, or two brothers but one brother that we are really close to, he has got two sisters and his mother, "There is no cancer in our family, so he couldn't possibly have cancer" and that's what it is, his own mother and two sisters and so we don't have anything to do with them, they don't care, they don't want to know about it do they? They just don't care. Out of sight, out of mind.

Bill also notes that his family's relationships and dynamics have been altered by his bowel cancer and colostomy:

> [My son's] a man in a big position in industry and he's quite full of himself even now. I'll be quite frank. You can't look at him sideways. You look at him sideways and he gets cross with you. As I said, he never ever came near me, the whole time I was in hospital ... My daughter was very supportive. Ah, but, ah, there's not the – the real the real depth of affection there either … All right, I'll tell you. I'll be quite frank. I have a lover, and she was very supportive of me … Yeah, yeah, more so than my family, my daughter, my wife, anybody else … Yeah, it really hurt me when my son wouldn't come anywhere near me. That - that - that - that really hurt that. And I thought I'd been a good father. I'd done

> everything. Still. You can't, you can't - you raise children and point them in the right direction. But what they bring home with as a result, you have no control over.

Even close partnerships can be strained and damaged. Sharon recalls the conflict between her and Mark in the first two years after Mark's treatment:

> And the fights ... It was, it was horrible. Our kids didn't want to be here anymore, did they? It was trying to live with somebody, and I was trying to look at it from Mark's point of view, it was really, really hard on me, really hard.

Lynn speaks of the gap between her and her husband since her colectomy and ileostomy:

> Sometimes you just want them to understand … [Sobbing] And they can't … And you just want them. You don't want to dwell on it, that it's been a bad experience [deep breath, regains composure, wipes eyes]…I feel, sometimes I just wished he would understand. And yet if he would give me too much sympathy, maybe I would, maybe it wouldn't be good for me.

G. Fatigue

Many of our narrators spoke directly or indirectly of fatigue as a problem in their daily lives. Jean, managing well after her surgery for bowel cancer, finds that she can no longer go bush-walking with her social club. She replaces her activities with more passive pursuits:

> I am not getting enough walking. But if I get tired then I am at home, and I think "This is no good. I can't sit here brooding with myself." I'll go and get on the train, go into town, or take a book and do the circle around and read my book on the way round from the city - into the city, around Hornsby and back to Concord West [suburbs in Sydney, Australia] … Or sometimes I'll go in and see a movie or something, you know.

Lynn finds, to her disappointment, that she is too fatigued to return to her work as a nurse after her colectomy and ileostomy:

> I went back, and of course as soon as they saw me on the scene, they were ringing me up. So I wasn't working full time, and I was doing a few shifts, and then I worked in the day surgery, but I was just so tired. I shouldn't have, I shouldn't have gone back at that stage. And I was just so, I was just so tired, and I thought, oh, well I should be getting better.

Mark tells of the illness and fatigue with which he lives since his surgery for bowel cancer, and of the ways in which they affect his life:

> The other morning I woke just feeling like shit, just didn't feel like going to work, I just felt sick. I just felt I wanted to stay home, but I got myself going, I got myself to work, and that's what some days are like. Some days are good, fine, I am flying through the day, other days I just don't feel like doing anything. Some days, weekends here, I get out of bed, and you know, I just couldn't be bothered. You know, I just want to go back to bed, and just snore … You know, I just feel like staying home, you know, just pottering around the garden. Sharon feels like going out, but virtually you have got to, when we go out I have got to feel a 100 per cent before we go anywhere.

Samantha Miles, responding to the Internet forum sponsored by the Australian Broadcasting Commission after the ABC's program *Surviving Survival*, notes that fatigue can be debilitating even for someone whose achievements seem to be high:

> I have had numerous achievements since my cancer experience (academic success, successful job, public recognition, etc) and here I sit hardly able to put one foot in front of the other…

Evan Handler tells us how the fatigue is in part engendered by a sense that action is pointless:

> I told her [his physician] how, after I got well from the transplant, for a long time, I couldn't get myself up off the couch. I had my health back, but I didn't feel like

> *doing anything.* I just felt, well - if my life doesn't depend on it, why bother?[9]

H. Sense of Ageing

Cancer presents sufferers with a stark view of the end of their lives. Most people will not have to confront that reality so suddenly. Most will have time to work toward an acceptance of their mortality. Cancer, particularly in those who are young, crams life experience into a short space. This may make some people 'feel their age', while others may feel old before their time. Lynn feels older than her years:

> No, it's not an excuse, it's just um, because I think I should be able to do everything, everything. It shouldn't make any difference, but then I think, it does. Physically I think I get tired, but I might be still tired because I am 57. But then I am not old either.

Anna, a school-girl when her liver cancer was treated, observes the rapid maturing she experienced because of her ordeal:

> …when you get cancer when you are a kid, or when you are a teenager, just the whole growing up thing is just blown out of the water really. You have to grow up like so quickly, and that's part of the alienation when you get back to school, is that you just feel so much older than these kids that are worrying about what their hair looks, and it's "Hello I don't have any hair, I'm not you know. I'm just focusing on getting myself to live and you're worried about what your hair looks like, or what to wear to the school social." I mean, it's just normal kids things that kids are going through, but you just feel like you can't relate to them when they are talking about stuff like that, you know.

Others may also be aware of this apparent ageing. Handler's physician talks to him about his "loss of innocence," and farewells him from her rooms by patting him on the back and saying "You take care - *Old Man.*"[10]

I. Aspiration/Achievement Mismatch

Cancer illness brings existential insights, changes in values, physical changes, fatigue and a sense of ageing. It is not surprising, therefore, that survivors of cancer may want to do things with their lives that they simply cannot achieve. Lynn, for example, seeks something meaningful to do in place of her nursing; but the replacement she finds fails to satisfy her aspirations to provide essential services for others:

> My friend who does Party Plan [a commercial party planning and catering service] said to me, "Oh well come and do Party Plan with me". So I do Party Plan, but my heart is not in it, I do it, and it's not like, and I have done quite well, but my heart is not, it's not the same as the sort of things that I am used to, and it is my nature, is my passion. … And so I am very confused at the moment…I sort of think, well *what am I supposed to do now?*

J. Loss of Future Memory

In discussing identity, we have elsewhere made the point that continuity of memory and of embodiment are important to our sense of identity.[11] Mental processes that we call memory assign meaning to past experiences, and interpret aspects of present experience. The same interpretative process projects into the future, assigning meaning to the plans and aspirations we may have. This meaning-making and interpretative continuity in our mental lives we call 'future memory.'[12] Helen reflects on the changes she notices in the way in which she looks to her future since her cancer:

> If somebody had come to me and said "Let's go away at Christmas next year", I really couldn't have really said yes. I could plan like say for three months, I knew it was Amanda's birthday, I'd think oh well, okay we can get birthday and Christmas. I couldn't think past that, so I kind of - I remember my local doctor coming down and having a talk to me and saying "Look just think *daily"*, you know? Just think every day. But then I thought "Oh god why is he telling me that? I am going to *die."* You know what I mean?

Bill also is explicit about the lack of meaning in his future:

> I'm just now tinged with regret of what I have had to put up with, and there is just nothing on the horizon, there is nowhere I can turn for the future.

Lynn seeks to restore meaning to her future by finding a cause to work for:

> I said to John, "If I don't work John, I am going to have to get into some cause or something, [laughter] I am going to have work for something."

K. Guilt, Accountability, Debt

Finally, survivors express senses of guilt, obligation, accountability and debt. These categories of feeling may be directed to families, other patients, the health system and its health care workers, even to society at large. Anna records her sense of guilt for having disrupted her family:

> I didn't feel alienated at all at home, I just felt pretty guilty actually for what was happening to my family. Because mum stayed with me for the whole time, and I've got three younger brothers and sisters, and I felt pretty bad that they were, I knew that they were having, because all kids do, have their growing problems and stuff like that, then mum just wasn't there for a year, she was with me the whole time, which put a lot of stress on dad and on the kids as well.

Bill feels a sense of obligation to return his personal experience and knowledge about his colostomy to others, even though he has never found the time to become a counsellor:

> I just, at times I thought maybe I should go and talk to people about this operation. I know that there's a Colostomy Association always asks if people will do this, but I, just like everything else, put it aside, put it aside. But my reaction, I repeat, if I can help anybody at all, in any sort of situation as far as counselling people, okay. I think I am qualified to talk in that respect, about the three aspects that we've spoken about. The surgery aspect, the mental trauma and the life that you've got to lead as a result.

Miles[13] is so aware of the social expectations that she wonders whether it might be easier if she became sick again:

> …why was I thinking that perhaps life would be easier if I got sick again? Not really sick, but … just a little bit. Just to take the pressure off. Just to give myself a bit of breathing space from a world that expected too much.

The categories listed above seem to offer a reasonably complete account of the phenomena experienced by survivors who report significant distress. They give an account, in other words, of the *phenomenology* of survivor distress. We have elsewhere developed theoretical models to explain these phenomena, and we will not review that material in this paper.[14]

6. The Downward Spiral

What we have said so far provides a phenomenology of PCD, and a partial explanation of mechanisms that may cause it. It fails, however, to account for the *dynamics* of the processes by which a particular point is reached. Emma's narrative describes a downward cycle of events, which culminate in an inability to complete her law degree, the loss of an apparently stable partnership, problems with other relationships, and tensions in her work environment.

A. Self-esteem

The narratives of Emma, Bill, Lynn and Mark give us insight into the state of diminished self-esteem reached by those who experience PCD, but they do little to *explain* what produces the state. Self-esteem theory has a long history, and self-esteem is clearly important to our daily functioning and our relationships.[15] Furthermore, self-esteem is the basis of the claims we make on other people for their love, support and respect. Loss of self-esteem reduces the sense that we can make such claims, which reinforces the loss of self-esteem.

At the same time, self-esteem is a slippery notion, and its constituents are contested.[16] William James, in his classic analysis of self-esteem, characterised it as the balance between a person's achievements and pretensions.[17] While this definition has gone out of favour, the tension between aspirations and achievements characterises something important, which we would term 'existential comfort'. Lynn's discomfort at her changed social role, and Bill's anger at his truncated social life both represent existential discomfort that results from an imbalance between what is wanted and what is achievable. An inability to adjust aspirations to realities can be a source of continuing personal dissatisfaction, and can contribute to a sense of continuing failure and inadequacy.

B. Self-efficacy

This raises the question of self-efficacy,[18] the confidence we have in our capacity to cope with particular contexts (e.g. social, working, emotional, cognitive, physical) in the future, on the basis of past experience and inherited and acquired skills and attributes. Self-efficacy is important to our sense of identity and well-being. There is little question that self-efficacy is diminished in those with PCD. People confronting the liminal experience take a new view of life. They value things differently, as Helen emphasises when she says 'I mean, if I wake up alive that's what's important to me now.' This kind of existential insight can profoundly change one's view of previous values, held without reflection before the cancer. This may modify, or even remove, the motivation to do certain kinds of work, or to seek certain friendships. The loss of motivation leads to diminished drive, diminished performance, and to loss of respect from others. At the same time, awareness of diminished performance and diminished respect reduce self-efficacy. This reflexive process is part at least of the downward cycle, contributing to the sense of lost continuity, loss of life-plan and life-meaning, loss of future memory, loss of significant relatedness, and perhaps to fatigue. But there are other forces at work. The downward cycle can be further understood in terms of theories of *well-being* and of *self-determination*.

C. Well-being

The literature on well-being has been reviewed in some detail by Ryan and Deci.[19] They point out that there are two strands of thinking about well-being, the *hedonic* and the *eudaimonic*. The hedonic, which concentrates on subjective well-being (SWB), claims that personal pleasure and satisfaction are the key elements for study.[20] The eudaimonic, emphasising psychological well-being (PWB), postulates that personal development is more important than pleasure. In characterising the components of PWB, Ryff and Keyes list six key categories: autonomy, personal growth, self-acceptance, life purpose, mastery and positive relatedness.[21] Each of these attributes may be seriously challenged by cancer illness. While the differences between hedonic and eudaimonic well-being are important for researchers, and demand different methods for their study, the link between them in daily living is close. Pleasure without development or development without pleasure is likely to become sterile and unsatisfying. It is difficult to imagine one without the other.

If we concentrate on the eudaimonic model, PWB leads to two further insights. The first is that PWB is linked to *personal expressiveness*, a state that Waterman has characterised as a balance between personal values and life activities.[22] This balance is close to what we have earlier referred to as 'existential comfort', and to what James called self-esteem. The imbalance between values and activities recorded by Lynn when she talks about the end of her nursing career is a cause of continuing distress.

D. Self-determination

The second insight is provided by *self-determination theory*.[23] Ryan and Deci have produced evidence that self-determination depends primarily on three basic psychological needs – autonomy, competence and relatedness. Clearly, the sense of being an independent moral agent, capable of choice, is important to our sense of who we are, and what degree of control we have over ourselves and the events we encounter. Equally, our sense of competence determines our self-efficacy, the sense we have of our ability to handle situations based on past experience and natural attributes. Relatedness, the sense of relationship to significant others, provides both support and satisfaction of basic needs. Autonomy, competence and relatedness together are essential for psychological growth, for cultural integration (the personal assimilation of cultural practices), happiness, vitality and well-being. As Ryan and Deci write:

> [C]ontextual and cultural, as well as developmental, factors continually influence the modes of expression, the means of satisfaction, and the ambient support for these needs, and it is because of their effects on need satisfaction that they, in turn, influence growth, integrity, and well-being at both between-person and within-person levels of analysis.[24]

Self-determination theory posits that satisfaction of the psychological needs for autonomy, competence and relatedness fosters both hedonic and eudaimonic well-being. There is a subtle and important relationship between the three needs. Feeling pressured to succeed, for example, leads to happiness at success, but not to vitality, whereas success in an autonomously chosen endeavour leads to both happiness and vitality.[25] There is evidence that the quality, rather than quantity, of relationships is important to well-being.[26] Good quality of relationships is hard to sustain or create when one feels a sense of lessened autonomy or of reduced competence. There is also a close link between physical health and well-being. Ryan and Frederick noted a correlation between subjective vitality, personal autonomy and relatedness, and a co-variation with physical symptoms.[27] This is hardly surprising, since physical symptoms reduce the sense of autonomy and diminish performance.

If we consider the relationship between these three basic needs, we can begin to understand the mechanism of the downward spiral of PCD. While the details will vary from person to person, the general pattern probably develops along these lines:

Cancer disrupts the valued order of a life, and causes a reordering of priorities and a reassessment of close relationships. The confrontation with death and the recognition of the frailty and finiteness of the body make some survivors into compulsory existentialists, aware that life has at best a fragile meaning. This means that motivation to do what seemed important before the cancer may change, and the drive to persist with old competencies may diminish. This may lead to diminished performance in familiar roles. This in turn leads to censure by others and self-censure made more severe by awareness of the disapproval of others.

At the same time, close friends may be re-evaluated. Some of their preoccupations may now seem trivial. Some, uneasy in the face of life-threatening illness, may seem to lack involvement and concern, or may fail to understand the nature of the cancer experience. Others may seem to demand a return to an old self lost because of the insights that cancer brings. New friends may be sought who have had similar experiences.

Cancer is an experience beyond our control. Its treatment demands the surrender of a significant part of our autonomy. Awareness of bodily fragility, of continuing symptoms after treatment, and of the need for medical follow-up for long periods, all reinforce the sense of lost autonomy.

Cancer illness and its aftermath, for some people at least, thus diminish autonomy, competence and relatedness. As competence diminishes, so does autonomy, because capacity for choice is reduced. Diminished autonomy leads to diminished self-regard, and diminution in the regard of others. Thus relatedness is also reduced. The losses in the three psychological needs are reflexively related, and cumulative. Their reflexive relationship constitutes a vicious downward cycle.

Fatigue, sadness, anxiety, fear of inadequacy and of failure, and a sense of alienation are common complaints, and may lead to diagnoses of depression or post-traumatic stress disorder (PTSD).

The reflexive relationship between autonomy, competence and relatedness is shown in Figure 1.

Williams has proposed a model of dysfunctional illness behaviour that may have some relevance for both further understanding of PCD and its amelioration.[28] He proposes that responses to illness are determined by three things – people's beliefs about their illnesses (illness representation), beliefs about themselves, others and the world (self-schema), and the interaction between their illness representations and self-schemata.

Further insight comes from self-discrepancy theory.[29] Higgins and colleagues have shown that discrepancies between the actual self, the ideal self and the 'ought self' (the self of duties and obligations) can lead to disturbances of affect in both the short and long term.[30] Discrepancy between actual and ideal selves leads to sadness and dejection; between actual and ought selves, to agitation, anxiety and fear. Cancer survivors may lose a significant parts of their sense of actual self, and yet retain senses of what they might be ideally and what they ought to be. They may therefore suffer a sense of discrepancy between the actual and the desired, and experience sadness, dejection *and* anxiety or fear. These are the components of PCD.

If these insights are true of the survival experience, both psychodynamic and cognitive methods might be applicable to the relief of PCD.[31] It also seems intuitively likely that personality will significantly determine survival experience. It would be of interest to know, for example, more about the predictive power of personality profiles, measured perhaps using the 'Big Five' factors of Costa and McCrae.[32]

E. Fatigue

It is worth while to comment further on the phenomenon of fatigue among survivors. While it is generally recognised that fatigue is an important symptom amongst those who have had cancer, its incidence, significance and mechanisms are all debated.[33] There are those who argue that it is no more common among cancer survivors than among controls. Nevertheless, it is a universal complaint among those with PCD.

It may be possible to shed some light on this observation by considering *vitality*. In their review, Ryan and Deci summarise the work of Ryan and Frederick:

> Ryan and Frederick (1997) assessed subjective vitality, a positive and phenomenologically accessible state of having energy available to the self, and used it as an indicator of eudaimonic well-being. They found that subjective vitality not only correlated with psychological factors such as personal autonomy and relatedness, but that it also covaried with physical symptoms. That is, more physical symptoms in a day predicted decreased energy and aliveness for that day, as did poor health habits such as smoking and fatty diets. They argued that vitality is a phenomenally salient variable that is affected by both somatic and psychological factors.[34]

In the context of survival, vitality *may* be inversely related to life-complexity. It requires emotional and cognitive work to restore the valued order represented by autonomy, competence and relatedness. These psychological needs become the bases for a renewed life plan, a reconstructed future memory and an adaptation to uncomfortable insights. Jordens and colleagues examined the concept of life-complexity and its reflection in 'hard-working' narratives.[35] If vitality is energy available for the self, it is logical to think that hard work committed to self-reconstruction may diminish vitality.[36] Certainly, Bill, Lynn and Mark – the three people with the most complex narratives and lives in the study of Jordens et al., and who reappear in the present study – are the ones who complain most of lack of vitality and energy for themselves. Bill has only his work, and has practically abandoned his social life. Lynn can no longer work as a nurse because she "was just so tired." Mark finds that he wants to "potter about in the garden," rather than take part in the social activities that his wife seeks.

7. Conclusions

Self-determination theory thus provides at least a partial explanation of the processes that lead to the state that we call PCD. While depression and PTSD may occur among survivors, the distress we have encountered so commonly does not satisfy the usual diagnostic criteria for these conditions. Most survivors manage to lead productive lives, and suicide is rare. Flashbacks, nightmares, and alexithymia are not usually part of the distress. There have been attempts to alter the diagnostic criteria for PTSD, so that the survivor state can be included, but it is not clear that this serves any useful purpose.[37] The condition we describe is one of existential distress, which can be troubling, and at times disabling. To call it psychopathology under a conventional label is to stigmatise people confronting the problems inherent in human life, albeit in a more intense way than most of us will encounter except toward the end of our lives.

Its remedy lies not with medications or psychoanalysis, but in understanding and identifying ways in which the vicious cycle can be broken. This may mean significant restructuring of a life, including the adjustment of aspirations, the development of new competencies, new work milieus, and changes in close relationships. Despite these apparently overwhelming demands, most survivors seem to come to terms with their distress, and lead productive, balanced, and even enriched lives. A small minority, however, may need psychological support and therapy. The present account of the components of the distress, and the processes whereby it develops, may be helpful to those who provide relevant support and therapy.

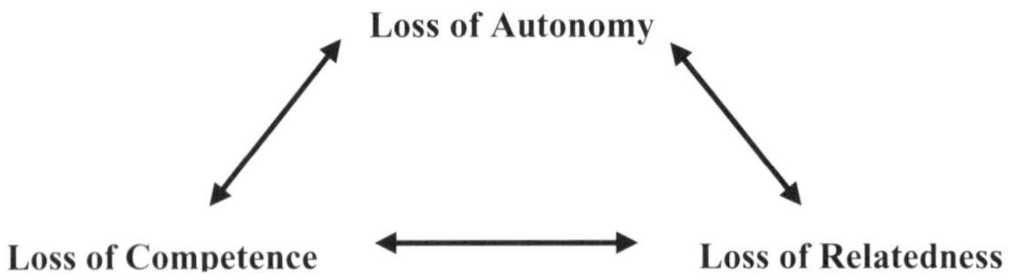

Figure 1
The constituents of the downward cycle. Loss of autonomy, competence and relatedness are reflexively related, and mutually reinforcing.

Notes

[1] Little, Jordens, Paul, Montgomery et al. 1998; Little, Jordens, Paul, Sayers et al. 1999; Little, Jordens, Paul, Sayers et al. 2000; Little, Paul, Jordens and Sayers 2000; Little, Sayers, Paul and Jordens 2000; Little, Sayers, Paul and Jordens 2000; Little, Jordens, Paul and Sayers 2001; Little, Jordens, Paul and Sayers 2002.
[2] Little, Jordens, Paul and Sayers 2001.
[3] Strauss and Corbin 1990.
[4] Buchanan 1994; Stone 1994; Canfield, Hansen, Aubrey and Mitchell 1996.
[5] Miles 1995;Miles 1997; Miles 2000.
[6] Handler 1996.
[7] Ibid., 257.
[8] Ibid., 272.
[9] Ibid., 277.
[10] Ibid., 278.
[11] Little, Jordens, Paul and Sayers 2001, 19-32 and Little, Jordens, Paul and Sayers 2002.
[12] Little, Jordens, Paul and Sayers 2001, 20-21, 99 and Little, Jordens, Paul and Sayers 2002.
[13] Miles 2000.
[14] Little, Jordens, Paul, Montgomery et al. 1998; Little, Jordens, Paul, Sayers et al. 1999; Little, Jordens, Paul, Sayers et al. 2000; Little, Paul, Jordens and Sayers 2000; Little, Sayers, Paul and Jordens 2000; Little, Sayers, Paul and Jordens 2000; Little, Jordens, Paul and Sayers 2001; Little, Jordens, Paul and Sayers 2002.
[15] Sabat, Fath, Moghaddam and Harré 1999.
[16] Robson 1988.
[17] James 1990 (1890), p. 200.

[18] Bandura 1995 and Bandura 1997.
[19] Ryan and Deci 2001.
[20] Diener and Lucas 1999 and Kahneman, Diener and Schwarz 1999.
[21] Ryff and Keyes 1995.
[22] Waterman 1993.
[23] (Ryan and Deci 2000)
[24] Ryan and Deci 2001, 146.
[25] Ibid.
[26] Ryff and Singer 2000.
[27] Ryan and Frederick 1997.
[28] Williams 1997.
[29] Higgins 1987.
[30] Higgins, Bond, Klein and Strauman 1986.
[31] Moretti and Higgins 1999, 214-216.
[32] Costa and McCrae 1992.
[33] Bush, Haberman, Donaldson and Sullivan 1995; Smets, Visser, Willems-Groot, Garssen et al. 1998; Loge, Abrahamsen, Ekeberg and Kaasa 1999; and Bower, Ganz, Desmond, Rowland et al. 2000.
[34] Ryan and Deci 2001.
[35] Jordens, Little, Paul and Sayers 2001.
[36] Ryan and Frederick 1997.
[37] Alonzo 2000.

Bibliography

Alonzo, A.A. "The Experience of Chronic Illness and Post-traumatic Stress Disorder: The Consequences of Cumulative Adversity." *Social Science and Medicine*, 50 (2000): 1475-1484.

Bandura, A., ed. *Self-efficacy in Changing Societies*. 1995, Cambridge University Press: Cambridge.

Bandura, A., *Self-efficacy: The Exercise of Control*. 1997, New York: W. H. Freeman and Company.

Bower, J.E., P.A. Ganz, K.A. Desmond, J.H. Rowland, B.E. Meyerowitz, and T.R. Belin. "Fatigue in Breast Cancer Survivors: Occurrence, Correlates, and Impact on Quality of Life." *Journal of Clinical Oncology*, 18, 4 (2000): 743-753.

Buchanan, S., *I'm Alive and the Doctor's Dead*. 1994, Grand Rapids, Michigan: Zondervan Publishing House.

Bush, N.E., M. Haberman, G. Donaldson, and K.M. Sullivan. "Quality of Life of 125 Adults Surviving 6-18 Years after Bone Marrow Transplantation." *Social Science and Medicine*, 40 (1995): 479-490.

Canfield, J., M.V. Hansen, P. Aubrey, and N. Mitchell. *Chicken Soup for the Surviving Soul*. 1996, Deerfield Beach, Florida: Health Communications, Inc.

Costa, P.T. and R.R. McCrae. "The Five-factor Model of Personality and its Relevance to Personality Disorders." *Journal of Personality Disorders*, 6 (1992): 343-359.

Diener, E. and R.E. Lucas. "Personality and Subjective Well-being." In *Well-Being: The Foundations of Hedonic Psychology*. Edited by D. Kahneman, E. Diener, and N. Schwarz, 213-219. Russell Sage Foundation: New York, 1999.

Handler, E. *Time on Fire: My Comedy of Terrors*. New York: Owl Books, 1996.

Higgins, E.T., R.N. Bond, R. Klein, and T. Strauman. "Self-discrepancies and Emotional Vulnerability: How Magnitude, Accessibility, and Type of Discrepancy Influence Affect." *Journal of Personality and Social Psychology*, 51 (1986): 5-15.

Higgins, E.T. "Self-discrepancy: A Theory Relating Self and Affect." *Psychological Review*, 94 (1987): 319-340.

James, W. *The Principles of Psychology*. Edited by M.J. Adler. Chicago: Encyclopaedia Britannica, 1990 (1890).

Jordens, C.F.C., M. Little, K. Paul, and E.-J. Sayers. "Life Disruption and Generic Complexity: A Social Linguistic Analysis of Narratives of Cancer Illness." *Social Science and Medicine*, 53 (2001): 1227-1236.

Kahneman, D., E. Diener, and N. Schwarz, eds. *Well-Being: The Foundations of Hedonic Psychology*. Russell Sage Foundation: New York, 1999.

Little, M., C.F.C. Jordens, K. Paul, and E.-J. Sayers: *Surviving Survival: Life After Cancer*. Marrickville: Choice Books, 2001.

Little, M., C.F.C. Jordens, K. Paul, and E.-J. Sayers. “Survivorship and Discourses of Identity.” *Psycho-Oncology*, 11 (2002): 170-178.

Little, M., C.F.C. Jordens, K. Paul, E.-J. Sayers, and D. Sriskandarajah. “Approval and Disapproval in the Narratives of Patients with Colorectal Cancer and their Carers.” *Health*, 3 (1999): 451-467.

Little, M., C.F.C. Jordens, K. Paul, E.-J. Sayers, and D. Sriskandarajah. “Face, Honor and Dignity in the Context of Colon Cancer.” *Journal of Medical Humanities*, 21 (2000): 229-243.

Little, M., C.F.C. Jordens, K. Paul, K. Montgomery, and B. Philipson. “Liminality: A Major Category of the Experience of Cancer Illness.” *Social Science and Medicine*, 47 (1998): 1485-1494.

Little, M., E.-J. Sayers, K. Paul, and C.F.C. Jordens. “On surviving Cancer.” *Journal of the Royal Society of Medicine*, 93 (2000): 501-503.

Little, M., E.-J. Sayers, K. Paul, and C.F.C. Jordens. “The Paradox of Survival: Cancer and its Aftermath.” *Journal of Pelvic Surgery*, 6 (2000): 287-290.

Little, M., K. Paul, C.F.C. Jordens, and E.-J. Sayers. “Vulnerability in the Narratives of Patients and their Carers - Studies of Colorectal Cancer.” *Health*, 4 (2000): 499-514.

Loge, J.H., A.F. Abrahamsen, Ø. Ekeberg, and S. Kaasa. “Hodgkin's Disease Survivors More Fatigued than the General Population.” *Journal of Clinical Oncology*, 17 (1999): 253-261.

Miles, S. “A Most Recidivist Remedy.” In *Agenda: Official Newsletter of Cancer and the Young Adult*. (1997): 4-7.

Miles, S. *At Least it's not Contagious*. St Leonards, Sydney: Allen & Unwin, 1995.

Miles, S. “Topic of Cancer.” In *Sydney Morning Herald*. Sydney, Australia. (2000): 32.

Moretti, M.M. and E.T. Higgins. "Own Versus Other Standpoints in Self-regulation: Developmental Antecedents and Functional Consequences." *Review of General Psychology*, 3 (1999): 188-223.

Robson, P.J. "Self Esteem: A Psychiatric View." *British Journal of Psychiatry*, 153 (1988): 6-15.

Ryan, R.M. and C.M. Frederick. "On Energy, Personality and Health: Subjective Vitality as a Dynamic Reflection of Well-being." *Journal of Personality*, 65 (1997): 529-565.

Ryan, R.M. and E.L. Deci. "On Happiness and Human Potentials: A Review of Research on Hedonic and Eudaimonic Well-being." *Annual Review of Psychology*, 52 (2001): 141-166.

Ryan, R.M. and E.L. Deci. "Self-determination Theory and the Facilitation of Intrinsic Motivation, Social Development, and Well-being." *American Psychologist*, 55 (2000): 68-78.

Ryff, C.D. and B. Singer. "Interpersonal Flourishing: A Positive Health Agenda for the New Millennium." *Personality and Social Psychology Review*, 4 (2000): 30-44.

Ryff, C.D. and C.L.M. Keyes. "The Structure of Psychological Well-being Revisited." *Journal of Personality and Social Psychology*, 69 (1995): 719-727.

Sabat, S.R., H. Fath, F.M. Moghaddam, and R. Harré. "The Maintenance of Self-esteem: Lessons from the Culture of Alzheimer's Sufferers." *Culture and Psychology*, 5 (1999): 5-31.

Smets, E.M., M.R. Visser, A.F. Willems-Groot, B. Garssen, A.L. Schuster-Uitterhoeve, and J.C. de Haes. "Fatigue and Radiotherapy: (B) Experience in Patients Nine Months Following Treatment." *British Journal of Cancer*, 78 (1998): 907-912.

Stone, B. *Cancer as Initiation: Surviving the Fire*. Chicago and La Salle, Illinois: Open Court, 1994.

Strauss, A. and J. Corbin. *Basics of Qualitative Research: Grounded Theory Procedures and Techniques*. Newbury Park, Ca: Sage, 1990.

Waterman, A.S. "Two Conceptions of Happiness: Contrasts of Personal Expressiveness (Eudaimonia) and Hedonic Enjoyment." *Journal of Personality and Social Psychology*, 64 (1993): 678-691.

Williams, C. "A Cognitive Model of Dysfunctional Illness Behaviour." *British Journal of Health Psychology*, 2 (1997): 153-165.

Notes on Contributors

Emma Sayers is the Survivorship Coordinator at the Centre for Values, Ethics and the Law Medicine, University of Sydney. In that role she facilitates the provision of research-based information and support to those experiencing difficulties in the aftermath of cancer treatment. She has also assisted cancer care organisations wishing to formulate new policy around survivorship issues and is actively involved in the education of health professionals who care for survivors. She is a coauthor of the Centre's book *Surviving Survival: Life After Cancer* published by Choice Books in 2001. She has degrees in Asian Studies and Law from the University of New South Wales.

John Miles Little (AM, MD, MS, FRACS) is Emeritus Professor of Surgery, University of Sydney, and Director of the Centre for Values, Ethics and the Law in Medicine, University of Sydney.

Life "In Limbo": Donor Families, Organ Recipients and their Experience in Germany

Vera Kalitzkus

Organ transplantation is a form of medical treatment that is almost practised worldwide. It uses human organs from either brain-dead patients or – in the case of kidneys, parts of the liver and the lung – living donors in order to safe the lives of patients or give them a chance to live without dialysis. Since the initial public upheaval after the first heart transplantations in the 1960s by Christian Barnard, in some fields organ transplantation today might be even considered a standard form of treatment. In Germany since the 1990s every year about 1000 patients in the state of brain-death become organ donors, around 4000 patients receive a transplant (including transplants from living donors).[1]

Yet, this biomedical technology is probing the boundaries in two existential fields: it blurs the formerly taken for granted demarcation between life and death and transgresses the boundaries between individual embodied selves. As both concepts are culturally defined and embedded in a historical context, the aim of this paper is to contribute to the understanding of how people experience and live with these vague boundaries in a specific socio-cultural setting.[2]

Death in Western societies is conceptually linked to the corpse, a lifeless body. As the philosopher Thomas Macho states, the corpse is necessary to realize the "facticity" of death.[3] Since the implementation of the so-called Transplantation Law in Germany in 1997 the state of brain death is legally recognized as defining the death of a person. This generates the paradox of a (biologically) "living corps," because the body of a patient in the state of irreversible coma (e.g. brain death) has to be kept on life support machines to enable its biological functioning. Without this intervention the body would soon die of cardiac arrest and the organs could not be used anymore for transplantation purposes. Before the emergence of the concept of brain death, those patients were still considered alive – although dying; now they are excluded from the community of the living, as sociologist Gesa Lindemann observes in her study on the shifting boundaries between the living and the dead.[4] Through the 'clinical gaze,' the bodies of brain-dead patients are transformed into objectifiable therapeutic tools, that can be used for the good of other patients.

But the body is more than just the biological material basis of our living selves. In Euro-American societies the body is intimately linked with the self of the person. It is saturated with the self and therefore not easily objectified. In this conception *one* self is linked to *one and only one* (living) body.[5] The term 'self' connotes here the aspect of the own consciousness and self-perception as an individual embodied ‘I’, especially in distinction from other selves. Deviations from that norm are considered to be pathologic. One example would be the case of multiple personality disorder, where a number of selves share one body; in the case of schizophrenia a person is not able any more to differentiate between his self and the selves of others or inanimate things and therefore can no longer experience his body as the basis of his individual self.

Given these social conditions and cultural concepts, I want to explore the following aspects:

1. How do ‘donor relatives’ experience the confrontation with brain death and the necessity of making the decision of donating the organs of a person they love?
2. How do organ recipients master the integration of another person’s organ in their own body and self? Furthermore, how do they cope with the fact, that there is a direct link between their prolonged life and the death of another person?
3. How do ‘donor families’ and organ recipients cope with the ‘relationship’ based on sharing a bodily substance and established through death.

My study is based mainly on narrative interviews from one to four hours with donor relatives and organ recipients in Western Germany. It was difficult to get into contact with donor families, as in Germany they seldom speak about their experience in public and are – with one exception – not organized in support groups. Most transplant centres I asked were not willing to cooperate in establishing contacts. I therefore turned to the option of announcing my project in newspapers, from which resulted the majority of the 21 interviews with 23 immediate next of kin of 19 organ donors. The sample is very diverse in terms of age and kinship relation of donor and relative. The interviews were conducted as soon as three months after the donor’s death to as many as twenty years afterwards. The relationship between kin and donor cover all next of kin relations (father, mother, child, spouse).

I contacted organ recipients via self-help organisations for transplant patients and many were very willing to co-operate. As one of my main concerns is about death and its ‘new face,’ I excluded living-related donation. The 19 narrative interviews on the recipient side comprise kidney, liver, heart- and heart-lung-transplant patients from age 24 till 65. One organ recipient interviewed had had the first transplant nineteen years ago, one patient less than a year ago. Five kidney recipients have had retransplants, two of them already a third.

The data from the interviews are supplemented by participant observation at meetings of self-help groups, national as well as international transplant sporting events (comparable to the Paralympics) and in a transplant unit and ICU of a university clinic in Germany. The heterogeneity of the empirical material enables insights into the complexity and diversity of the experience of patients and relatives. My aim was to identify common features in the wide range of experience, enabling conclusions about general culturally conditioned problems of organ transplantation. In order to do so I applied the following analytical perspective.

1. The 'Clinical Gaze' Versus the Lay Perspective

The analysis of the dialectical relationship between cultural concepts and the individual lived experience is based on the theoretical distinction between the *body* ("Körper") and the *lived body* ("Leib"). I define *body* in this context as a biomedically defined object, in contrast to the individual experienced, subjective *Leib* or *lived body* (which implies emotions, feelings, bodily sensations etc.).[6] It is important to note, that the *lived body* is not untouched by cultural conditioning. On the contrary, that which comes up as feelings and sensations from the core of our being and which seems to be so 'natural' and unquestionable is also culturally conditioned, as Gesa Lindemann points out.[7]

In the context of organ transplantation one has to look at the self in relation to the body. For social anthropologist Anthony Giddens the self – especially under conditions of high modernity – is not given and unchangeable, but has to be confirmed and reflexively fostered by the individual. In conditions of high modernity, the body is actually far less 'docile' than ever before in relation to the self, since the two are intimately coordinated within the reflexive project of self-identity. The body itself – as mobilised in praxis – becomes more immediately relevant to the identity the individual promotes.[8]

Giddens defines self-identity as the self that is understood from the individual according to his or her biographic reflexively.[9] This is done via the body: "Experiencing the body is a way of cohering the self as an integrated whole, whereby the individual says 'this is where I live.'"[10] Organ transplantation raises questions about whether the body is the 'home' of the individual self, whose continuity according to Giddens also secures the continuity of the self-identity.[11] After transplantation, an organ that is intimately connected with the self of another individual demands a new 'home' in the body of the recipient. The individual self has to react to this existential challenge, in order to maintain itself. The close connection between the body and the self even survives death. This raises the question, whether donor relatives are able to abstract the biologically functioning body of the brain-dead patient from his/her *lived body* (*Leib*), and conceptualise the harvested organs as pure biological material.

Transplant medicine operates in the area of tension between the *body* as objectifiable and therefore alienable thing on the one hand, and the *lived body* as constitutive for the individual self on the other. The medico-professional side focuses primarily – if not totally – on the objectifiable body and treats human transplants as a common good. According to the dominant transplant perspective, once detached from the context of the original body there is no longer any connection between the organ and the self, of which it had been a constituent part. Only by the detachment of the biologically still living body from the self of the brain dead person can one justify this massive intrusion into the dying process and the transplantation of organs between individual human beings. In this perspective human transplants are conceptualised in the same way as artificial organs or spare parts and stripped of all aspects of self or the lived body.

In contrast, the public discourse conceptualises transplants as a "gift of life" and therefore organs are partly personalized. "How nice, that you gave away your heart! Would you like to do it again after your death?," one could read on huge posters in Germany 1997/1998 on public advertising boards. These posters pictured a young couple in tender embrace at a rail way station. They were part of an organ donation campaign by the German Federal Centre for Health Education ("Bundeszentrale für gesundheitliche Aufklärung") in order to promote organ donations. The poster draws on the cultural metaphoric meaning the body and its organs have – especially the heart as the centre of our self identity and seat of emotions. Thus organ transplants are turned from a mere biological 'spare part' into a very personal gift.

This increases the discrepancy between the biomedical perspective and those of the lay people in contact with organ transplantation. As both concepts are promoted in public, patients and relatives are torn between these two conflicting concepts in their struggle to cope with and make sense of their experience. In the narratives of donor relatives and organ recipients one finds most of the time alongside the aspects of the *body* also aspects of the *lived body* (*Leib*) – the body saturated by the self. This impedes the detachment and alienability of organs, even more so as organ transplantation is unavoidably connected with the shifting of the boundaries between individual embodied selves on the one hand and between life and death on the other.

This raises the question of the extent to which patients and donor relatives are able to conceptualise organs as alienable things and rid the body of the organ donor from all aspects of the self. With these thoughts I want to turn to the experience of my interview participants and show, how they cope with these conflicting concepts and the confrontation with illness, grief and death.

2. Between Life and Death: The Experience of Donor Relatives

> Rationality, however, is challenged in the face of sudden death and body dismemberment, and feelings of unease sometimes creep back in. (Margaret Lock)[12]

Organ donation is promoted as the ultimate gift, destined to give meaning to an otherwise meaningless death (even more so as there are quite often young victims and sudden deaths involved with donation). This – the public discourse has it – could console the bereaved family and help them to get over their loss. But the official discourse about organ donation can be characterized as romantic, following sociologists Renée Fox and Judith Swazey, because it glosses over major areas of conflict for donor families.[13] The kind of death necessary to procure organs usable for transplantation is hardly talked about in public, nor are the implications of organ donation for the bereaved families.

In Germany the donation process is organized according to the informed consent regulation: either one can decide and document their wishes or relatives are requested to do so on behalf of the individual. In the majority of the cases, relatives have to decide whether or not to consent to the removal of organs. In recent years, only about three to four percent of the donors had documented their decision in writing.[14] As a result, relatives must provide the consent to donate their loved ones organs typically under emotionally extreme conditions: at the moment at the ICU (Intensive Care Unit), when they are confronted with the message of a mostly sudden death.

Causes of death can bc cither traumatic (caused by accidents) or atraumatic (for example caused by brain infarct, tumours or aneurysms). In Germany atraumatic causes of death of organ donors outnumber the other causes accounting for over 70%.[15] To remove organs suitable for transplantation, the donor has to be in the state of brain death. Brain death is defined as

> the irreversible arrest of the functioning of the whole brain, including the brainstem, while the functioning of the heart-lung-circulatory-system is still sustained via life-support machines and artificial respiration.[16]

Brain death is only to be understood intellectually and to be proved by medical technology. The sensual experience via the *lived body* confronts the relatives with all signs associated with life, but not with death. A patient in the state of irreversible coma cannot be distinguished from any other comatose patient: her body is warm, the chest is heaving, the heart beat can be felt – although only because of the life-support machines. Also the severity of the head injury often cannot be estimated from the outside. A mother of a 15-year-old boy, who died after a skiing accident, told me:

> There was no change to be seen. We were sitting there [at his bed in the ICU], holding his hands, caress him. His body was warm. How should we realize, that he's supposed to be dead? I had the experience, that after getting the news of his death, this knowledge disappeared again. And I kept on sitting there, praying and hoping, that he surely would open his eyes again. I couldn't imagine it otherwise. (translated by the author)

My interviews with donor relatives clearly showed, that brain death is not an intellectual problem in the first case, but a problem of perception. The knowledge based on the natural sciences about the body is not congruent with the perception of the *lived body* (*Leib*), through which the other is perceived. Both concepts are contradictory. Because relatives at the ICU are confronted with the signs of life but not of death, they are insecure and full of doubts. As other studies have demonstrated, even medical professionals and nurses who work directly with brain-dead patients experience this uncertainty concerning the status of a brain-dead patient.[17]

Relatives have to say their last farewell, while the patient still looks alive. This can lead to feelings of guilt and betrayal for having abandoned the loved person in her most vulnerable and desperate hour. This is especially true when parents of young children consent to the donation of organs.

The period of time from brain death diagnosis until the end of the organ removal is an additional burden for the bereaved. This period can last from a few to 24 hours, sometimes even longer. This can lead relatives "to wait for the phone call, that now she is really dead," as a 28-year old woman told me about the death of her mother. "Really dead" in this context means that the body of the brain-dead person has turned into a corpse in the traditional sense and can be experienced as a corpse on the sensual level. One donor father put it in the following words: "My son has died two deaths." The first death refers to the brain death, the second death to the one after organ removal.

Organ transplantation interferes severely with the farewell of a dying person. It deprives donor relatives of comprehending the dying of their beloved one, which many of them regret afterwards. Instead they are confronted with a new face of death that is not congruent with traditional cultural interpretation schemes. They experience death as fragmented, divided between 'brain death' and the 'traditional' form of death after organ removal. This fragmentation gives rise to severe doubts about the 'real moment' of death. The fragmentation of death is even pushed further as the transplanted organs biologically live on in the body of the recipients. Some donor relatives talked about their belief that part of the organ donor's self still lives on in the body of the recipient. This shows that in their perception even after death the removed organ – an intimate part of the body – is closely linked to the self of the donor. Seen in the light of the *lived body* (*Leib*), the organs can be said to be in some sense the prolongation of the donor's self. In other words, the connection between the organ and the organ donor is not severed with its removal out of the body. To some donor relatives, this is consoling; to others – especially if they had traumatic experiences in the clinic – this could be a painful thought. One mother told me:

> I don't believe the relatives, who say, that they are comforted by that thought. Maybe for them it is helpful to endure the painful experience. I cannot imagine that, … it's too grotesque. What has my son's heart to do in another person's body? For me it's unbelievably painful. It doesn't allow me to think, that somebody could have been helped by that. That exceeds my capacity. Before my direct experience I thought like many others, that somebody's life could be saved. But if one is experiencing it directly, it seems to be so grotesque, that something that belongs so individually and personally to another person should be exchangeable. For me it's so absolutely painful, I can't be consoled by that. (translated by the author)

The analysis of my material shows, that for a little more than half of the relatives, who were confronted with brain death at the ICU, the organ donation meant an additional burden and quite often a very painful experience. Most of the relatives, who were not confronted with their loved one in the state of brain death, judge their donation experience in retrospect as positive. For the bereaved understanding of and coping with this new form of death constitutes the major problem in the donation process. In this respect organ donation quite often would be more correctly termed as a sacrifice of the bereaved for the good of total strangers than as just a mere act of charity and goodwill.

3. Fighting to Survive: The Experience of Organ Recipients

The official discourse on organ transplantation is promoting the image of a "second life," a "rebirth" after the transplantation. German brochures to educate the public about organ donation portray happy and agile transplant recipients, who state that they are "healed" by the transplant. Especially athletically engaged transplant recipients talked about their new bodily abilities and power. "I'm healthy," they proudly say and want to show to the public that the outcome of a transplantation is not a condition of decay, but a state of health worthwhile living for.

This is remarkable given the fact that the (still) life long immune-suppressive medication they have to take in order to prevent the rejection of the organ has severe side effects. Organ transplantation does not cure the patient, but leads to chronic illness. Elaborate regular medical check-ups (involving also painful and strenuous procedures such as biopsies) are needed to secure the recipients' fragile state of health. Only regular medical tests can detect a life-threatening chronic rejection. The fear of rejection, and therefore the fear of dying, is a dominant element in the life after transplantation. As one recipient put it, they live under a sword of Damocles. Not being able to sense this fatal threat can lead to an alienation from the body and loss of trust in it (as their own body and the transplant are working 'against' them). The relation of the patient to their body as well as the bodily sensations in the lived body are changed after a transplantation. A 32-year old heart-recipient told me, "One is never really healthy again, because one can never again deal with oneself, ones body or ones surroundings in a normal and natural way" (translated by the author).

My interview participants always stressed their huge gratitude towards the organ donor and his relatives. But they are never able to express this gratitude directly, as they do not receive any information about the donor's identity. The possibility to transmit a personal, but still anonymous letter of thanks to the donor relatives via transplant centres is seldom known among the patients and also not encouraged by the transplant centres in Germany.[18] To show their happiness and gratitude, many organ recipients engage in self-help-groups and support other patients and the promotion of organ donation.

Concerning their donor, organ recipients mostly state that they do not feel guilty about his or her death because the donor 'would have died anyway.' Still, the fact that their life is causally connected to the death of another person is a burden for these patients, that is especially pertinent during the time on the waiting list for a transplant. The transplant is inseparable from death: their own death as well as that of the donor. This can lead to a denial process in order to go on living. A 37-year old kidney recipient stated:

> I don't know of any patient, who really has problems with the transplanted organ. For that, I believe, the difference of quality of life between dialysis or life with a transplanted kidney is too huge. I believe that this is completely split off, because, it just cannot be! One cannot come to the conclusion, that this [the transplant]

> is not possible, it is just not possible. Because it would be suicidal (translated by the author).

There are many hints that transplant patients shy away from a confrontation with the transplant or the donor. Some do not want to look at the ultrasound picture of the new organ. One kidney recipient told me that she shrinks back from examining the organ by touch as this would confuse and unsettle her. Because of the underlying cultural conceptions as outlined above, the integration of an organ is a task that patients have to cope with on the physical as well as on the mental level,. This is true despite of the fact that in my conversations, organ recipients told me they do not have any problems with the integration of the new organ and described – according to the dominant medical model – the heart as "just a pump," other organs as "spare parts."

The question about the organ is intricately connected to the problem of self-identity. To distance themselves from questions of their social surrounding about a possible identity alteration after organ transplantation, they describe the condition after transplant "as just as before." With that, they also voice their longing for a sense of normalcy and continuation in their lives. But what if psychical aspects of the donor connected with the organ remained? Only few organ recipients claim to have concrete memories of their donor. Psychoneuroimmunologist Paul Pearsall talked to more than 74 transplant patients, 23 of them heart recipients, who claim to have 'inside' knowledge about their donor.[19] Claire Sylvia for example stated in her report about her heart transplantation:

> Sometimes I had the feeling, that somebody else was with me and that in some not clearly definable way my sense of I has turned into some kind of we. Although I couldn't sense this additional presence all the time, it sometimes felt almost as if I shared my body with two souls.[20]

Statements like this are severely criticised by the medical profession and other transplant recipients, because they point towards a dimension that, according to the medical and dominant social discourse, cannot possibly exist. They touch the innermost centre of our self-understanding. I do not intend to make any statement about the "real" causes for these sentiments. But the cultural perspective can contribute to the understanding of what cultural models patients refer to in order to make sense of their experience.

4. Conclusion

Transplantation medicine is at the forefront of the quest to conquer death. But instead of conquering death, this medical technique is (yet) totally dependent upon death, and tries to snatch away the last glimpses of life. Although one could speak of a consolation and exchange with death, because of its use for the good for the living, there is a kind of cultural amnesia about where the organs for transplantation come from. The public unwillingness to accept death leads to conflicts in the lives of people directly involved with organ transplantation.

Donor relatives are not adequately appreciated for the sacrifice they give to society. Instead, they still seem to be the "forgotten side" in the transplantation process. Their needs are often neglected in the clinical procedure as well as afterwards, for example in overcoming difficulties in the grieving process. In the imagination of bereaved relatives the corpse is still saturated with the self of the person, who died. For some, the donation has a consoling effect in the grieving process, for others – especially those confronted with brain-death and/or negative experience in the clinic – the organ donation has been an additional burden.

Organ recipients know that they owe their "second life" to the death of another person. They have to live with the overwhelming sense of debt towards the donor and his/her relatives. In addition to coping with the negative side effects after the transplantation on the physical level, they have to react on a psychological and emotional level to the threat the transplanted organ causes to their self. To publicly acknowledge this task of overcoming the culturally caused difficulties would be a relief for them, instead of adding additional guilt, if they might not be able to live up to the promise of the success story of organ transplantation.

Organ transplantation is limited not so much by its technical dimension, but by the human factor involved. Even with the highest donation rate possible, the organs usable for transplantation wouldn't meet the demand of the transplantation medicine. Apart from this, a limitation is caused by what humans are able to cope with and what they are willing to endure for their own or another person's survival.

Notes

1. Deutsche Stiftung Organtransplantation (eds.), *Weniger Transplantationen, leichter Rückgang bei der Organspende*. Press information, 30 January 2001.

2. The results of this research on organ transplantation constitute my dissertation and are published under Vera Kalitzkus, *Leben durch den Tod. Die zwei Seiten der Organtransplantation. Eine medizinethnologische*

Studie. (Frankfurt a.M./New York: Campus, 2003). The study was part of a larger research project sponsored by the German Research Foundation (Deutsche Forschungsgemeinschaft) and conducted at the Institut für Ethnologie at the University of Göttingen, Germany, under the chair of Prof. Brigitta Hauser-Schäublin. In this project we also looked at reproductive technologies. The results are published in Brigitta Hauser-Schäublin, Vera Kalitzkus, Imme Petersen, Iris Schröder, *Der geteilte Leib. Die kulturelle Dimension von Organtransplantation und Reproduktionsmedizin in Deutschland* (Frankfurt a. M./New York: Campus, 2001).
3. Thomas Macho, *Todesmetaphern. Zur Logik der Grenzerfahrung.* (Frankfurt a. M.: Suhrkamp,1987), 408-409.
4. Gesa Lindemann, *Die Grenzen des Sozialen. Zur sozio-technischen Konstruktion von Leben und Tod in der Intensivmedizin.* (München: Fink, 2002). An analysis about the German debate in historical perspective is given by Claudia Wiesemann. "Defining Brain Death: The German Debate in Historical Perspective." In *Coping with Sickness: Medicine, Law and Human Rights*, edited by John Woodward and Robert Jütte, Sheffield: Europ. Assoc. for the History of Medicine and Health Publication, 2000.
5. Nancy Scheper-Hughes and Margaret Lock, "The Mindful Body : A Prolegomenon to Future Work in Medical Anthropology," *Medical Anthropology Quarterly (1)*, 1987, 16-17.
6. A term coined by Drew Leder "Medicine and Paradigms of Embodiment," *The Journal of Medicine and Philosophy* 9 (1), 1984, 29-44.
7. Gesa Lindemann, "Das soziale Geschlecht unter der Haut," *KEA – Zeitschrift für Kulturwissenschaften*, 7, 1994, 12. For a good etymological derivation of "Körper" und "Leib" see Thomas Ots, "The Silenced Body – the Expressive Leib: on the Dialectic of Mind and Life in Chinese Cathartic Healing," in *Embodiment and Experience. The Existential Ground of Culture and Self*, edited by Thomas J. Csordas, 116-117. Cambridge: Cambridge University Press, 1996. Concerning the distinction between the *body* and the *lived body* see Thomas J. Csordas, "Embodiment as a Paradigm for Anthropology," *Ethos*, 18 (1), 1990, 5-47; Nick Crossley, "Merleau-Ponty, the Elusive Body and Carnal Sociology," *Body and Society*, 1 (1), 1995, 43-63; Bernhard Waldenfels, *Das leibliche Selbst. Vorlesungen zur Phänomenologie des Leibes* (Frankfurt a. M.: Suhrkamp, 2000).
8. Anthony Giddens, *Modernity and Self-Identity. Self and Society in the Late Modern Age* (Cambridge: Polity Press, 1991), 218.
9. Ibid., 244.
10. Ibid., 78.
11. Ibid., 55.

12. Margaret Lock, *Twice Dead. Organ Transplants and the Reinvention of Death* (Berkeley et al.: University of California Press, 2002), 207.
13. Renée Fox and Judith Swazey, *Spare Parts: Organ Replacement in American Society* (Oxford: Oxford University Press, 1992).
14. Deutsche Stiftung Organtransplantation (ed.), *Organspende und Transplantation in Deutschland 1999* (Neu-Isenburg: Deutsche Stiftung Organtransplantation, 2000), 2002, 14.
15. Ibid., 16.
16. Hans-Peter Schlake and Klaus Roosen, *Der Hirntod als der Tod des Menschen* (Neu-Isenburg: Deutsche Stiftung Organtransplantation, 1995), 13. Translation by the author.
17. Ulrike Baurheitel and Anna Bergmann, *Herzloser Tod. Das Dilemma der Organspende* (Stuttgart: Klett-Cotta, 1999); Linda F. Hogle, *Recovering the Nation's Body. Cultural Memory, Medicine, and the Politics of Redemption* (New Brunswick/New Jersey: Rutgers University Press, 1999); Hans Walter Striebel, Jürgen Link, ed., *Ich pflege Tote. Die andere Seite der Transplantationsmedizin* (Basel: Recom, 1991).
18. This is true despite of the fact, that years ago a major organisation of dialysis patients and kidney recipients (*Dialysepatienten Deutschlands e.V.*) launched a campaign to encourage letter of thanks to the donor relatives.
19. Paul Pearsall, *The Heart's Code: the True Stories of Organ Transplant Patients and What they Reveal about Where We Store our Memories* (New York/London: Thorsons), 1998.
20. Claire Sylvia, *Herzensfremd. Wie ein Spenderherz mein Selbst veränderte* (Hamburg: Hoffmann und Campe, 1998). Translated by the author.

Bibliography

Baurheitel, Ulrike and Bergmann, Anna. *Herzloser Tod. Das Dilemma der Organspende*. Stuttgart: Klett-Cotta, 1999.

Crossley, Nick. “Merleau-Ponty, the Elusive Body and Carnal Sociology.” *Body and Society*, 1, 1 (1995): 43-63.

Csordas, Thomas J. “Embodiment as a Paradigm for Anthropology.” *Ethos*, 18, 1 (1990): 5-47.

Deutsche Stiftung Organtransplantation (ed.). *Organspende und Transplantation in Deutschland 1999*. Neu-Isenburg: Deutsche Stiftung Organtransplantation, 2000.

Deutsche Stiftung Organtransplantation (ed.). *Weniger Transplantationen, leichter Rückgang bei der Organspende.* Press information, 30 January 2001.

Fox, Renée and Swazey, Judith. *Spare Parts: Organ Replacement in American Society*. Oxford: Oxford University Press, 1992.

Giddens, Anthony. *Modernity and Self-Identity. Self and Society in the Late Modern Age*. Cambridge: Polity Press, 1991.

Hauser-Schäublin, Brigitta, Vera Kalitzkus, Imme Petersen and Iris Schröder. *Der geteilte Leib. Die kulturelle Dimension von Organtransplantation und Reproduktionsmedizin in Deutschland.* Frankfurt a. M./New York: Campus, 2001.

Hogle, Linda F. *Recovering the Nation's Body. Cultural Memory, Medicine, and the Politics of Redemption*. New Brunswick/New Jersey: Rutgers University Press, 1999.

Kalitzkus, Vera. *Leben durch den Tod. Die zwei Seiten der Organtransplantation. Eine medizinethnologische Studie*. Frankfurt a.M./ New York: Campus, 2003.

Leder, Drew. "Medicine and Paradigms of Embodiment." *The Journal of Medicine and Philosophy*, 9, 1 (1984): 29-44.

Lindemann, Gesa. "Das soziale Geschlecht unter der Haut." *KEA – Zeitschrift für Kulturwissenschaften*, 7, 1994, 1-12.

Lindemann, Gesa. *Die Grenzen des Sozialen. Zur sozio-technischen Konstruktion von Leben und Tod in der Intensivmedizin*. München: Fink, 2002.

Lock, Margaret. *Twice Dead. Organ Transplants and the Reinvention of Death*. Berkeley et al.: University of California Press, 2002.

Macho, Thomas. *Todesmetaphern. Zur Logik der Grenzerfahrung.* Frankfurt a. M.: Suhrkamp, 1987.

Ots, Thomas. "The Silenced Body – the Expressive Leib: on the Dialectic of Mind and Life in Chinese Cathartic Healing." In *Embodiment and Experience. The Existential Ground of Culture and Self*, edited by Thomas J. Csordas, 116-136. Cambridge: Cambridge University Press, 1996.

Pearsall, Paul. *The Heart's Code: the True Stories of Organ Transplant Patients and What they Reveal about Where We Store our Memories*. New York/London: Thorsons, 1998.

Scheper-Hughes, Nancy and Lock, Margaret. "The Mindful Body: a Prolegomenon to Future Work in Medical Anthropology." *Medical Anthropology Quarterly*, 1 (1987): 6-41.

Schlake, Hans-Peter and Roosen, Klaus. *Der Hirntod als der Tod des Menschen*. Neu-Isenburg: Deutsche Stiftung Organtransplantation, 1995.

Sharp, Leslie A. "Organ Transplantation as a Transformative Experience: Anthropological Insights into the Restructuring of the Self." *Medical Anthropology Quarterly*, 9, 3 (1995): 357-389.

Striebel, Hans Walter and Link, Jürgen (ed.). *Ich pflege Tote. Die andere Seite der Transplantationsmedizin*. Basel: Recom, 1991.

Sylvia, Claire. *Herzensfremd. Wie ein Spenderherz mein Selbst veränderte.* Hamburg: Hoffmann und Campe, 1998.

Waldenfels, Bernhard. *Das leibliche Selbst. Vorlesungen zur Phänomenologie des Leibes*. Frankfurt a. M.: Suhrkamp, 2000.

Wiesemann, Claudia. "Defining Brain Death: the German Debate in Historical Perspective." In *Coping with Sickness: Medicine, Law and Human Rights*. Edited by John Woodward and Robert Jütte. Sheffield: Europ. Assoc. for the History of Medicine and Health Publ., 2000.

Note on Contributor

Vera Kalitzkus completed her PhD in Cultural Anthropology at the University of Göttingen (Germany) in 2002. She has been a lecturer on the cultural construction of death and dying at the University of Göttingen and now joined the Society for Promoting Communication in Medicine (Gesellschaft zur Förderung Medizinischer Kommunikation e.V.) working in a project on "Salutogenesis in General Practice" in collaboration with the Department of Medical Psychology, University of Göttingen.